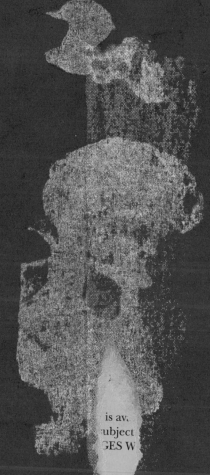

is av...
...ubject
...GES W

Plastic and Reconstructive Surgery

MOSBY'S PERIOPERATIVE NURSING SERIES

Plastic and Reconstructive Surgery

Nancymarie Fortunato, RN, BA, BSN, MEd, RNFA, CNOR, CPSN
Clinical Nursing
Cleveland Clinic Foundation
Cleveland, Ohio;
Educational Services for Professionals
Ashtabula, Ohio

Susan M. McCullough, RN, BSN, CNOR
Clinical Nursing
Cleveland Clinic Foundation
Cleveland, Ohio;
Educational Services for Professionals
Ashtabula, Ohio

with 450 illustrations

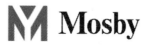

St. Louis Baltimore Boston Carlsbad Chicago Naples New York Philadelphia Portland
London Madrid Mexico City Singapore Sydney Tokyo Toronto Wiesbaden

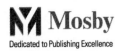
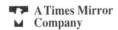

A Times Mirror
Company

Publisher Nancy L. Coon
Editor Michael S. Ledbetter
Developmental Editor Nancy L. O'Brien
Project Manager Dana Peick
Production Editor Jeff Patterson
Composition Specialist Wendy Bellm
Designer Amy Buxton
Manufacturing Manager Don Carlisle
Cover Photo Nancymarie Fortunato

A NOTE TO THE READER:
The author and publisher have made every attempt to check dosages and nursing content for accuracy. Because the science of pharmacology is continually advancing, our knowledge base continues to expand. Therefore we recommend that the reader always check product information for changes in dosage or administration before administering any medication. This is particularly important with new or rarely used drugs.

Printed in the United States of America
Composition by Mosby Electronic Production
Lithography/color film by Accu-Color, Inc.
Printing/binding by Von Hoffmann

Mosby, Inc.
11830 Westline Industrial Drive
St. Louis, Missouri 63146

ISBN 0-8151-3305-7

Contributors

Martin A. Phillips III, RN, BSN, CNOR
Director, Perioperative Services
Marymount Hospital
Garfield Heights, Ohio
*Chapter 3 Plastic and Reconstructive Surgery
        Practice Settings*

Ruth Bakst, RN, RNFA, CNOR
Perioperative Educator
St. Luke's Medical Center
Cleveland, Ohio
Chapter 10 Breast Surgical Procedures

Consultants

Brian W. Davies, MD
Plastic and Reconstructive Surgery
Akron, Ohio

Patricia E. Chapek, RN, BA, CNOR
Clinical Nursing
Cleveland Clinic Foundation
Cleveland, Ohio

Patti Houck, RN, RNFA, CNOR
Registered Nurse First Assistant
Plastic and Reconstructive Surgery
Akron, Ohio

M. Jane Rua, RN, BSN, JD
Jeffries, Kube, Forrest, and Monteleone, Co LPA
Cleveland, Ohio

Patricia Seymour, RN, MS
Administrator, Educational Services for Professionals
Ashtabula, Ohio

Reviewers

Terri Goodman, RN, BSN, MA, CNOR
Manager, Professional Education
Johnson & Johnson Medical, Inc.
Arlington, Texas

Cecil A. King, RN, BSN, MS (C), CNOR
Assistant Nurse Manager
University of Washington Medical Center
Seattle, Washington

Kathleen Lunday, RN, MSN, CNOR
Instructor, Nell Hodgson Woodruff School of Nursing
Emory University
Atlanta, Georgia

Rosemary Ann Roth, RN, MSN, CNOR, CNAA
Administrator, Surgical/Perinatal Services
The Genesee Hospital
Rochester, New York

Vicki Suster, RN, BSN
Clinical Support Specialist
PHS Mt. Sinai Medical Center
Cleveland, Ohio

Laurel A. Wiersema-Bryant, RN, MSN, CS
Clinical Nurse Specialist
Barnes-Jewish Hospital
St. Louis, Missouri

Denise L. Witt, AAS, BSN, MA
Assistant Professor
Nassau Community College
Garden City, New York

Dedicated to our wonderful families,
dear colleagues, and loving supporters

Preface

The objective of this textbook is to conceptualize plastic surgery for perioperative nurses, surgical technologists, and other caregivers at a baseline level. Practices and techniques vary between surgeons and facility types, but the goals for restoration of form and function are the same. Plastic, or aesthetic, surgery is fundamental to the beautification of physical form, which is what the patient sees after the procedure is completed.

Part 1 provides information that is fundamental to all plastic surgery patients, such as the following:
- Foundations, including photography, equipment, and instrumentation
- Features of a plastic surgery facility
- Perioperative caregiver roles
- Anesthesia considerations
- Psychosocial aspects of plastic surgery patients
- Skin anatomy and physiology
- Wound management

The purpose of Part 1 is to establish common ground and describe specific conceptual aspects of the plastic surgery process and environment. A short chronologic history of plastic surgery ranging from early recorded history to the present provides baseline information essential to all procedures. An emphasis is placed on the importance of clinical photography and how the perioperative nurse can help set the stage and snap the pictures as necessary. A systematic method of photo styling is important to the usefulness of the final prints.

Instrumentation common to most plastic surgery procedures is pictured as single generic units. Each facility has its own combination sets stemming from a base set with individual surgeon's preference items added as desired. Basic anesthetic techniques are described, and specific patient selection considerations identified for safe administration of anesthesia during the surgical procedure.

Team roles and credentials in the planning of care stress the importance fo the nursing process and holistic perioperative patient care. Professionalism and voluntary certification are explained and encouraged. This information is useful criteria by which to develop performance evaluations.

The psyche of the patient seeking aesthetic surgery is explored. The perioperative nurse should assess the patient for motive and realistic expectations. Proper psychologic and physiologic preparation can help the patient adapt to changes and avoid disappointment caused by unrealistic expectations. Understanding why the patient desires surgical intervention can be helpful when setting attainable goals. Psychologic considerations for pediatric and geriatric patient care are included. Safe positioning, prepping, and skin marking are described. Care of the patient's incisions and the process of wound closure and healing are detailed for enhanced clinical understanding.

Part 2 describes and categorizes plastic surgical procedures according to location of the anatomy, such as the following:
- Surface: Skin surface, grafts, flaps, and burns
- Subsurface: Liposuction, abdominoplasty, injectables, implants, hand
- Head and neck: Facelift, nose, ear, hair
- Breast: Anatomy, physiology, pathophysiology, reconstruction, augmentation, reduction

Selected surgical procedures are explained and illustrated in each chapter. Many plastic and reconstructive procedures use the same or similar techniques, although the actual site may vary. In the interest of avoiding repetition, representative procedures are depicted in this text. Appropriate anatomy and physiology for each surgical procedure is explained in detail. Perioperative patient care for each procedure is included.

Plastic and reconstructive surgical nursing is challenging and rewarding. The completed process is like watching an evolving work of art personified by the patient's reaction to his or her new look.

Acknowledgements

This text was made possible through the patience and assistance of our dear colleagues, contributors, and consultants. We are particularly thankful to Dr. Brian W. Davies who provided most of the clinical photographs. He kindly allowed his beautiful Akron, Ohio clinic to be an example of a free-standing facility and offered his expertise and knowledge without hesitation. His caring rapport with his patients serves as a positive example for us all.

We are grateful to the library staff at the Cleveland Clinic Foundation for their assistance during the research phases of this book.

Many thanks to all the manufacturers, who supplied photos of instrumentation, equipment, and supplies,

Special thanks to Michael Ledbetter, nursing editor, and Nancy O'Brien, developmental editor, for their patience and assistance with the production of this work.

Contents

Foundations of PLASTIC AND RECONSTRUCTIVE SURGERY

1 History and Fundamentals of Plastic and Reconstructive Surgery

Many techniques used today in plastic and reconstructive surgery are based on practices and procedures that have been developed throughout history.

EARLY PLASTIC SURGERY

The earliest recorded plastic surgery procedures were documented in the Edwin Smith papyrus and the Ebers papyrus written in Egypt around 1800 BC. This ancient document describes the healing of wounds after treatment with sugar and honey. Dressings saturated with this mixture in an emulsion of animal fat exhibited antibacterial qualities and promoted uncomplicated healing. Later writings showed that the Egyptians were concerned with an aesthetic result and closed wounds with early forms of suture and linen strips. Evidence of dermabrasion has been found. Mummified remains have been discovered that have lacerations with intact suture material. The Egyptians were the first to develop practice specialties.

Skin flaps were common in India and are documented as early as 700 BC by Sushruta in *The Samhita*. Flaps were taken from the forehead and cheeks for reconstruction of the nose. Nasal amputation was a common form of punishment for infidelity or criminal acts. Alcoholic drinks were used as anesthetic agents. Physicians in India were among the first to use insect jaws as wound closure clips. References are also made to asepsis and the need to remain clean.

The ancient Greek physician Hippocrates (480-377 BC) described the importance of allowing a wound to heal on its own for the best results. Most of the wounds observed by Hippocrates were battle-induced injuries, such as arrow puncture sites. He did not view surgery as a specialized discipline but as a secondary, low-skill treatment.

Homer documents that wounds were irrigated with wine and allowed to heal by secondary intention. Cautery was used for bleeding. Primary closure was performed with horse hair and cotton threads. The Greeks were the first to document the need for assistants, adequate lighting, and appropriate instrumentation.

The Romans further refined the use of suture ligatures and skin flaps. Celsus (25-50 AD) developed advancement flaps and island pedicle grafts. Galen (130-200 AD) founded the basics of wound repair that are currently used today. He supported tendon repair, trimming approximated wound edges, and placing primary incisions in natural skin lines. Galen taught that wounds could not heal unless they became supperative. He believed that foul smelling exudate meant that the wound was beginning to heal.

The Renaissance of the fourteenth century continued into the sixteenth century. Education and shared knowledge of the sciences brought about improved surgical technique. Ambroise Paré (1510-1590), while in military service as a medic, observed the treatment of gunshot wounds. The standard of care was to pour boiling oil into the wound. During one particular battle the supply of oil was depleted, so he dressed the wounds with room temperature cooking lard. He was surprised to find that the soldiers treated with boiling oil became infected and the others treated with lard were healing without complications. Paré found that ligatures and butterfly strips preserved the viability of tissue when used for hemostasis better than cautery. He often coated wounds with turpentine, which demonstrated an antibacterial effect. Paré went against popular tradition of the time and wrote that the patient should be treated humanely regardless of societal position, that wealthy and poor patients should be treated the same. This belief was unpopular for many centuries but has become the cornerstone for medical and nursing practice of modern times.

DEVELOPMENT OF MODERN PLASTIC AND RECONSTRUCTIVE SURGERY

The seventeenth to nineteenth centuries brought about monumental advances in surgical technique and the survival rate after the procedure. Major discoveries included the function of blood, methods of transfusion, germ theory, and microscopy. Anesthesia, x-ray examination, and endoscopy were added to the surgical arena during the twentieth century.

These landmark events supported the development of modern plastic and reconstructive disciplines as they are practiced today.

Technologic strides have been made in wound healing based on historic procedures. Tissue flaps are commonly transferred from one area of the body to another. Portions of flaps, such as muscle layers, can remain vascularized in situ after transfer. Reconstruction of the breast is accomplished with myocutaneous flaps that look and feel as natural as the original tissue. The underlying structure of a body part can be modified for form or functional purposes. The surface can be altered by lasers, tattoos, and dermal/epidermal mechanical and chemical procedures. The result is successful because of wound closure techniques, specialized instrumentation, and careful attention to sterile technique.

Aesthetic Versus Reconstructive Surgery

Form follows function and function follows form. In the realm of aesthetic surgery, the functional appeal is closely mirrored by the visual form. Aesthetic surgery involves improving or enhancing appearance by altering the shape of facial structures and skin, sculpting body contours, and "perfecting" natural body features. Aesthetically, patients who seek surgical intervention for beautification or appearance also may be seeking healing of the psyche. Patients who are unhappy with their appearance are not able to deal with the world as confidently as they would if they felt positive about themselves. Self image can improve after aesthetic surgery causing a better quality of life. Historically, more females have sought aesthetic intervention, but recently the number of males undergoing aesthetic procedures has increased. Formerly thought of as procedures of the wealthy, aesthetic surgery is now sought by individuals from all socioeconomic backgrounds.

Reconstructive surgery is performed to create, replace, restore, or repair natural body parts. The result of a disfiguring injury, congenital defect, or radical surgical procedure can impact an individual throughout his or her entire life. Reconstructive procedures can create functional body parts, such as digit creation or transfers for appositional grasping and palate reinforcement for eating. In addition to creating functional parts, the psyche benefits from reconstruction (Fig. 1-1).

Throughout history, humans have regarded deformed offspring as undesirable and possibly evil. Even with nonlethal deformities, many of these infants were destroyed or abandoned in the wilderness. This is not unlike activities in other mammalian species. Most often, the male would destroy any unusual offspring in an effort to provide more food for the healthiest of the litter. In some cultures, breech presentations, twin births, and infants born on unlucky days were considered evil. The

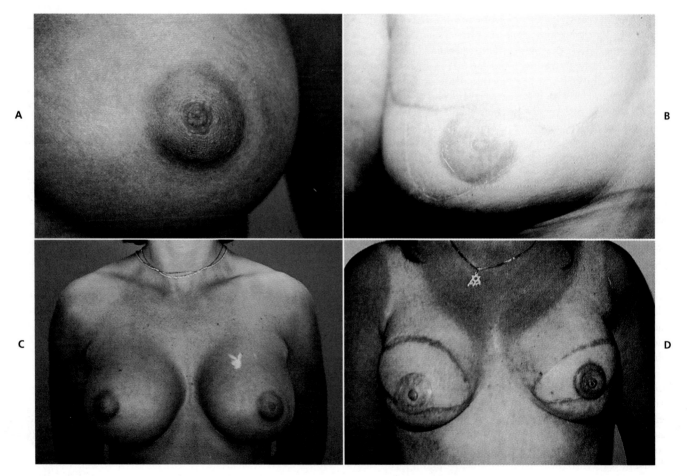

Fig. 1-1 Aesthetic vs. reconstructive plastic surgery. (*Courtesy Brian W. Davies, MD.*)

belief in reincarnation and afterlife influenced the practice of infanticide. In times of famine, cannibalism was practiced. The weaker and deformed children were fed to the stronger and more healthy children of the family. A deformed child was thought to be an omen of the devil or the product of bad karma. Some cultures thought that a deformed child was a punishment for bad parents. In some regions the mother was put to death with the child as atonement for the perceived transgression. This was particularly true if the infant resembled some type of monster or mythical being.

Monstrosities were historically categorized as (1) those with too much, such as extra digits; (2) those with missing parts, such as limbs; and (3) those with complete duplications, such as an extra limb or the case of complete Siamese twins. Although through history these children were regarded as freaks, in modern society they are considered human children of human parents. The question of compatibility with life is taken into consideration when planning a reconstructive procedure.

Clinical Photography in Plastic and Reconstructive Surgery

The use of photography in plastic surgery has been valuable in planning care and monitoring chronologic changes in the patient's condition. The images, whether still photos (referred to as prints or slides) or videos, are taken before, during, and after any aesthetic or reconstructive surgical procedure. Each print or slide is made to correspond to life-size proportions and may be derived from video sequences utilizing stop-action or pause. Some facilities may have a professional photographer on staff. In smaller practice settings, the perioperative nurse or first assistant may be responsible for clinical photography (Box 1-1).

Before any photographs or videos are made, the patient should sign a consent form and, in some settings, may need to sign a release for use of the material as a teaching tool. When used as a teaching tool, the photo or video image should not unnecessarily reveal the patient's identity. Regardless of informed consent, the patient's privacy is important. Some facilities have a formal studio and darkroom (Fig. 1-2) wherein the patient can be photographed in complete privacy. Jewelry, makeup, and clothing can be a distraction and should be removed if possible.

If a controlled environment is not available, background and foreground clutter should be covered or focused out before the photograph is taken. In the operating room (OR), the area should be squared off with clean sterile towels. Blues, grays, and greens provide the best photographic background contrast. Black is stark and may diminish fine lines or definition in pigmented tissue. Bloody instruments and sponges should not be included in the photo. During an educational session, these photos or videos may be seen by the patient or other lay public.

Uniform, life-size views of the patient should be established according to a standard technique. As a "working model" of the patient, these photographs are essential to planning, patient teaching, and documentation. Standard views for each procedure should be established. These views should include body posture, angulation of features, and distance from the lens and should be reproducible for serial photographic sessions to document staged procedures. Alteration of the view may distort the

---

Box 1-1 **Nursing Considerations in Clinical Photography**

PREPARE THE PATIENT
Obtain informed consent
Set realistic expectations
Provide patient privacy
Prepare positioning for serial images
Document site of specimen and identity of subject

PREPARE EQUIPMENT
Check film speed
Install fresh batteries in camera
Provide source of augmented lighting as needed
Fully charge power packs for flash
Clean lenses

PREPARE ENVIRONMENT
Prepare lighting
Remove clutter from foreground and background
Protect self and equipment from body substances
Prevent contamination of sterile field
Position cables and cords safely

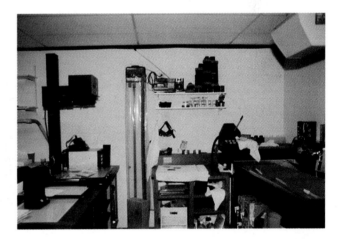

Fig. 1-2 Clinical onsite darkroom.

---

approach, creating a risk for overcorrection or undercorrection of the body part. Photographs of children who will be having staged reconstructive procedures over a period of time (perhaps years) should take growth patterns into consideration when planning photo sessions (Fig. 1-3). Comparison with photos of siblings or the parents when they were young may help with creating the series.

The planning phase of the surgical procedure is based in part on photographs of the surgical site before it is altered or restored. Measurements are carefully made of the existing tissue, and translucent overlays are drawn to demonstrate projected changes (Fig. 1-4). The markings on the overlay correspond to proportionate modifications and form a maplike template. This template enables the surgeon and the patient to make decisions about

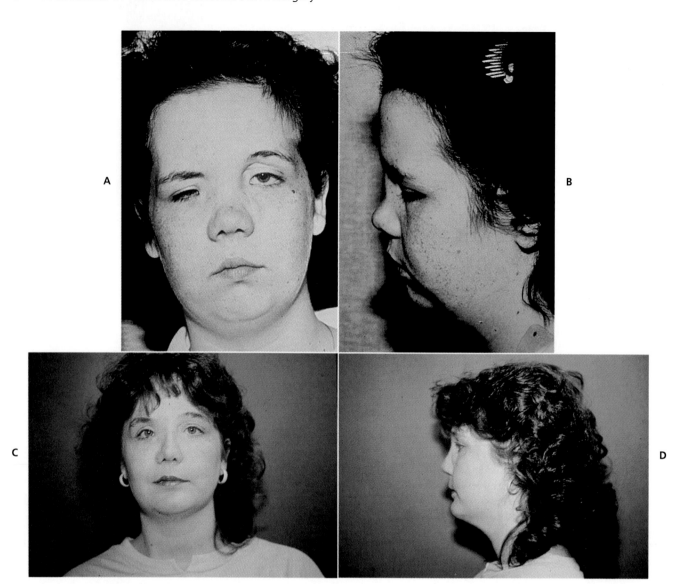

Fig. 1-3 Example of plastic and reconstructive surgery for congenital deformity. (*Courtesy Brian W. Davies, MD.*)

how to proceed with the surgical procedure. Every attempt should be made to maintain realistic expectations about results (Figs. 1-5, 1-6, and 1-7).

Equipment

A 35 mm single lens reflex (SLR) camera with a motor drive is optimal for producing the photographic record. The motor drive enables the photographer to expose 2.5 frames per second without distortion caused by stopping to advance the film between shots. A tripod is also useful for stabilization of the camera during the session. Many office-based settings have darkroom capabilities on the premises.

Lighting is important to the clarity, depth of field, and accuracy of the image. It is measured by a hand-held light meter or by a meter contained within the camera via through-the-lens (TTL) metering. TTL can be set to control strobe flash units directly in synchronization with the shutter of the camera. Flash

units may be free standing, attached to a "hot shoe" on the camera, or on a ring light encircling the lens. The level of lighting directly affects the quality of the photograph.

Lenses come in sizes ranging from 7.5 mm to 1600 mm. An adjustable 85 to 105 mm lens may work well for some clinical photography. Zoom lenses are not used often because it is difficult to record a consistent image for serial photographs. The amount of light that enters the lens is controlled by adjusting the aperture, referred to as the *f-stop*. Smaller numbers on the f-stop adjustment admit more light through the lens. Larger numbers minimize the opening of the aperture to limit the amount of light exposure. F-stops range between f/1.4 and f/32 depending on the type of lens used. The rate of speed at which the aperture opens is measured in seconds and fractions of seconds ranging from 1 second to 1/1000th of a second. The f-stop is set to open only to a certain degree for a prescribed period of time to create a photograph.

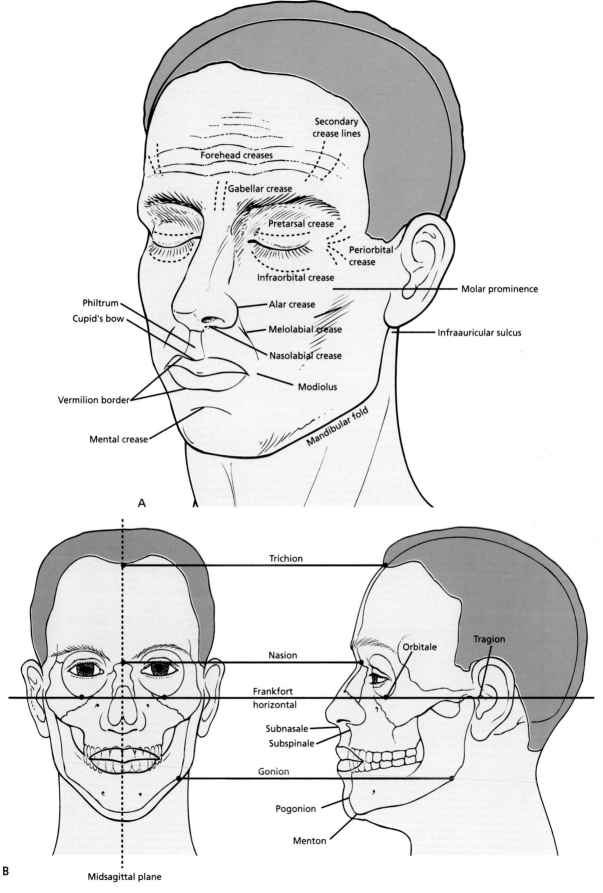

Fig. 1-4 A, Important landmarks and creases of the face. **B,** Anthropometric landmarks essential for measuring facial bony structures.

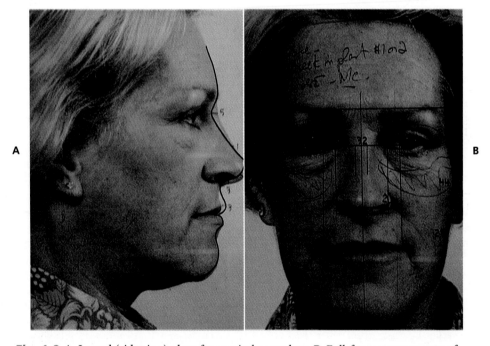

Fig. 1-5 A, Lateral (side view) plans for chin augmentation. **B,** Full-face measurements of planned changes. (*Courtesy Brian W. Davies, MD.*)

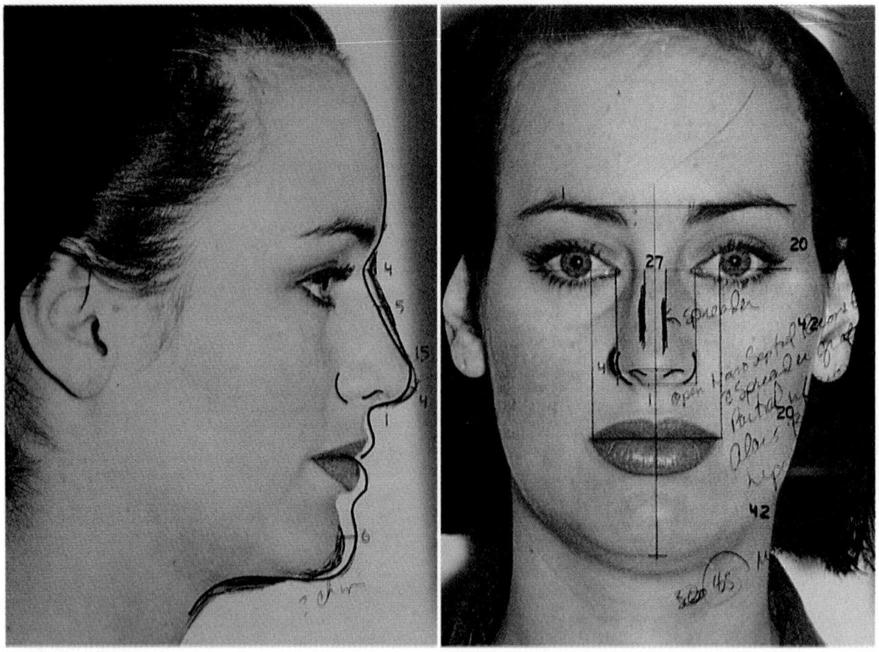

Fig. 1-6 A, Lateral (side view) plans for surgical procedure. **B,** Full-face measurements of planned changes. (*Courtesy Brian W. Davies, MD.*)

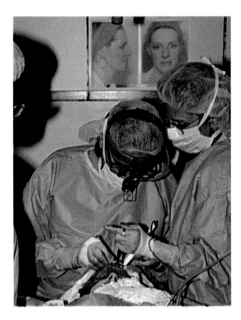

Fig. 1-7 Preoperative photographs are prominently displayed for reference during the surgical procedure. (*Courtesy Brian W. Davies, MD.*)

Macroimages can be made with a 50 to 100 mm lens when close-ups of smaller anatomic features are necessary. These appear larger than life-size without much depth of field. This can be compensated for by a smaller aperture and a longer exposure time. High-magnification photography is usually done with a tripod and a shutter release cable to minimize vibration. Ring lights are useful for macrophotography because they cast no shadows. Close-up lens attachments and extension tubes are available and can increase the image beyond a 1:1 ratio. These are helpful when photographing small features of excised specimens. A graduated marker, ruler, or size-perspective object, such as an instrument tip, can be placed in the foreground to demonstrate the actual size of the specimen.

The depth of field is defined by the amount of foreground and background included with the photographed subject. Smaller f-stops increase the depth of field in the photograph. More details are clearly visible. Many manufacturers have developed cameras that are equipped with aperture priority, program, and high-speed program modes that, when activated, automatically set the light exposure through the lens for the correct amount of exposure time. Autofocus equipment is also available in combination with automatic settings.

Filters may interfere with the accuracy of the image because of optical density. The light exposure is decreased, and longer exposure times may be needed. The f-stop should be decreased by 1.0 or more if a filter is used. This may help to compensate for the light modifications. Polarizers eliminate reflections of nonmetalic surfaces. If used, a smaller aperture (higher numbered f-stop) is needed. This is referred to as "stopping down" the lens.

Slide film is used most often for recording aesthetic and reconstructive procedures. Prints can be made from slides for specific needs, such as life size models with overlays to depict "before and after" procedural plans of care. Film speed is measured in units

referred to as International Standards Organization (ISO) and is selected for use according to the amount of light available for imaging. Lower speeds require more light exposure. Film speeds range between 25 to 1000 ISO. In clinical photography, lower speeds are used because they are more clear and have less grain. ISO 25 slide film is optimal for clinical use and produces the best results. ISO 25, 64, and 100 are most commonly used. Higher-speed films are more light sensitive and require less light exposure to create the image. The result is more grain and less clarity. Color film is useful for making slides for presentation or publication. It is also used to document pigmented lesions and is generally more interesting for educational sessions. Black-and-white film is available for use in incandescent lighting or daylight and is useful when texture or shading gradient is the main feature of the subject.

In areas of functional mobility, such as the jaw, the use of videography may be helpful in creating a plan for reconstruction based on anatomic motion. Still prints can be made of specific poses that will be useful in the reconstructive process. The video, when played in slow motion, may give clues as to other functional defects that may go unnoticed in real-time viewing. Some types of video imaging and endoscopic photography can be computer enhanced to project progressive changes through graphic application. Images can be stored on diskette or compact disc (CD). Still prints can be selectively printed for inclusion in the permanent record. Some computer-enhanced images may be misleading to patients and may lead to unrealistic expectations of the surgical procedure.

Other Considerations

Photographs or videos may be used for legal documentation of trauma, reconstruction of congenital or acquired defects, procedural practices, or validation of the need for surgery to an insurance provider. Photographs provided by the patient also can be useful during the preoperative assessment. In reconstruction, photos of pretrauma features can serve as a guide for development of the intraoperative plan of care. Photos of genetic family members may also provide structural information.

During the photography session, consideration for infection control and maintenance of the sterile field is important. The camera and related equipment should be protected from body substance exposure. Cords and cables should not be draped over the sterile field. Care should be taken in the darkroom to avoid chemical exposure. Used solutions and developer should be disposed of properly. Some solutions contain metallics that should not be disposed of in municipal sewage systems. Silver salvage devices are commercially available.

The American Society of Plastic and Reconstructive Surgeons (ASPRS) is an excellent resource for information about standardization in clinical photography. The Plastic Surgery Educational Foundation (PSEF) sponsors workshops on photography for perioperative caregivers. Refer to the following for more information:

ASPRS/PSEF
444 East Algonquin Road
Arlington Heights, IL 60005-4664
1-800-766-4955, ext. 404

Instrumentation

Plastic surgery requiring incisional or excisional procedures is performed with the same or similar instrumentation as minor procedures in other services. This is because most plastic surgeries are performed with smaller, more precise, concealed incisions. A basic plastic instrument set (Fig. 1-8) with delicate scissors, pickups, forceps, and retractors is the baseline set to which additional, more specific instruments can be added. Few large instruments are used unless a large flap, such as in abdominoplasty, is raised. When needed, longer, wider, and heavier instruments such as those used in general surgery are added to the basic set. See Figures 1-9 through 1-27 for select individual instruments and Figures 1-28 through 1-30 for microinstrumentation.

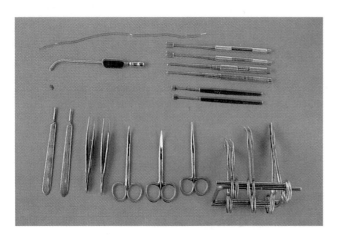

Fig. 1-8 Basic plastic instrument set. *Left top,* Killian suction stylet; Killian suction tube. *Right top,* two Joseph skin hooks, double; two Joseph skin hooks, single; two Bair (Rollet) retractors, 4-prong. *Bottom: left to right,* two Bard Parker knife handles, No. 3; two Castroviejo suturing forceps, wide handles, with tying platforms, 0.5 mm teeth; plastic scissors, sharp, curved; one strabismus scissors, slightly curved; Stevens tenotomy scissors, straight; Backhaus towel forceps, small: two Halstead mosquito forceps, curved; Johnson needle holder, smooth jaw; Webster needle holder, diamond jaw. *(From Brooks-Tighe:* Instrumentation for the operating room, *ed 4, St Louis, 1994, Mosby.)*

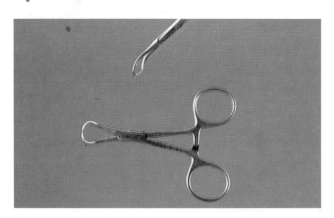

Fig. 1-9 Small Backhaus towel clip. *(From Brooks-Tighe:* Instrumentation for the operating room, *ed 4, St Louis, 1994, Mosby.)*

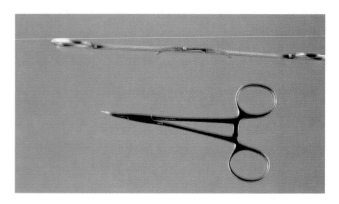

Fig. 1-10 Halstead curved mosquito forceps. *(From Brooks-Tighe:* Instrumentation for the operating room, *ed 4, St Louis, 1994, Mosby.)*

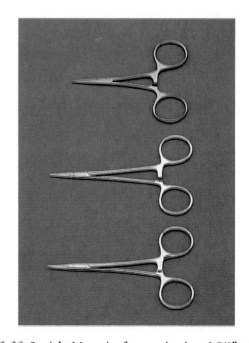

Fig. 1-11 Straight Mosquito forceps titanium 3 7/8", straight Mosquito stainless 5', straight Mosquito 6 3/8'. *(Courtesy Scanlon, International, St Paul, Minnesota.)*

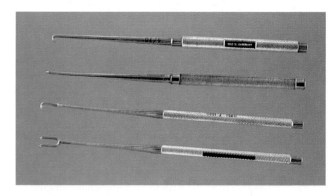

Fig. 1-12 *Top,* Joseph skin hook retractor, single. *Bottom,* Joseph skin hook retractor, double. *(From Brooks-Tighe:* Instrumentation for the operating room, *ed 4, St Louis, 1994, Mosby.)*

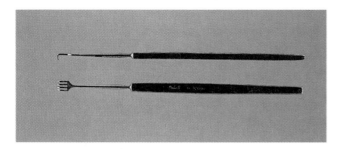

Fig. 1-13 Blair-Rollet 4-prong retractor. *(From Brooks-Tighe:* Instrumentation for the operating room, *ed 4, St Louis, 1994, Mosby.)*

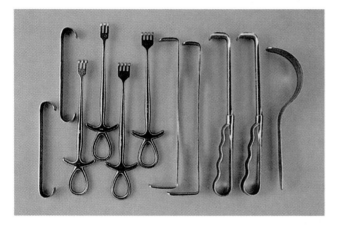

Fig. 1-14 Assorted retractors used in plastic surgery. *(From Brooks-Tighe:* Instrumentation for the operating room, *ed 4, St Louis, 1994, Mosby.)*

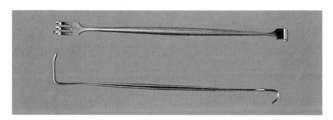

Fig. 1-15 Senn-Kanavel retractor. *(From Brooks-Tighe:* Instrumentation for the operating room, *ed 4, St Louis, 1994, Mosby.)*

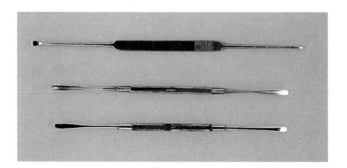

Fig. 1-16 Periosteal elevators. *(From Brooks-Tighe:* Instrumentation for the operating room, *ed 4, St Louis, 1994, Mosby.)*

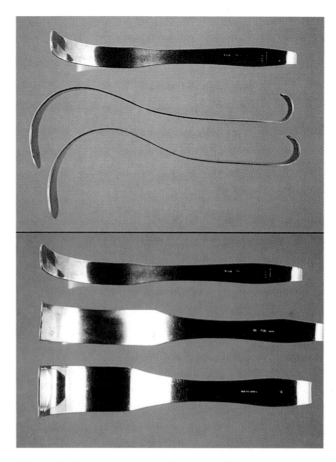

Fig. 1-17 Deaver retractors of various widths for larger flaps. *(From Brooks-Tighe:* Instrumentation for the operating room, *ed 4, St Louis, 1994, Mosby.)*

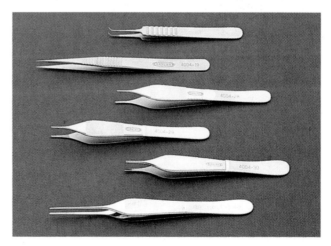

Fig. 1-18 Forceps. *Top to bottom,* 45 angled jeweler's forceps, straight jeweler's forceps, Adson forceps with 1:1 teeth, Adson forceps with 1:1 teeth 1.2 mm, Adson-Brown tissue forceps with side teeth, Broli-Adson forceps with diamond dust tips. *(Courtesy Scanlon, International, St Paul, Minnesota.)*

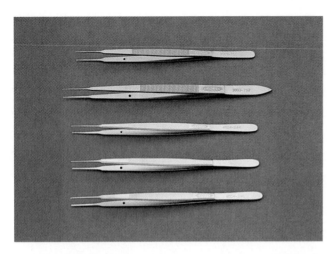

Fig. 1-19 Gerald forceps. *Top to bottom,* Titanium diamond dust ring tips 7′, titanium diamond dust ring tips 8′, stainless diamond dust ring tips 7′, delicate 1:2 teeth 7′, 1 mm diamond dust 7′. *(Courtesy Scanlon, International, St Paul, Minnesota.)*

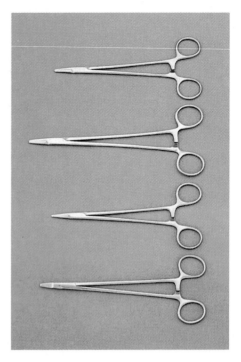

Fig. 1-21 Needle holders. *Top to bottom,* Mayo-Hegar 7 1/8′ diamond dust jaw, Mayo-Hegar 8 5/8′ diamond dust jaw, DeBakey 7 1/8′ diamond dust jaw, DeBakey 8 5/8′ diamond dust jaw. *(Courtesy Scanlon, International, St Paul, Minnesota.)*

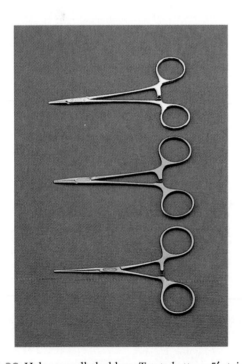

Fig. 1-20 Halsey needle holders. *Top to bottom,* 5′ stainless, 5′ diamond dust jaw, 5′ titanium. *(Courtesy Scanlon, International, St Paul, Minnesota.)*

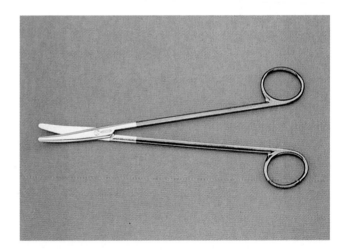

Fig. 1-22 Curved Metzenbaum scissors 7′ stainless. *(Courtesy Scanlon, International, St Paul, Minnesota.)*

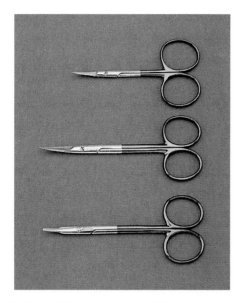

Fig. 1-23 Curved Jabaley scissors 4 3/4', curved Jabaley scissors 5', straight Jabaley scissors 5'. *(Courtesy Scanlon, International, St Paul, Minnesota.)*

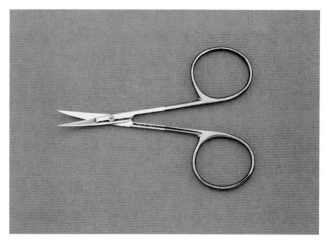

Fig. 1-26 Curved Iris scissors 4'. *(Courtesy Scanlon, International, St Paul, Minnesota.)*

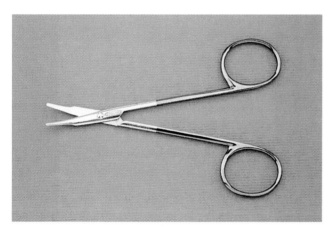

Fig. 1-24 Curved Stevens tenotomy scissors 4 5/8'. *(Courtesy Scanlon, International, St Paul, Minnesota.)*

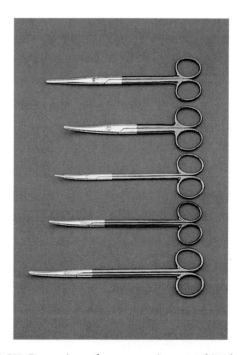

Fig. 1-27 Comparison of common scissors used in plastic surgery. Straight Mayo scissors 6 3/4', curved Mayo scissors 6 3/4', curved Stevens tenotomy scissors 7', curved Metzenbaum scissors 7', curved Metzenbaum scissors 8'. *(Courtesy Scanlon, International, St Paul, Minnesota.)*

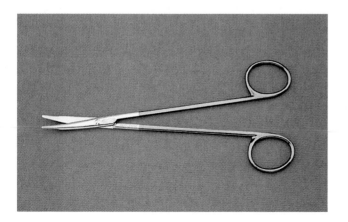

Fig. 1-25 Curved Stevens tenotomy scissors 7'. *(Courtesy Scanlon, International, St Paul, Minnesota.)*

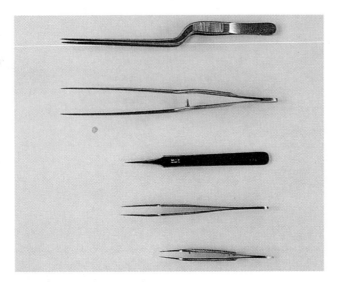

Fig. 1-28 *Top to bottom,* 2 Yasargil micro forceps, bayonet shaft: side view, front view; 2 jeweler's forceps: side view, front view; 1 Castroviejo suturing forceps. *(From Brooks-Tighe: Instrumentation for the operating room, ed 4, St Louis, 1994, Mosby.)*

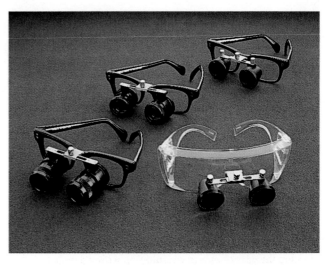

Fig. 1-30 Magnifying loupes. Some plastic surgeons use microinstruments for procedures that do not require the use of a microscope. Surgical loupes can provide sufficient magnification for procedures requiring delicate tissue handling, such as in neurological or vascular repair. *(Courtesy Scanlon, International, St Paul, Minnesota.)*

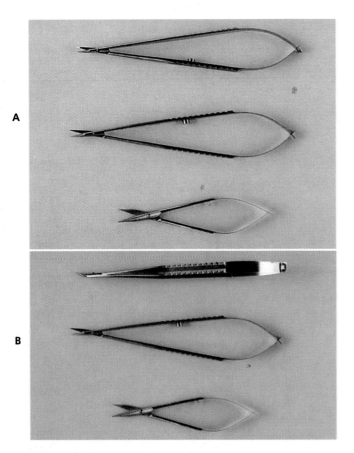

A

B

Fig. 1-29 A, *Top to bottom,* 1 Westcott tenotomy scissors, curved; 1 Westcott tenotomy scissors, straight; 1 Vannas capsulotomy scissors. **B,** *Top to bottom,* 1 Westcott tenotomy scissors, curved, side view; 1 Westcott tenotomy scissors, straight; 1 Vannas capsulotomy scissors. *(From Brooks-Tighe: Instrumentation for the operating room, ed 4, St Louis, 1994, Mosby.)*

Bibliography

American Society of Plastic and Reconstructive Surgical Nurses: *Core curriculum for plastic and reconstructive surgical nursing,* ed 2, Pitman, New Jersey, 1996, ASPRSN.

Bennett RG: *Fundamentals of cutaneous surgery,* St Louis, 1988, Mosby.

Carr J et al: Making use of photography in the assessment of injuries, *Nursing Times* 87(44):30, 1991.

Ellenbogen R et al: Achieving standardized photographs in aesthetic surgery, *Plast Reconstr Surg* 86(5):955, 1990.

Halpin-Landry JE: Documenting wounds through the camera's eye, *Nursing* 24(12):58, 1994.

Harris ES, Morgan RF: Thomas Dent Mutter, MD: early reparative surgeon, *Ann Plast Surg* 33(3):333, 1994.

Marlenga B, Parker-Conrad JE: Knowledge of occupational hazards in photography, *AAOHN J* 41(4):175, 1993.

Smoot EC III, Higgs J: Photographing the patient with burns for medical documentation, *J Burn Care Rehabil* 15(5):434, 1994.

Starr P: *The social transformation of American medicine,* New York, 1982, Basic Books.

Wentz MG: Clinical photography simplified: developing a personal set of uniform views, *Plast Surg Nurs* 15(4):211, 1995.

2 Members of the Plastic and Reconstructive Surgery Team

The perioperative plastic and reconstructive surgical team consists of the perioperative nurse, the registered nurse first assistant (RNFA), and the plastic surgeon. Together they develop the plan of care in consultation with the patient. Other disciplines of caregivers such as surgical technologists and physician assistants may contribute to patient care. The plastic and reconstructive surgery team may be found in institutional settings, office-based surgical suites, and free-standing ambulatory centers. As a team, in combination with qualified anesthesia providers, they strive to improve the way a patient looks, functions, and subjectively feels (Fig. 2-1). For some patients, the restoration of function is the focus of care. For others, beautification is the main objective. Regardless of the motivation for the procedures, the team assists the patient to set attainable goals and outcomes that are critical to the success of the surgical procedure.

Professional organizations, such as the American Society of Plastic and Reconstructive Surgeons (ASPRS) and American Society of Plastic and Reconstructive Surgical Nurses (ASPRSN) have developed standards by which to measure patient care outcomes (see Appendix). Surgeons and nurses who belong to these groups have met membership requirements and have taken an additional stride in professionalism.

PERIOPERATIVE NURSE IN PLASTIC AND RECONSTRUCTIVE SURGERY

The professional perioperative nurse provides the link between caregivers and patients through the nursing process (Fig. 2-2). Although the patient is directing most of his or her attention to the surgical procedure and the outcome, the perioperative nurse helps the patient view the plastic and/or reconstructive process in realistic terms. A multidisciplinary collaborative effort may include a social worker or clinical psychologist who can help the patient work through multistage reconstructive procedures. The patient's family or significant others also may be involved with the development and implementation of the plan because they may be involved with postoperative care. The perioperative nurse maintains continuity by coordinating all aspects of patient care through a holistic approach.

The plan of care is initiated and followed to completion by the perioperative nurse. The plan is structured around the intended surgical procedure and the standard activities of the operating surgeon, and it is tailored to the needs, problems, or health considerations of the patient. Development of the plan begins with the initial preoperative interview and initial nursing assessment. The surgeon or the RNFA performs a preoperative history and physical examination to provide baseline data. The perioperative nurse establishes the appropriate nursing diagnoses

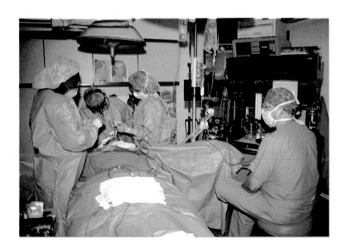

Fig. 2-1 Teamwork in the intraoperative phase of care.

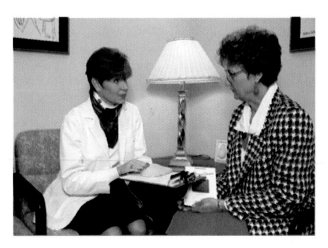

Fig. 2-2 Initial preoperative interview. *(From Potter:* Basic nursing, *ed 3, St Louis, 1995, Mosby.)*

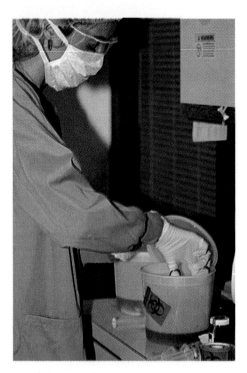

Fig. 2-3 Circulating nurse preparing surgical specimen while wearing appropriate personal protective attire.

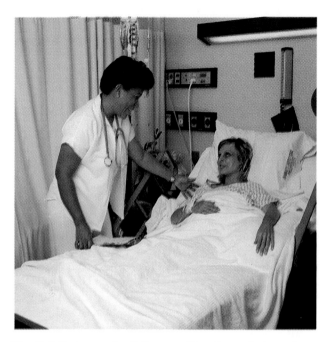

Fig. 2-4 Postoperative follow-up. *(From Potter:* Basic nursing, *ed 3, St Louis, 1995, Mosby.)*

and identifies expected outcomes. Specific preoperative, intraoperative, and postoperative interventions are individualized in consideration for the entire perioperative cycle, including remote postoperative care (Fig. 2-3). Postoperatively, the perioperative nurse evaluates the plan and measures the attainment of desired outcomes (Fig. 2-4).

Professionalism in plastic and reconstructive surgical nursing can be demonstrated through additional voluntary credentialing. Certification by examination in plastic and reconstructive plastic surgical nursing is available to registered nurses in plastic surgery practice through the Plastic Surgical Nursing Certification Board (PSNCB) (Fig. 2-5). Plastic surgery nursing practice can consist of staff, assisting, administrative, teaching, or research roles. The examination is composed of objective questions and is designed to test the nurse's ability to synthesize the nursing process and apply biopsychosocial science to patient care. Established in 1989, eligibility for certification and recertification in plastic surgery nursing includes the following:

- Licensure as a registered nurse in the United States or Canada
- Minimum of 2 years of experience in plastic surgery nursing within 5 years of the application process
- Hours in plastic surgical nursing practice equaling 50% of total hours worked in a 2-year period within 5 years of the application process

Credentialing as a certified plastic surgery nurse (CPSN) is valid for 3 years. At that time the credential may be renewed by reexamination or continuing education. Recertification may be attained by the contact hour method. A total of 45 contact hours are required in a 3-year period. This is divided into 30 hours specific to plastic and reconstructive surgical nursing and

15 hours of nursing topics of choice. The certification/recertification process is available to members of the ASPRSN at a reduced rate. Membership in the ASPRSN also includes a subscription to the quarterly journal, Plastic Surgical Nursing. See Figure 2-6 for a sample ASPRSN certificate. Information about membership, certification, and recertification can be obtained from the following:

American Society of Plastic and Reconstructive Surgical Nurses
East Holly Avenue
PO Box 56
Pitman, New Jersey 08071-0056
(609) 256-2340
http://www.inurse.com/~asprsn

RNFA IN PLASTIC AND RECONSTRUCTIVE SURGERY

A perioperative nurse may be credentialed to perform in the expanded role as a plastic and reconstructive first assistant in the perioperative setting. Credentialing as an RNFA includes attendance at an accredited program as recommended by the Association of Operating Room Nurses (AORN). RNFA program length and design vary according to state requirements. Eligibility for entrance to a RNFA program generally includes the following:

- Registered nursing license in the state of practice
- Perioperative certification, CNOR with 24 months of perioperative nursing experience
- Proficiency in scrub and circulating role (Fig. 2-7)
- Basic knowledge of anatomy and physiology
- Cardiopulmonary resuscitation (CPR)/Basic Life Saver (BLS) certification (may vary between states and facilities)
- Ability to perform in stressful situations

Plastic Surgical Nursing Certification Board

hereby attests that

Nancy Marie Fortunato

having successfully fulfilled the Education, Practice, and Written Examination Requirements merits the Designation

Certified Plastic Surgical Nurse

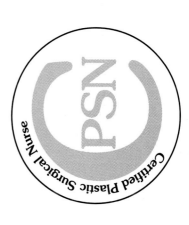

Valid through June 1999

Margaret Shirer, BS, RN, CPSN
President
Plastic Surgical Nursing
Certification Board

Fig. 2-5 Certified Plastic Surgical Nurse certification.

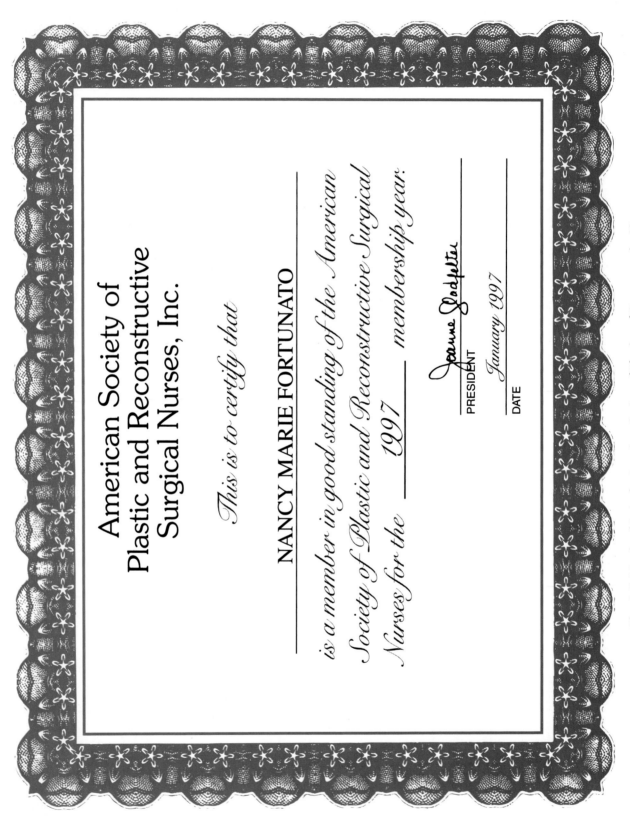

Fig. 2-6 Membership in the American Society of Plastic and Reconstructive Nurses.

National Certification Board:
Perioperative Nursing, Inc.

Confers upon

Nancymarie Fortunato

Certification I.D.

941907

Certification for Professional Achievement in
Perioperative Nursing Practice

1994 to 1999

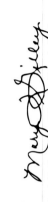

President, National Certification Board: Perioperative Nursing, Inc.

Secretary, National Certification Board: Perioperative Nursing, Inc.

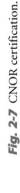

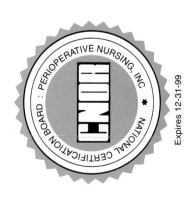

Expires 12-31-99

Fig. 2-7 CNOR certification.

- Ability to recognize safety hazards in perioperative environment and initiate correction
- Letters of reference from specified colleagues and surgeons
- Professional liability insurance

Some states require Advanced Cardiac Life Support (ACLS) certification. Pediatric Advanced Life Support (PALS) certification is advised where the practice is comprised mainly of pediatric patients. The RNFA provides professional care to the surgical patient throughout the perioperative experience. Credentialing is also required in the facility of practice. Each facility has its own particular method of credentialing and granting practice privileges. The scope of practice of the RNFA is defined by each individual state's nurse practice act. RNFA programs based on the AORN *Core Curriculum for the RN First Assistant* (1994) are designed to prepare the perioperative nurse for the role of RNFA, including education and experience in the following:

- Pharmacology
- Legal aspects of the role
- Emergency protocol
- Surgical anatomy
- Psychomotor skills associated with first assisting
- Wound management
- Physical assessment and history taking

In the preoperative environment, the RNFA performs physical assessment and documents the history and physical for the permanent record. This role may be performed in a hospital, office-based practice, or other clinical site. Pertinent data are reported to the primary surgeon. Preoperative tests pertaining to the intended procedure may be ordered or performed at this time. Previous test results are reviewed and documented to establish a baseline. Patient teaching may be initiated by the RNFA, and the patient's responses may be included in the plan of care. Expected outcomes may be identified and defined for the patient in realistic terms.

The RNFA provides assistance in the preparation of the patient before entrance to the surgical suite, such as skin marking, clinical photographic record, and other routine preparation. The RNFA may initiate routine orders that are cosigned by a physician or surgeon.

In the intraoperative environment, patient care performed by the RNFA includes positioning, skin preparation, and draping according to the needs of the surgeon to facilitate the procedure. Care is taken to avoid positioning-related injury. The skin prep is performed according to the surgeon's preference. If the skin is marked with incision lines preoperatively, care is taken to avoid completely washing the markings away. Skin markers are commercially available that withstand the rigors of the surgical skin prep. Some surgeons create linear skin scratches or wheals as incisional guides. Others use materials such as methylene blue or indigo carmine on a stylus. Drapes are placed carefully to expose only the surgical site.

The RNFA does not concurrently function as a scrub nurse while in the first assisting role because undivided attention must be paid to the surgical field. During most procedures, the RNFA is positioned across from the surgeon (Fig. 2-8). One or both may be wearing a headlight and loupes. Flip-up loupes are useful because the depth of field is altered for superficial suturing and

tissue handling. Intraoperatively, the RNFA performs such tasks as the following:

- Providing exposure of the surgical site
- Tissue handling
- Suturing
- Using instrumentation
- Providing hemostasis
- Closing tissue and skin

At the conclusion of the procedure, the RNFA may initiate routine orders as cosigned by the attending surgeon. The RNFA in the postoperative environment may provide follow-up care of drains, sutures, dressings, and wounds. This role may be performed in the hospital, office-based practice, or other clinical setting. The RNFA provides patient care in a collaborative milieu under the guidance and supervision of the attending surgeon. The RNFA practices the art and science of the nursing process in an expanded perioperative role and is prohibited from doing the following:

- Performing the actual procedure or the intended role of a surgeon
- Practicing as an RNFA before attaining state credentialing and requirements
- Prescribing medication

Since 1993, the Certification Board Perioperative Nursing (CBPN) (formerly known as National Certification Board: Perioperative Nursing, Inc) has offered the opportunity for voluntary certification by examination for the RNFA. As of January 1, 1998, eligibility for certification as an RNFA (CRNFA) includes the following:

- CNOR (maintained concurrently with CRNFA)
- Proof of satisfactory completion of a formal, college-affiliated RNFA program based on the AORN's Core Curriculum

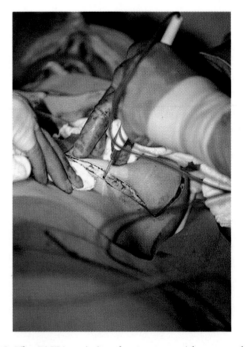

Fig. 2-8 The RNFA assisting the surgeon with a procedure by applying traction and countertraction to the incision.

for the RN First Assistant that awards college credit or a certificate of RNFA status on completion

- Documentation of 2000 practice hours in the RNFA role (candidate may include clinical internship hours incorporated within 600 preoperative and postoperative patient care hours and 1400 intraoperative patient care hours as an RNFA); 500 hours of RNFA practice must be within 2 years of the application for the certification examination
- Bachelor of Science in Nursing (BSN) (required after 2000)

The CBPN is an independent certifying body that has its roots in the AORN but is incorporated as a separate organization. RNFA recertification may be attained by reexamination or attendance at 150 contact hours specific to the practice of the RNFA in addition to 150 contact hours needed to maintain CNOR status. A total of 300 contact hours is needed in a 5-year period for recertification (CNOR and CRNFA) by the contact hour method. A convenient method for combined CNOR and CRNFA recertification is being developed by the CBPN.

PLASTIC AND RECONSTRUCTIVE SURGEON

Credentialing of the plastic and reconstructive surgeon is not governed by state law. Any physician with a medical degree can claim to be a plastic surgeon. A plastic surgery specialist has completed at least 3 years in a residency program that provided experience in many aspects of plastic and reconstructive procedures (Fig. 2-9). The ASPRS has developed standards to promote quality in the care of plastic and reconstructive surgery patients. Membership in the ASPRS is available only to plastic surgeons who are certified by the American Board of Plastic Surgery (ABPS). Eligibility for certification includes the following:

- Graduation from an accredited medical school
- 3 years in a general surgery residency program
- 2 years in an approved plastic and reconstructive surgery residency program
- 2 years in a plastic and reconstructive surgery practice
- Written and oral examinations
- Acceptance by the ABPS for high standards and ethics by peer review
- Continued education

Patients are advised by the ASPRS to interview two or three plastic surgeons before making a selection for their procedure. Surgeons may be recommended by friends, perioperative nurses, local hospitals, medical societies, and professional specialty organizations. Some surgeons charge a fee for their time for this interview. Information patients are prompted to evaluate includes the following:

- Educational preparation
- Residency
- Board certification
- Qualification for desired procedure
- Personality and willingness to answer questions
- Fees and payment policies
- Perioperative follow-through and confidentiality
- Risks and benefits
- Anesthesia
- Potential expected outcome in realistic terms

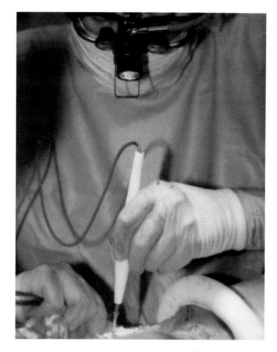

Fig. 2-9 Plastic and reconstructive surgeon.

Ethical plastic and reconstructive surgeons are willing to take the time to work with each patient's individual needs. Developing a trusting rapport and establishing realistic outcome expectations is reassuring to the patient and is beneficial to the result of the procedure. The patient will be more compliant with the perioperative regimen ensuring the best possible result. Complications can be kept to a minimum. A satisfied patient is the best advertisement. For more information on plastic surgeon credentialing, contact the ASPRS at 1-800-635-0635.

Bibliography

Anderson LG: The Nordstrom's of medical practices, *Plast Surg Nurs* 15(3):172, 1995.

Atkinson LJ, Fortunato NM: *Berry and Kohn's operating room technique,* ed 8, St Louis, 1996, Mosby.

Association of Operating Room Nurses: *AORN standards and recommended practices for perioperative nursing,* Denver, 1996, AORN.

Association of Operating Room Nurses: *Core curriculum for the RN first assistant,* ed 2, Denver, 1994, AORN.

Gruendemann BJ, Fernsebner B: *Comprehensive perioperative nursing,* Boston, 1995, Jones & Barlett.

American Society of Plastic and Reconstructive Surgeons: *How to choose a qualified plastic surgeon,* Arlington Heights, Ill, 1993, ASPRS.

Maksud D, Moncada G: Managed care: concepts and issues, *Plast Surg Nurs* 15(1):42, 1995.

Meeker MH, Rothrock JC: *Alexander's care of the patient in surgery,* ed 10, St Louis, 1994, Mosby.

Phippen ML, Wells MP: *Perioperative nursing practice,* Philadelphia, 1994, WB Saunders.

Rothrock JC: *The RN first assistant: an expanded perioperative nursing role,* ed 2, Philadelphia, 1993, JB Lippincott.

Strzyzewski NM: The cycle of perioperative nursing care for plastic surgery patients, *Plast Surg Nurs* 15(2):78, 1995.

3 Plastic and Reconstructive Surgery Practice Settings

FREE-STANDING PLASTIC AND RECONSTRUCTIVE SURGERY CENTER

According to the American Society of Plastic and Reconstructive Surgeons (ASPRS), most plastic and reconstructive procedures are performed in outpatient settings. Over 58 percent of outpatient procedures are performed in free-standing facilities, such as physicians' offices or surgicenters. This trend has increased because the costs associated with outpatient surgery are significantly less than hospital costs. Factors such as competitive pricing, less complex admission procedures, and improved anesthetic methods have directly affected an increase in patient volume.

Most plastic and reconstructive surgeons have combined hospital and free-standing surgicenter privileges and work in both settings. Complex procedures such as reconstruction after serious trauma can be initially performed in a hospital setting. Supplemental procedures such as scar revision can be performed in a free-standing center by the same surgeon.

KEY ELEMENTS FOR A SUCCESSFUL FREE-STANDING PROGRAM

Careful planning is essential to the operation of the free-standing center. Each component is integral to the smooth operation of the daily activities. One objective for a free-standing facility is time efficiency. The patient's admission, surgical procedure, postsurgical care, and discharge should take minimal time. However, streamlining should not endanger safety or quality of care. Main operational categories to consider include location, structural, administrative, and patient-care issues.

Location

The free-standing surgery center should be located at an easily accessed site (Fig 3-1). It should be close to main highway systems and convenient roads. Consideration should be given to nearby hospital support in the event of an emergency. Outlying regions may need to consider air transport support if a hospital is not within a reasonable ambulance transport distance.

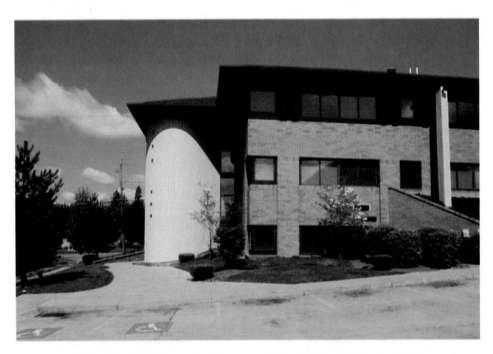

Fig. 3-1 Ambulatory plastic surgery clinic of Brian W. Davies, MD.

Contracts may be established with transport and supporting facilities.

Parking should include a plan for patient pick-up and drop-off points. Handicap and short-term parking areas should be identified near the main entrance. Federal, state, and local statutes indicate that curbs should not hinder access routes. Delivery vehicles and supply trucks should have parking allotted in the rear of the building. Storage rooms could be designed near the point of delivery to decrease the time spent in handling supplies. Personnel parking should be designated away from the main entrance. Closer parking spots should be reserved for patients and their families.

Physical Plant Structure

Efficiency in design facilitates the flow of patient care. Consideration should be given to functional activities such as patient check-in and processing, preoperative and postoperative care, supply, and equipment. Separate and distinct areas should be designated for patient reception, administrative processing, supplies, clean and dirty instrumentation, equipment, and record keeping. Patient care areas should be planned for comfort, safety, privacy, and utility. The Association of Operating Room Nurses (AORN) standards, recommended practices, and guidelines should be consulted for the design of traffic flow and restricted, semirestricted, and unrestricted areas.

Regional building codes reflect the number and type of emergency exit doors. Placement of fire extinguishers and fire alarm systems are mandated by the office of the local fire marshal. Cost containment is a consideration, but minimizing expenses too steeply in design can create the need for further expenditure in the future if more space must be added for growth and expansion.

Preoperative patient care areas should include dressing rooms with lockers for storage of personal effects. Patients should be instructed to not bring valuables to the center. Stretchers and lounge chairs should be provided for patient comfort. When local anesthesia is used the patient may return to this area for a brief period of observation before discharge. A postanesthesia area is needed for patients who have had significant amounts of sedation and/or general anesthesia (Fig 3-2). Cardiac and respiratory monitoring and resuscitative equipment are required for these areas. Personnel staffing these areas should be competent in the use and interpretation of monitoring equipment and cardiopulmonary resuscitation (CPR) and certified at a minimum of the Basic Lifesaver level. Advanced Lifesaver certification is preferred. Consideration should be given to patients who may need more time for postanesthesia recovery. Referral to a hospital or free-standing recovery center may be necessary. Lavatories for patient use should be close to the preoperative and postoperative care areas. Some facilities have shower rooms available for patients who are returning for next-day dressing changes. Face-lift patients may have their hair washed, dried, and styled on site at their first postoperative check-up. An area designated as a mini salon is nice for teaching skin care after resurfacing procedures (Fig 3-3).

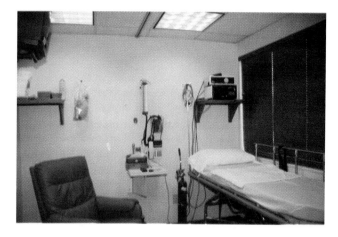

Fig. 3-2 Postprocedural recovery area.

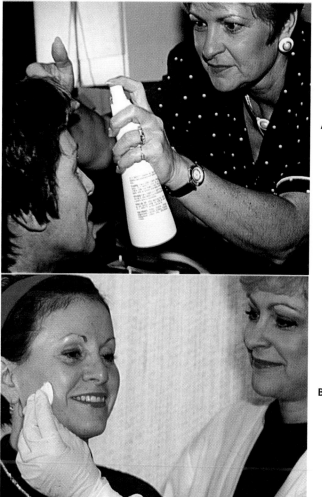

Fig. 3-3 Staff consultants teach patient how to care for new improved self. *(Courtesy Brian W. Davies, MD.)*

The operating room of a free-standing center should be situated away from distractions and noise. It should measure at least 18 × 18 feet, especially if general anesthesia is used. The operating bed should be positioned in the center of the room for ease of patient access from all sides, which is useful in the event of an emergency. The doorway should be large enough to accommodate a transport stretcher and emergency equipment. The hallway should be wide enough for passage of an emergency transport team if patient transfer is necessary.

Interior materials used in the structure should be planned for durability and function. Vinyl wall covering is easiest to clean and less expensive to periodically replace than ceramic tile. Neutral-toned linoleum floor tile is easy to clean and looks attractive. The floor surface should be resistant to staining by blood, skin marking, and prep solutions. Drapes should be avoided if there are windows. Vinyl miniblinds are easier to clean and maintain on a daily basis than fabric curtains. Blues and greens are peaceful shades for decor. Lighter colors enhance room lighting. Flame-resistant materials should be used throughout the facility (Fig 3-4).

Lighting and electricity

Three-pronged (grounded) electrical outlets should be positioned strategically throughout the room. Baseboard outlets are useful for low-to-the-ground equipment such as lipectomy suction and operating bed plugs. Waist-level plugs are useful for endoscopy light sources and related equipment. Adequate numbers of electrical outlets for monitors and anesthesia equipment are generally positioned out of the main traffic path at one end of the room. Extension cords are discouraged because the connections can come loose. The number of electrical outlets may vary according to permissible

units in building codes. Line isolation monitoring and ground fault interruption systems should be in place.

Ceiling-mounted surgical lights are useful for illuminating the field during the procedure. Centrally located, mounted lighting allows for versatility in room setup. Some procedures require the use of headlamps. Fiberoptic varieties are lightweight. Light sources for these units generate various amounts of noise from the cooling fans. Quieter models are recommended for noise control in smaller operating rooms. Fluorescent lights are commonly used but can be irritating to the eyes. Patient skin tones are better monitored in lighting that closely resembles natural daylight. Some lighting systems can make the patient's skin tones appear gray or yellow. This can alter the intraoperative appearance of tissue flaps during assessment for capillary refill. Lighting can also affect the quality of intraoperative photography.

Storage and space efficiency

Storage cabinets in each operating room (OR) should be closed units. Sliding doors eliminate space needed for clearance of doors that swing open. The surface should be smooth and durable, such as stainless steel or heavy formica. Supplies that may be needed immediately should be available in small numbers in the OR. The bulk of these supplies should be kept in a clean storage room adjacent to the OR to prevent inadvertent contamination.

Instrumentation in the OR should be limited to the sets immediately needed for the case. Sterile instrument sets should be kept in a clean, dry, environmentally controlled area to maintain sterility. Sterile instruments and supplies should be kept separate from contaminated instruments. Event-related sterility policies should be in place.

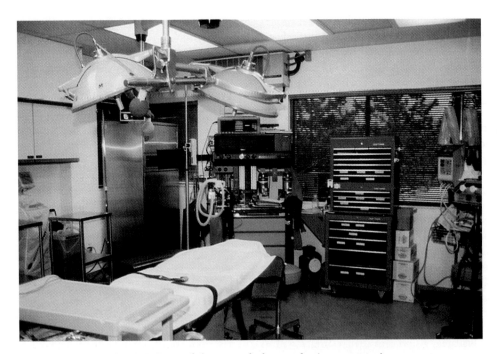

Fig. 3-4 State-of-the-art ambulatory plastic surgery suite.

Many free-standing centers use customized disposable drape packs. Storage of the packs can create problems with space if ordered in excess quantities. Disposable and reusable supplies can be stored together after sterilization.

Instrument processing

Instruments should be processed according to current AORN standards, recommended practices, and guidelines. Provisions should be made for terminal processing and cleaning before instruments are wrapped for sterilization. Clean and dirty instrument areas should be separated and clearly marked. Outsourcing of instrument processing is another option. Before sending instruments out to an independent processor, a washer-sterilizer should be used to remove gross debris and contaminants. Prevention of cross contamination is essential for infection control.

Personnel areas

Lounges and dressing rooms should be provided for staff. Some facilities provide a washing machine and dryer for uniforms. Smaller free-standing centers may also wash and dry OR linens on site. Appropriate containment procedures and safety guidelines for on-site laundry facilities should be followed.

Administrative Issues

Organizational formats apply to free-standing surgery centers much in the same way they apply to large hospital surgical services departments. The organizational chart should include a decision-making hierarchy, management structure, workforce design, maintenance, and patient flow support services. Protocol should be clearly defined and adhered to by all personnel at the facility.

Policies

Clarification of expected behaviors, routines, and activities should be outlined by policies that are reviewed and updated on a regular basis. The standard of care in a free-standing center is not measured differently than the standard of care in a hospital setting. Policies and procedures should be reviewed yearly and updated as needed.

Personnel performance descriptions

Performance descriptions should be documents that outline the minimal expected behaviors of the patient care staff. These behaviors are measured by performance appraisals. Specific competencies should be developed to measure performance.

Documentation

All aspects of patient care should be documented. Most centers have standardized forms for recording information throughout the preoperative, intraoperative, and postoperative phases of care. AORN standards, recommended practices, and guidelines provide rationale and interpretive statements that can guide the content of recorded patient data. Documentation should reflect adherence to policy and procedure.

Other forms of documentation necessary include personnel files, financial book keeping, inventory logs, and routine patient files. Computerized programs integrate administrative and financial activities such as staff scheduling, patient registration, billing, and inventory control.

Contracted services

Preoperative laboratory tests, x-ray examinations, scans, and workups can be performed at a local laboratory or hospital testing center. Contracted services with a nearby testing center are more economical than duplicating facilities within close proximity. Pharmaceutical supplies can be outsourced and maintained by a service. Externally operated environmental services may be considered.

Some free-standing centers have photographic darkroom facilities on site. Although the start-up costs may seem high, the need for instant contour measurement templates justifies the investment. Valuable time could be lost by parceling out the photographic work. Time is lost during the processing period. On-site photography facilities expedite surgical planning. Before, during, and after photographs are useful in the documentation process. The value of photography in the success of the procedure is recaptured in the satisfied customer.

Reimbursement considerations

Financial aspects include patient charges. Most of these charges are based on standardized coding procedures that are accepted and understood by most health insurance providers. These standardized codes are a uniform descriptive language of diseases and procedures. Diseases are categorized in International Classification of Diseases: 9th Revision with Clinical Modifications (ICD-9-CM) codes. This collection is updated every 10 years with input by physicians and insurance providers. Procedures are categorized in current procedural terminology (CPT) codes. This collection is updated annually by the American Medical Association in consultation with specialty groups, such as the ASPRS. Both ICD-9 and CPT codes are used for each patient. It is important to assign the correct codes to each patient for correct reimbursement. Advance approval by some insurance providers is required. More recent forms of reimbursement include ambulatory surgery groupings (ASGs). This form resembles diagnostic related groups (DRGs) but is specific to same day procedures without an overnight stay.

Many procedures are not covered by insurance providers. Patients who pay out-of-pocket expenses for aesthetic procedures may need to provide a percentage-based down payment followed by a payment schedule. Terms of the agreement should be discussed before the procedure is performed.

Accreditation

Voluntary certification and accreditation may be attained through several independent organizations, such as the Joint Commission on Accreditation of Healthcare Organizations (JCAHO), the Accreditation Association for Ambulatory Health Care, and the American Association for Accreditation of Ambulatory Surgery Facilities. Each organization has an established set of standardized criteria that is "scored" by on-site reviewers. Written standards are available from these organizations for purchase in preparation for the reviewer's visit. Scoring criteria include but are not limited to the following:

- The physical plant meets accepted standards for structural safety, and compliance with building codes, infection control, and routine maintenance is established.
- Administrative policies and procedures for risk management, personnel competency, patient care issues, and continuous quality improvement are in place and reviewed periodically.
- Personnel education, qualifications, and credentials are documented and validated.
- Patient care activities are monitored and documented. Patients' rights are protected.
- Emergency preparedness is documented and practiced at regular intervals.
- Aseptic and sterile practices are monitored and maintained within the standard of care.
- Procedures performed on site are appropriate and approved for the facility.
- Documentation of patient care and practices surrounding patient care is clear and precise. Document storage and retrieval is appropriate for the type of facility.

Accreditation by one or more specialty-focused organizations can be a valuable credential. Consumer awareness groups advocate shopping around for quality care and frequently rely on professional organizations for referral to a facility. Much publicity is based on certification of services and some measurement of meeting or exceeding the standard of care for a free-standing facility.

Patient Care Issues

Patient care in a free-standing center should be provided within the same standard of care as hospitals and large facilities. Issues such as infection control, asepsis, and sterilization are monitored. Appropriate attire is worn in restricted areas, and personal protective gear is worn as necessary. Specimen handling and storage is documented and delivered to pathology services in a timely manner. Refrigeration and chemical fixation may be needed to preserve specimen integrity. Provisions should be made for immediate transport of frozen sections or fresh tissue assays.

Patient satisfaction is the best advertisement for referral business. Postoperative surveys can provide information for improvement of services. A follow-up phone call to the patient 24 to 48 hours postoperatively enhances the relationship between personnel at the facility and the patient. This call can reveal information about the patient's condition, answer any additional questions, confirm postoperative visits, and convey a sense of caring. Discussion content should be documented in the patient's record. Comments for improvement of service should be referred to quality improvement personnel.

Emergency preparedness

Patient care in a free-standing facility does not have a comparable level of immediate back-up support that a hospital can provide. Many procedures are performed under variations of local anesthesia. The risk of complications may be less than the risk associated with general anesthesia, but it has a significant potential for patient injury or death. General anesthesia is commonly used and carries its own series of potential complications.

Emergency preparedness should include policies and procedures for emergency situation management, such as cardiopulmonary arrest, malignant hyperthermia, excessive blood loss, and other unforeseen patient decline.

Policies and procedures should be in place that outline the course of action to be taken if a patient is having an untoward physiologic response to a medication or procedure. Transport protocol should be in place for transfer to an emergency treatment facility, such as a local hospital emergency room. Some free-standing facilities utilize a community-based emergency medical service (EMS) or 9-1-1 services for emergency transport to a hospital. The emergency transport service and the potential receiving hospital identified in the protocol should be notified that they are incorporated in the plan of emergency care.

Security issues

Visitors to the facility should be clearly identified. Entrance to patient care areas should be restricted to authorized personnel. A buzzer-release door latch should be in place to prevent entrance beyond the reception area. Expensive equipment, medications, and other valuables could be targeted for theft by intruders. Policies and procedures should be in place that define security of the building during and after business hours. Door alarm systems with electronic police alert mechanisms are recommended for use after hours.

SUMMARY

The design and construction of a self-contained, free-standing facility is different than a hospital-based surgical suite. Although the physical plant is different, the standards of care and provision of service are the same. AORN standards, recommended practices, and guidelines should be incorporated into the policies and procedures of the facility. JCAHO and other accrediting organizations provide additional guidance in providing safe, effective, and efficient patient care.

Bibliography

Association of Operating Room Nurses: *Standards, recommended practices, and guidelines,* Denver, 1997, AORN.

Atkinson LJ, Fortunato NM: *Berry and Kohn's operating room technique,* St Louis, 1996, Mosby.

Bruce P: Off-site preadmission unit supports hospital ambulatory surgical unit, *J Post Anesth Nurs* 8(4):262, 1993.

Burden N: Telephone follow-up of ambulatory surgery patients following discharge is a nursing responsibility, *J Post Anesth Nurs* 7(4):256, 1992.

Covell CA, Walton RP: "Amb-Track": development of a surgicenter model within a main operating room, *AORN J* 59(6):1257, 1994:

Goodman T, editor: *Core curriculum for plastic and reconstructive surgery,* ed 2, Pitman, New Jersey, 1996, American Society of Plastic and Reconstructive Plastic Surgery.

Meikle SM, Dresen SD: The use of local area networks in day surgery department, *J Post Anesth Nurs* 9(4):232, 1994.

Pierce LA: Planning ahead for emergencies, *Plast Surg Nurs* 14(3):178, 1994.

Ruberg RL, Smith DJ: *Plastic surgery: a core curriculum,* St Louis, 1994, Mosby.

Swan BA: A collaborative ambulatory preoperative evaluation model: implementation, implications, evaluation, *AORN J* 59(2):430, 1994.

Tabbush V, Swanson G: Changing paradigms in medical payment, *Arch Intern Med* 156(4):357, 1996.

4 Anesthesia Considerations for Plastic Surgery Patients

Anesthesia for plastic surgery is comparable with the administration of anesthesia for any other surgical procedure. The same risks and benefits can be appreciated. Many surgical procedures in all disciplines are performed on an outpatient basis. Plastic surgery is commonly performed in free-standing facilities.

The choice of anesthetic is based on the type and length of the surgical procedure and physiologic and psychologic condition of the patient. Preoperative assessment for the plastic surgery patient should include the following:

- Reason for the procedure
- Age, height (in inches), weight (in pounds and kilograms)
- Patient's perception of outcome
- Objective data
- Subjective data
- Medical and surgical history
- Anesthetic history
- Family history
- Current medications
- Social history
- Allergies

Determination of anesthetic use is made collaboratively among the patient, surgeon, and/or anesthesia provider. Intraoperative pain control is also a consideration. Perioperative nurses who specialize in plastic and reconstructive surgery should be familiar with the drugs used for anesthesia and the potential risks involved. Anesthesia methods vary in complexity and may include one or a combination of the following:

- None
- Local infiltration
- Intravenous conscious sedation (IVCS)
- Monitored anesthesia care (MAC) (formerly referred to as attended local anesthesia)
- Regional block (specific nerve area, spinal, or epidural)
- General

LOCAL ANESTHESIA

The refinement of same-day and outpatient surgery has popularized the use of local anesthesia for many surgical procedures involving a limited surgical site. Local anesthesia has continued to be a popular practice, and it has proven to be beneficial for the patient who desires a satisfactory means of perioperative pain control and a shorter recovery period. Surgeons prefer to use local anesthetics whenever possible because the associated risks are limited and the cost advantages are attractive to the patient (Fig. 4-1).

Patients receiving local anesthetics during a surgical procedure should be closely monitored for adverse effects and changes in physiologic status. An IV access site may be advised in some patients. The patient should be observed for heart rate and rhythm, respiratory rate, blood pressure, skin color and temperature, and mental status. Recommended monitoring equipment should include but is not limited to the following:

- Electrocardiogram (ECG) monitoring equipment
- Pulse oximeter to measure blood oxygenation
- Automatic blood pressure monitor or a sphygmomanometer with a stethoscope

A perioperative nurse should be assigned to monitor the patient receiving local anesthesia. This nurse should not be simultaneously performing circulating duties. Familiarity with the necessary equipment used for patient monitoring is essential. Monitoring personnel should be able to interpret results displayed by the monitoring devices. Vital signs and patient responses should be documented before the procedure begins, at each administration of anesthetic agent, every 10 to 15 minutes during the procedure, at the conclusion of the procedure, and before the patient is discharged from the operating room (OR) to another department. Additional vital signs may be taken and recorded as necessary. Resuscitative equipment along with the various drugs used during an emergency should be immediately available. The entire plastic surgery team should be

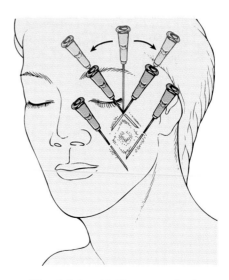

Fig. 4-1 Local infiltrate anesthesia.

familiar with emergency protocol and the use of emergency equipment. Institutional policies and procedures should be available for review by the team.

Local anesthetics are categorized as amino amides or amino esters. Table 4-1 illustrates the most common forms of local infiltration anesthetic agents. Many of these are also used for regional nerve blocks, epidurals, and spinal anesthesia. Dosages cited are without additive epinephrine unless otherwise indicated. Maximum dosages can be slightly higher when epinephrine is added. Higher amounts listed are used for peripheral nerve blocks.

Additives include epinephrine or hyaluronidase. Epinephrine is added to cause vasoconstriction and minimize bleeding. Local anesthetics with added epinephrine are not used on digits, penile tissue, or tissue with impaired circulation. Hyaluronidase is a bovine testicular enzyme that causes tissue fiber changes that permit enhanced absorption of the local anesthetic. This additive is not compatible with heparin or epinephrine. Sodium bicarbonate buffers the solution, improves dispersion into tissues, and decreases the pain of infiltration.

Adverse reaction to local anesthetic agents may begin with subjective changes in the patient. Any complaint of change in mental activity, numbness of the tongue, dizziness, tinnitus, confusion, and/or heightened anxiety can be early warning signs of a possible allergic reaction and should be reported to the surgeon immediately. Objective observation may reveal slurred speech, increased pulse rate, tachycardia, dysrhythmia, dyspnea, hypotension, pallor, diaphoresis, and/or restlessness. Initial measures include ensuring an open airway, providing oxygen, starting IV access (if not already in place), and monitoring the patient's cardiovascular status. An anesthesiologist should be called to assist as needed. Dosages are calculated as percentages of drug in solution. An example of dosage calculation for lidocaine is shown in Table 4-2.

Differentiating between toxicity and allergic reaction may be difficult. Careful monitoring of objective and subjective data can alert the OR team to a pending crisis. Table 4-3 illustrates the difference between toxic and allergic reactions to local anesthetic medication.

Postoperatively, the patientís vital signs and condition should be monitored for a minimum of 30 minutes before discharge from the facility. Additional analgesia during this time helps relax the patient and prepare him or her for discharge instructions. The patient should be cautioned about driving, operating dangerous machinery, and making major decisions while under the influence of analgesic medication. Discharge criteria as outlined by most facilities include but are not limited to the following:

- Stable vital signs
- Minimal complaints of pain or nausea
- No complications such as bleeding or adverse reaction to drugs
- Taking fluids or food by mouth
- Ambulatory with minimal assistance
- Voiding at least once after the procedure
- Someone to transport the patient home as needed

Tumescent Technique

The *tumescent technique* is a recent technique developed by dermatologic plastic surgeons. It dramatically improves the effects of local anesthetics by permitting anesthesia of the skin and subcutaneous tissues using direct infiltration rather than a proximal nerve block. By using large amounts of a dilute 1.0% or 0.50% lidocaine solution with epinephrine 1:100,000 in physiologic saline, the tumescent technique produces firmness, or *tumescence*, of targeted fatty areas.

The tumescent technique is successful with liposuction procedures. With the appropriate instrumentation, the tumescent

Table 4-1 **Local Infiltration Anesthesia**

GENERIC NAME	CONCENTRATIONS AVAILABLE	MAXIMUM DOSES
AMINO AMIDE ANESTHETICS		
Bupivacaine hydrochloride	0.25% to 0.50%	200 mg 400 mg block
Dibucaine hydrochloride	0.05% to 0.1%	30 mg
Etidocaine hydrochloride	0.50 % to 1.0 %	300 mg or 4 mg/kg 400 mg or 5.5 mg/kg w/epinephrine
Lidocaine hydrochloride	0.50 % to 4.0 %	300 mg or 4.5 mg/kg 500 mg or 7 mg/kg w/epinephrine
Mepivacaine hydrochloride	0.5 % to 2.0 %	500 mg or 7 mg/kg
Prilocaine hydrochloride	1.0 % to 3.0 %	600 mg
AMINO ESTER ANESTHETICS		
(More reactions are possible)		
Chloroprocaine hydrochloride	0.50 % to 3.0 %	800 mg or 11 mg/kg 1000 mg or 14 mg/kg w/epinephrine
Cocaine hydrochloride	4.0 % or 10 %	200 mg or 4 mg/kg
Procaine hydrochloride	0.50 % to 2.0 %	600 mg 14 mg/kg w/epinephrine
Tetracaine hydrochloride	1.0 % to 2.0 %	20 mg
ADDITIVES		
Hyaluronidase	150 U/ml	
Sodium bicarbonate	Standardized solution	1:10
Epinephrine hydrochloride	1:1000 1:100,000 1:200,000	

Table 4-2 **Dosage Scale for Lidocaine Calculation**

PERCENTAGE OF DRUG	MILLIGRAMS PER CC
0.50 %	5 mg/cc
1.0 %	10 mg/cc
2.0 %	20 mg/cc

Table 4-3 **Comparison of Toxic Reaction with Allergic Reaction to Local Anesthetic Drug**

TOXIC REACTION	ALLERGIC REACTION
	(Not common with amide)
Symptoms vary depending on the drug	Immediate generalized body reaction
Dizziness, somnolence, paresthesia, vomiting, visual problems, speech problems, muscle twitches, tremors, seizures, unconsciousness, coma	Sense of uneasiness, agitation, paresthesia
Decreased breathing rate and depth	Erythema, urticaria, wheals, pruritis
VASOVAGAL	
Dysrhythmia, bradycardia, vasodilation, hypotension, myocardial depression, cardiac arrest	Coughing, sneezing, wheezing, bronchospasm, hypotension, hypovolemia, vasodilation, cardiovascular collapse, cardiac arrest
TREATMENT	
Supportive, need for IV access, Trendelenberg position, diazepam for treatment of muscular contractions, airway management	Especially with ester type: airway management, IV fluids, epinephrine, diphenhydramine, and steroids as needed

technique permits liposuction of large volumes of fat with minimal narcotic analgesia or IVCS. Some patients require no additional intraoperative medication.

Recent clinical studies of the absorption pharmacokinetics of lidocaine used during the tumescent technique have shown a peak plasma concentration level that occurs approximately 12 to 14 hours after the start of infiltration. This permits a higher dosage of lidocaine than previously believed safe for use. This prolonged anesthesia of skin and subcutaneous tissue is probably a result of exposing sufficient lengths of sensory axons to marginal blocking concentrations of lidocaine.

Postoperative discomfort is minimal because the surgical site remains partially anesthetized up to 18 hours after surgery. Additional postoperative analgesia is not usually needed. (See Tumescent Infusion in Chapter 8.)

INTRAVENOUS CONSCIOUS SEDATION

Pharmacologic agents can be given to produce IVCS. A patient under conscious sedation will have a depressed level of consciousness but is able to retain the ability to independently maintain a patent airway and respond appropriately to verbal commands.

The perioperative nurse who administers IV drugs, monitors, and cares for a patient who is receiving IVCS should have the appropriate knowledge and skill associated with pharmacology, anatomy and physiology, potential complications, monitoring techniques, and resuscitation procedures. No other responsibilities should be assigned that would cause him or her to leave the patient unattended. Developing the plan of care for a patient undergoing IVCS includes anticipation of potential complications and intervention if there is an undesired physiologic response. Monitoring practices are defined by institutional policy and procedure and should require more than basic, minimal competency to perform.

The ideal IVCS produces amnesia, antiemetic effects, and relaxation with decreased anxiety. A calm atmosphere with minimal noise and activity enhances the patient's experience

resulting in minimal medication usage. Drugs and average doses commonly used for sedation include the following:

Diazepam (Valium)	2.0 mg to 10 mg
Lorazepam (Ativan)	0.40 mg/kg (2.0 mg maximum dose)
Midazolam (Versed)	0.15 mg/kg amnesia for 40 minutes
	0.20 mg to 0.25 mg/kg amnesia for 1 to 2 hours
	0.30 mg/kg unconsciousness (5.0 mg maximum dose)

Narcotics given in combination with these three sedatives produce hypnosis. Narcotics are administered with caution because they can produce prolonged central nervous system depression leading to respiratory depression. Examples of commonly used narcotics for adults include the following:

- Fentanyl (Sublimaze) 0.05 to 0.1mg IV
- Meperidine hydrochloride (Demerol) 75 to 100 mg IV
- Morphine sulfate 4.0 to 10 mg IV
- Ketamine (Ketalar) 0.5 to 2.0 mg/kg IV (administered by an anesthesia provider)

Ketamine can produce vivid and sometimes unpleasant dreams and even bizarre hallucinations. Diazepam is frequently used to decrease the effects that can often occur weeks after the administration of ketamine.

IV access is maintained throughout the perioperative course. The patient is continuously monitored throughout the procedure and during the postoperative or postanesthesia phase. Emergency precautions should include provision of personnel certified in Advanced Cardiac Life Support (ACLS) to manage the patient's airway, intubate if necessary, and perform advanced cardiopulmonary resuscitation (CPR).

MONITORED ANESTHESIA CARE

MAC is administered by an anesthesia provider such as an anesthesiologist or certified nurse anesthetist (CRNA) (Fig 4-2). A local anesthetic agent is injected at the surgical site by the surgeon, and sedation is administered by the anesthesia provider. This form of anesthesia care is usually provided for patients

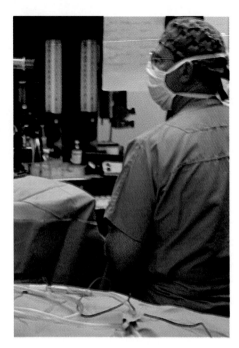

Fig. 4-2 The nurse anesthetist is an important member of the plastic and reconstructive surgical team.

with multiple physiologic conditions such as diabetes, severe hypertension, kidney disease, or other major organ failure. Age-extreme and apprehensive patients also benefit. MAC allows the surgeon and OR team to focus their attention on the surgical procedure. The anesthesia provider supplements the local anesthetic with IV medications that provide systemic analgesia and depress the patient's autonomic nervous system responses.

The anesthesia provider monitors the patient's vital functions and titrates additional IV medication to maintain an optimal physiologic and psychologic state in the patient.

REGIONAL ANESTHESIA

Regional anesthesia produces a loss of sensation to a circumscribed area with an anesthetic solution. Local anesthetic agents are injected directly into a specific area surrounding nervous tissue. Sensory impulses are blocked. The duration of the block depends on the type of anesthetic used for infiltration. Regional anesthesia is used for high-risk patients. Many patients prefer a regional block because it provides anesthesia to a wide area without altering consciousness. Regional anesthetic effects are time-limited and not recommended for procedures that may exceed the effective duration of the block.

Patient evaluation and preparation for regional anesthesia are similar to those scheduled for general anesthesia. A complete history and physical examination as well as laboratory evaluations are an important part of the patient preparation. Contraindications to regional anesthesia include allergy to a local anesthetic, peripheral infection, peripheral vascular disease, peripheral neuropathy, and any blood dyscrasias such as sickle cell anemia. Oral diazepam (Valium) may be given preoperatively, followed later by an IV supplement if more sedation is desired.

Regional anesthesia is useful for surgical procedures involving limbs, deep tissue, or organ systems below the diaphragm. Complications of regional blocks are usually the result of inadvertent intravascular injection or an overdose of the local anesthetic. Rarely, nerve damage may occur from trauma by the needle or compression from the volume of local anesthetic. Other complications are related to the site of injection and absorption of the medication and may include infection, air embolism, pneumothorax, paralysis, parasthesia, and systemic collapse.

Spinal Anesthesia

Spinal anesthesia is categorized as a major conduction block of the spinal nerve roots via the subarachnoid space of the meninges. A local anesthetic solution is injected intrathecally into the subarachnoid space to block pain sensation below the level of the diaphragm without the loss of consciousness. Surgical anesthesia extends from the xyphoid to the length of the lower extremities. The uptake of local anesthetic is determined by the weight of the drug and the rate of diffusion into the adjacent nervous tissue. Benefits of spinal anesthesia include reduction in blood loss and reduced metabolic stress. The anesthetics of choice include lidocaine, tetracaine, and bupivacaine without preservatives.

Epidural Anesthesia

Epidural anesthesia is useful for procedures involving the lower abdomen, pelvis, perineum, and lower extremities. Anesthetic solution is injected into the epidural space located between the ligamentum flavum and the dura mater and spread in all directions between the loose tissue structures that occupy this space. Bupivacaine 0.25% without preservative is frequently used.

Complications of spinal or epidural anesthesia

Sympathetic and parasympathetic nerve blockage can lead to profound physiologic changes such as hypotension, cardiovascular depression, and respiratory distress. Another potential complication is the postdural headache caused by decreased cerebrospinal fluid (CSF) pressure resulting from leakage of CSF through the needle hole in the dura. Characteristics of a postdural headache include but are not limited to tinnitus, diplopia, and frontal or occipital headache. Nausea and vomiting may accompany severe headache. Analgesics, bedrest, and hydration relieve most of the symptoms.

Peripheral Nerve Block

A wide variety of peripheral nerves can be effectively blocked by injecting local anesthetic around them to produce adequate surgical anesthesia. This form of regional anesthesia is often used for procedures of the upper extremities and provides the inhibition of conduction in the nerve fibers of the peripheral nervous system.

Minor nerve blocks are performed for procedures involving single nerve entities such as the ulnar and radial nerves at the wrist and the anterior or posterior tibial nerves at the ankle. Major nerve blocks involve those procedures in which multiple nerves or a nerve plexus, such as the brachial plexus, stellate ganglion, intercostal nerves, or celiac plexus, are anesthetized.

Onset and duration of a block are related to the type of drug used, its concentration, its volume, and additives such as epinephrine.

Bier block

The German surgeon August Bier developed the technique of single limb injection anesthesia and reported its use from 1908 through 1910. In 1970, the name *Bier block* was applied to the use of IV regional anesthesia used for surgery of the forearm and hand.

The Bier block is performed by IV injection of lidocaine or bupivacaine without epinephrine through a small-gauge IV catheter in the dorsum of the hand. A tourniquet is applied to the upper arm, the extremity is exsanguinated with an Eshmarch bandage, and the tourniquet is inflated 30 to 70 mm Hg higher than the systolic value of the blood pressure. Average tourniquet pressure for an upper extremity is 250 mm Hg to 300 mm Hg. Anesthetic medication is injected into the IV catheter and allowed to perfuse into the tissue. Reinjection may be performed after 90 minutes. Systemic toxicity can occur if the tourniquet fails or is released prematurely within 40 minutes of the IV injection.

Axillary nerve block

The axillary approach to the brachial plexus is the safest and simplest to perform. This technique reduces the risk of complications such as pneumothorax. With the axillary technique, the nerves are anesthetized around the axillary artery. The median and musculocutaneous nerves lie above the artery. The ulnar and radial nerves lie below and slightly posterior to the artery. Complications of the axillary block technique are rare but may include neuropathy, hematoma, and intravascular infection.

GENERAL ANESTHESIA

Complex and prolonged plastic surgical procedures require general anesthesia. This can be administered for inpatients or outpatients. Patient and surgeon preference are also factors.

The anesthesia provider reviews the patient's health history before administering a general anesthetic. General anesthesia is a means of providing unconsciousness, analgesia, muscle relaxation, and control of autonomic reflexes. The anesthesia provider maintains the lightest level of anesthesia in the brain that is compatible with operating conditions. Inhalation agents and IV injection of drugs control the patient's physiologic responses. Maintenance of homeostasis requires careful monitoring and careful administration of anesthesia. Table 4-4 describes examples of anesthetic drugs used for general anesthesia.

The perioperative nurse should remain at the patient's side during induction to provide reassurance to the patient and to assist the anesthesia provider as needed. This will help reduce the patient's apprehension. After induction, the anesthesia provider will indicate when the level of anesthesia is safe for patient positioning and preparation.

After the surgical procedure is complete, the patient is transferred to the postanesthesia care unit (PACU) for postoperative monitoring and assessment. A complete report is given by the anesthesia provider and circulator that should include the type of procedure, intraoperative activities, postoperative monitor-

Table 4-4 **Examples of General Anesthetic Medications**

INJECTABLE AGENTS	INHALATION AGENTS	MUSCLE RELAXANTS
Thiopental sodium	Halothane	Succinylcholine
Methohexital sodium	Enflurane	Vecuronium
Propofol	Isoflurane	Atracurium
Ketamine hydrochloride	Desflurane	Pancuronium
Fentanyl	Methoxyflurane	Tubocurarine chloride
Sufentanil citrate	Nitrous oxide	

ing devices needed, and postanesthesia patient care orders. Ambulatory surgery patients need to meet a certain physiologic level of recovery before discharge. These criteria are defined by institutional policy and closely parallel the criteria described earlier in this chapter under local anesthesia.

ANESTHETIC CONSIDERATIONS FOR THE PEDIATRIC PLASTIC SURGERY PATIENT

Pediatric patients having plastic surgical repairs often have multiple anatomic problems that require a multidisciplinary team approach to perioperative care. A coordinated team effort among the anesthesiologist, the surgeon, the perioperative nurse, and the rest of the surgical team is essential. Knowledge of the child's physiologic condition, the intended surgical procedure, and the desired outcome enable the anesthesia provider to individualize an anesthetic plan of care for the specific needs of each child. Examples of pediatric procedures requiring special anesthetic consideration include surgical repair of craniofacial anomalies such as cleft palate and lip, mandibular advancement, neck and thoracic reconstruction, and genitourinary neoconstruction. Pediatric plastic surgical procedures are challenges for the anesthesia provider because they involve maintaining an airway despite irregular facial shape, monitoring cardiovascular function between manipulations of the surgical team, and monitoring urine output during genitourinary procedures.

Induction of anesthesia in the pediatric patient is accomplished by intramuscular, intravenous, or inhalational methods. Rarely, rectal instillation may be necessary. A parent or guardian is often permitted to stay at the child's side to provide comfort during induction. After the child is asleep, the parent is escorted to the family waiting room. The perioperative nurse should periodically update the family about the progress of the procedure.

Care is taken to prevent excessive external pressure on the soft tissue of the anterior neck during intubation that could cause edema leading to airway obstruction. In situations where a child presents with a difficult airway, continuous positive airway pressure (CPAP) is supplied through the bag or mask ventilation and can often stent the obstructed upper airway. Although maintaining oxygenation is critical to all patients, pediatric patients have a high metabolism and increased oxygenation needs as a result. Pulse oximetry is crucial for observation of oxygen saturation. For pediatric patients undergoing cleft lip or palate repair, nasotracheal intubation is necessary.

Intraoperative position changes can dislodge the endotracheal tube. Uncuffed endotracheal tubes are used in patients up to 8 years of age because the pressure of the cuff can cause tissue necrosis. Careful positioning of the head and neck is important to avoid kinking of the endotracheal tube.

At the end of the surgical procedure, as consciousness begins to return, the anesthesia provider assesses the child's strength and ability to breath spontaneously and the return of purposeful movement. Pediatric patients often develop laryngospasm and are usually extubated only when awake to prevent airway occlusion.

POTENTIAL COMPLICATIONS OF ANESTHESIA

After head and neck surgery and flap reconstruction, it is imperative that the patient awaken without excessive coughing or movement. Hypotensive anesthesia may be used for procedures where blood loss may be extensive, such as with reduction mammoplasty and flaps. Agents commonly used in plastic surgery are sodium pentothal, nitrous oxide, enflurane, and various narcotics. Halothane is often the choice of agent in children.

Malignant Hyperthermia

Malignant hyperthermia (MH) was first identified as an anesthesia-related patient syndrome with familial tendencies in 1960. It has been defined as a chain reaction of abnormalities triggered in susceptible individuals by commonly used anesthetic agents and is classified as a hypermetabolic disorder of skeletal muscle. It is believed that susceptible patients possess a genetic pre-disposition for the development of the disease. In an acute episode of MH, muscles contract, metabolism increases, and calcium cannot reenter the sarcoplasmic reticulum.

The perioperative nurse should have a fundamental understanding of MH syndrome. The signs of MH include muscle spasm, a sudden rise in blood pressure, tachycardia, cardiac dysrhythmias, elevated end-tidal CO_2, tachypnea, metabolic and respiratory acidosis, cyanosis, myoglobinuria, and elevated body temperature. In some patients, elevated temperature is a late or absent sign. Known MH triggering agents are succinylcholine and halogenated inhalation anesthetic agents.

Successful treatment starts with early recognition of the syndrome followed by quick removal of the causative agent. Hyperventilation with 100% oxygen, immediate administration of dantrolene sodium, and aggressive cooling are first-line treatment options. Monitoring of CO_2 levels, frequent arterial blood gases, electrolyte monitoring, and urine output are all necessary.

Other causes of a similar collection of symptoms, neuroleptic malignant syndrome, are being studied. Potential drugs in question are Haldol and phenothiazines. Conditions such as heat exhaustion and extreme stress have produced similar symptoms in susceptible individuals. Dantrolene is effective in treating hypermetabolic, muscle heat-related crises similar to MH.

Bibliography

Algren CL, Algren JT: Pain management in children, *Plast Surg Nurs* 14(2):65, 1994.

American Society of Plastic and Reconstructive Surgical Nurses: Position statement on the role of the registered nurse (RN) in the management of patients receiving IV conscious sedation for short-term therapeutic, diagnostic, or surgical procedures, *Plast Surg Nurs* 12(1):32, 1992.

Atkinson LJ, Fortunato NM: *Berry and Kohn's operating room technique,* ed 8, St Louis, 1996, Mosby.

Benumof JL, Saidman LJ: *Anesthesia and perioperative complications,* St Louis, 1992, Mosby.

Canini BG et al: Epidural and spinal anesthesia, *Clinical anesthesia,* Philadelphia, 1991, JB Lippincott.

Galinske M: Malignant hyperthermia: a review, *Plast Surg Nurs* 15(1):30, 1995.

Klein JA: The tumescent technique: anesthesia for modified liposuction technique, *Derm Clin* 8(3):425, 1990.

Martin TJ: Physician-administered office anesthesia, *Clin Plast Surg* 18(4):877, 1991.

May SE, Schatzman B: *Anesthesia secrets,* Philadelphia, 1996, Hanley & Balfus.

Meeker MH, Rothrock, JC: *Alexander's care of the patient in surgery,* ed 10, St Louis, 1995, Mosby.

Meyer-Paholis E: Pediatric postanesthesia care, *Plast Surg Nurs* 14(2):92, 1994.

Mottura AL: Local anesthesia for reduction mammoplasty for outpatient surgery, *Anesth Plast Surg* 16(1):309, 1992.

Rogers MC: *Current practices in anesthesiology,* St Louis, 1992, Mosby.

Ruberg RL, Smith DJ: *A core curriculum: plastic surgery,* St Louis, 1994, Mosby.

Stehling LC: *Common problems in pediatric anesthesia,* ed 2, St Louis, 1992, Mosby.

Strzyzewski NM: The cycle of perioperative nursing care for the plastic surgery patient, *Plast Surg Nurs* 15(2):78, 1995.

Tobin M, Stevenson GW: Anesthetic consideration for the pediatric plastic surgical patient, *Plast Surg Nurs* 14(2):71, 1994.

Wetchler BV: *Anesthesia for ambulatory surgery,* ed 2, Philadelphia, 1990, JB Lippincott.

5 Patient Care Considerations in Plastic and Reconstructive Surgery

PSYCHOSOCIAL ASPECTS

According to the American Society of Plastic and Reconstructive Surgeons (ASPRS), the most common aesthetic procedures include liposuction (Fig. 5-1), blepharoplasty (Fig. 5-2), breast augmentation (Fig. 5-3), rhinoplasty (Figs. 5-4 and 5-5), and rhytidectomy (Fig. 5-6). Most patients undergoing these procedures range between 20 and 60 years of age. Social stigmas comparing beautification with vanity have diminished because physical attractiveness is openly glamorized by the media. In higher economic social circles, aesthetic surgery is common.

Improved body image benefits the patient emotionally and psychologically. Research has shown that patient perceptions vary according to the established norms of current societal views of beauty. Support by the patient's family is an important aspect. Significant others play a role in the successful adaptation to a changed appearance. The patient may feel saddened if friends and family fail to notice a change or improvement in physical appearance. Conversely, significant others may be critical of the result, causing depression in the patient.

Immediately after the operation, family and friends may be repulsed by the sight of bruising and swelling associated with some procedures. Later, after healing begins, a spouse may resent a mate's improved appearance and exhibit jealousy. The patient could look so vastly different that the spouse feels estranged. Potentially, a patient may make lifestyle changes based on a newly created appearance.

A patient can experience other undesirable outcomes as well. Postoperative infection (Fig. 5-7) can cause poor wound healing and scarring. The presence of infection can cause extrusion of a prosthetic device or necessitate its removal. The patient can simply be dissatisfied by the result. Perhaps the shape or configuration of the change is not up to expectations. Dissatisfaction can be caused by unrealistic expectations.

Text continued on p. 35

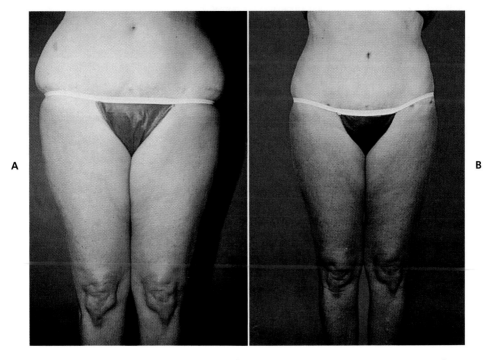

Fig. 5-1 Female pattern fat distribution for liposuction. **A,** Preoperative. **B,** Postoperative. *(Courtesy Brian W. Davies, MD.)*

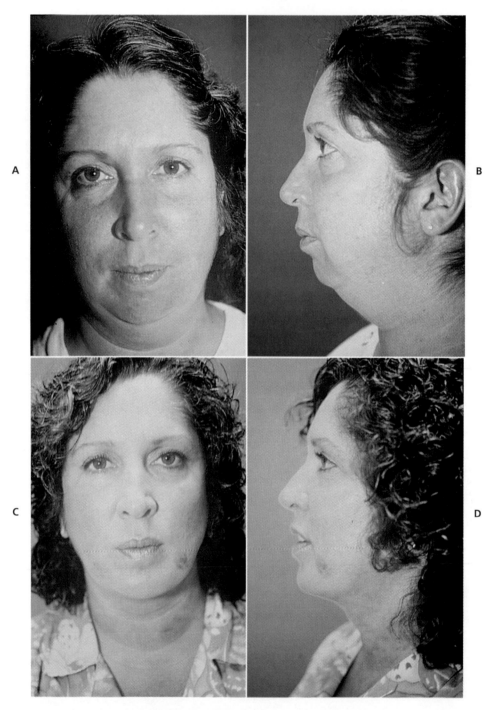

Fig. 5-2 Bilateral blepharoplasty and anterior neck suction-assisted liposuction. **A and B,** Preoperative. **C and D,** Postoperative. *(Courtesy Brian W. Davies, MD.)*

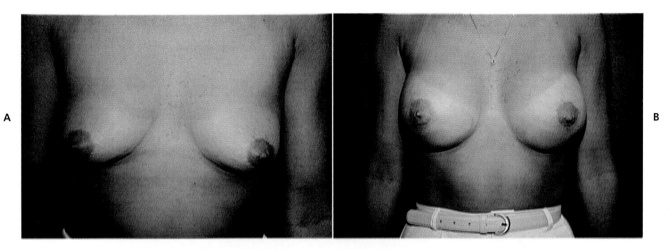

Fig. 5-3 Breast augmentation. **A,** Preoperative. **B,** Postoperative. *(Courtesy Brian W. Davies, MD.)*

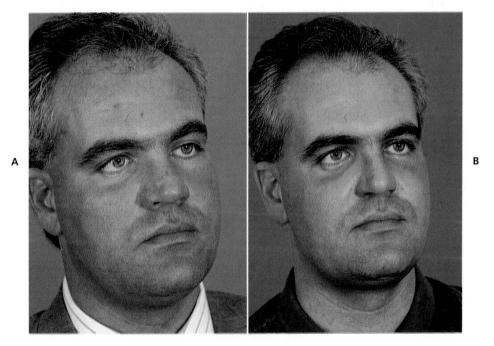

Fig. 5-4 Rhinoplasty. **A,** Preoperative. **B,** Postoperative. *(Courtesy Brian W. Davies, MD.)*

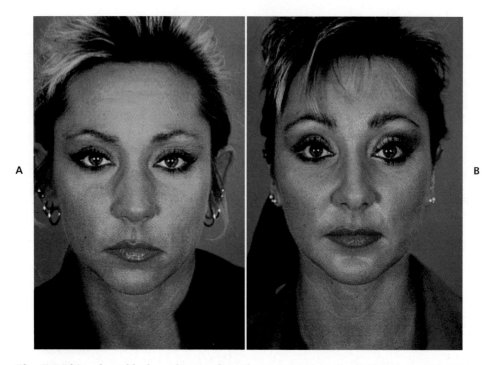

Fig. 5-5 Rhinoplasty, blepharoplasty, and otoplasty. **A,** Preoperative. **B,** Postoperative. *(Courtesy Brian W. Davies, MD.)*

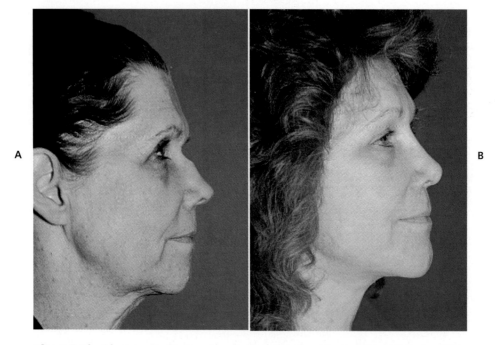

Fig. 5-6 Rhytidectomy. **A,** Preoperative. **B,** Postoperative. *(Courtesy Brian W. Davies, MD.)*

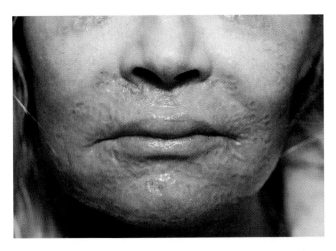

Fig. 5-7 Herpes simplex type I infection after facial resurfacing procedure. *(Courtesy Brian W. Davies, MD.)*

Patient selection and preparation are important aspects of the preoperative process. Outcome identification should reflect the actual realm of possibilities, including a result that is less than perfect.

Some patients can become addicted to plastic surgery. Often described as insatiable, they may seek surgical alteration of multiple body contours, facial features, and modification of secondary sex characteristics. Some individuals will request surgical procedures for every portion of his or her body. Little thought is given to the possibility of an undesired outcome. They commonly have unrealistic expectations and questionable motives for altering their appearance. Extreme requests for multiple procedures should be viewed with caution. The average patient may desire two or three types of procedures. Patients who have had multiple surgical procedures may desire to make other changes to their physical appearance, such as hair color (Fig. 5-8). Females may undergo breast alterations, such as augmentation, reduction, or mastopexy. Males may have procedures to enhance penile size and scrotal turgor. Either sex may desire liposuction of the abdomen, hips, thighs, neck, or upper arms. Patients who never seem satisfied with any result and continue to seek physical surgical alteration beyond reason should be referred for psychiatric evaluation and counseling.

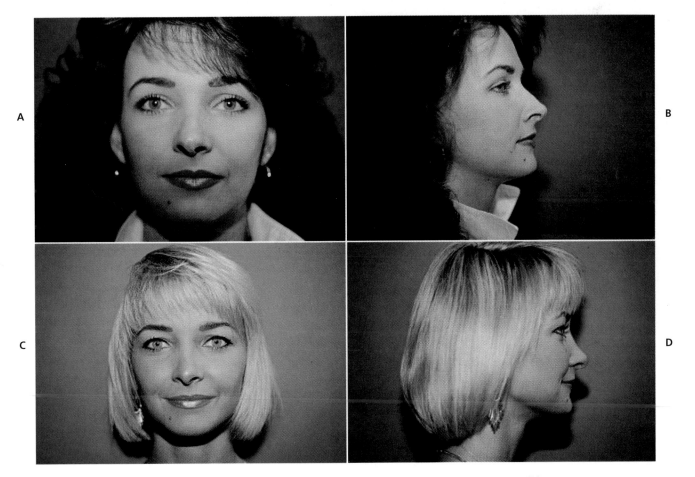

Fig. 5-8 Some patients change entire appearance after facial aesthetic surgery. Browlift, rhinoplasty, and blepharoplasty. **A and B,** Preoperative. **C and D,** Postoperative. *(Courtesy Brian W. Davies, MD.)*

Reconstructive procedures can restore self-esteem and confidence. Traumatic injuries can be physically mutilating and cause the patient to withdraw from society. Although some residual deformity may remain, restoring as much form and function as possible helps the patient reenter society with a more positive outlook. Resection or amputation for disease often requires combined medical and surgical intervention (Fig. 5-9). Reconstruction helps the patient adjust physically, but emotionally he or she may adopt a defeated attitude if psychological support is not provided. Women with breast cancer were studied, and the findings revealed that a positive attitude contributed to a longer survival rate.

Referral to social service agencies such as cancer survivor groups or rehabilitation facilities supports the patient through feelings of depression and grieving. These feelings may persist after reconstruction, and referral to the appropriate social service agency is advised.

Body Image

Body image is important regardless of age. Body image is the personal concept of self that is reflected to the outside world and conveys a sense of personal well-being. It is in part both reality and idealism. Specific perceptions evolve during developmental stages and phases identified by psychologic researchers such as Erikson and Piaget. Body image at any given age may be a learned phenomenon as perceptions of self and others. External influences include interaction with superiors, peers, and subordinates. Other influences include clothing designers, product advertisers, and celebrities. Internal influences include past and present sensory stimuli, emotional contacts, and cognitive awareness.

Alteration in body image may involve the change of function or appearance (Box 5-1). Self perception is distorted, causing anxiety and a sense of self-depreciation. Some patients go through mourning and phases of loss. Plastic and reconstructive procedures can help minimize body image alterations.

PEDIATRIC CONSIDERATIONS

Pediatric patients undergoing plastic or reconstructive procedures usually have congenital defects or have experienced a disfiguring trauma. Malformation is not always synonymous with mental retardation. A severely disfigured child can have normal or above-average intelligence. Conversely, a handsome child can be extremely retarded. Communication with any pediatric patient should be primarily patient-centered, not parent-centered. Speaking in terms that the child can comprehend and making body motions that are not startling enhance the relationship with trust. Including the parents in the conversation is also important because they can provide needed information about the child's history. The parents are essential to informed consent.

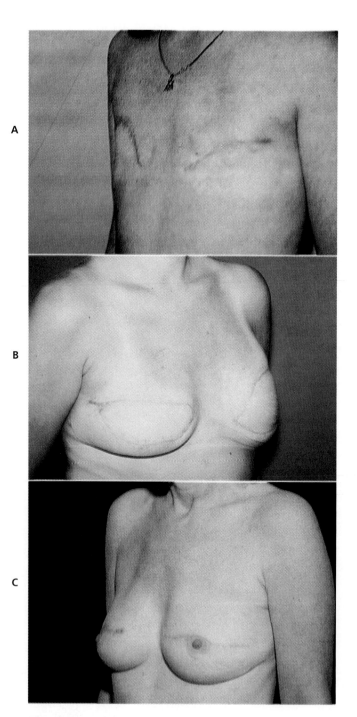

Fig. 5-9 Breast reconstruction. **A,** Preoperative. **B and C,** Postoperative. *(Courtesy Brian W. Davies, MD.)*

Box 5-1 **Body Image Alterations**

Altered appearance
Altered activities of daily living (ADL)
Altered mobility
Altered communication
Altered function
Altered comfort
Altered form
Altered vocation
Altered socialization

Infants and children have various levels of vulnerability according to developmental stage, support system, and understanding. The plan of care should include consideration for psychosocial and physiologic differences on an individual level. Chronologic age or body size should not be confused with cognition. A large child may be emotionally immature, though appearing older than his or her years. A small 6 year old may have greater stability than a teenager. Developmental acceleration or delay can influence how well a child copes with hospitalization.

Pediatric Response to Hospitalization

Repeated hospital admissions can affect the child's reaction to the perioperative environment. Some children respond positively because they understand much about the hospital environment. Some of these children may not need any form of premedication because their anxiety levels are manageable. Others demonstrate fear and acting-out behaviors because they sense separation and remember unpleasant physical effects. The fearful, anxious child should be encouraged to bring a favorite blanket or toy to the operating room (OR). Some facilities permit parents to remain with the child through induction of general anesthesia as a comfort measure. The child and parents should be reunited as soon as possible after the procedure. The fears expressed by children in the perioperative environment are related closely to developmental stage (Box 5-2).

Physiologic Considerations of the Pediatric Patient

The primary physiologic systems support is based on body size and configuration. Airway patency support includes the right size mask and/or endotracheal tube. Usually an uncuffed tube is used for children under 8 years of age to prevent damage to narrow areas of the airway. A small infant is an obligate nose breather. The tongue is large in proportion to the mandible until 2 years of age. The larynx is difficult to visualize because the epiglottis is floppy. The chest is more compliant and therefore more easily collapsed. Small infants desaturate quickly and must be monitored for blood oxygen saturation.

Fluid balance and body temperature are closely monitored. Sponges are weighed, and urine is measured. Body temperature is important because hyperthermia can cause sweating with resultant unmeasurable fluid loss. Excess blankets can absorb lost fluid as perspiration. Oxygen consumption increases with

body temperature because respiration increases in an effort to blow off heat. Fluid is lost in the exhaled breath. Preferred methods of warming include forced warm air and radiant lighting. Inadvertent hypothermia can result from evaporation of surface moisture.

Children less than 2 years of age may be fed breast milk 4 hours preoperatively without any serious side effects. Formula-fed children may be fed 6 hours preoperatively with additional clear fluids 4 hours before the surgical procedure. Older children may have solid food up to 8 hours preoperatively.

GERIATRIC CONSIDERATIONS

After the age of 50 or 60 years, rejuvenation of physical appearance may be sought to enhance job retention or prospects. Drooping eyelids and sagging jowls can give the appearance of being tired or angry. Facial tightening and resurfacing procedures can diminish effects of aging skin that disguise a youthful, more energetic spirit (Fig. 5-10). Some older patients desire facial rejuvenation to attract a mate. Fewer aesthetic procedures and more palliative or restorative procedures are performed in the aging population. This is age-related and usually applies to postretirement years. Some elective procedures, such as face lifts, may be cost prohibitive for this group. Necessary procedures, such as flaps or grafts to cover ulcerated areas, may be covered in part by insurance or Medicare.

As a patient becomes older, his or her skin looses much elasticity, and aesthetic results may be adversely affected. Other influences include vascular changes, loss of subcutaneous fat and tissues, and generalized diminished healing capabilities. Subsurface layers may not provide a foundation for sculpting with liposuction or tightening of fascial supports. Muscle fibers decrease in number, and tendons become coarser causing decreased range of motion. Bones become more brittle as demineralization causes osteoporitic conditions.

Physiologic Considerations of the Geriatric Patient

Elderly patients frequently have comorbid conditions such as diabetes or heart disease. These conditions often predispose geriatric patients to complications involving wound healing and circulatory status. Factors such as diminished range of motion or altered tissue perfusion significantly impact the plan of care. Careful assessment, planning, and implementation can help provide the best possible outcome. Determining a preoperative baseline of physiologic and systemic conditions, functional health patterns, and expected outcomes can serve as an early warning of potential adverse results. Evaluation of patient outcomes and responses should be documented in a retrievable form.

POSITIONING OF PATIENTS FOR PLASTIC AND RECONSTRUCTIVE PROCEDURES

After the patient is anesthetized, he or she is placed in the appropriate position for the surgical procedure. Bony prominences and pressure points are padded to prevent neurovascular injury and pressure sores. If local anesthesia is used, the patient can help

---

Box 5-2 **Childhood Fears**

Separation from family
Pain
The unknown
Bodily mutilation
Needles and tools
Loss of friends
Loss of control
Death

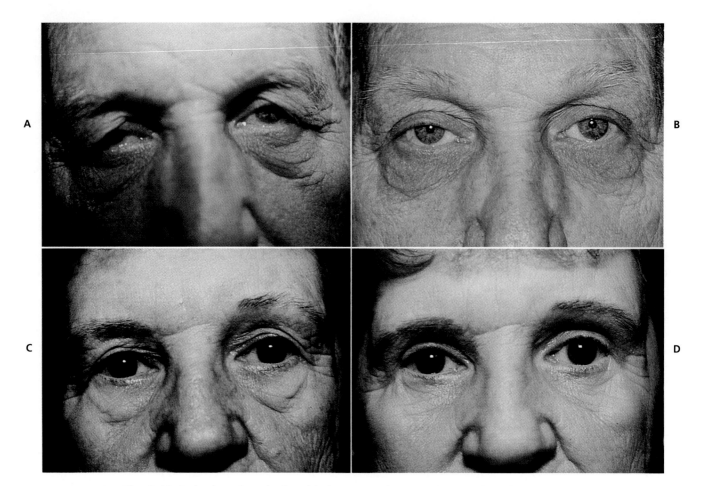

Fig. 5-10 Geriatric patients look and feel younger after procedures such as blepharoplasty. **A and B,** Male, preoperative and postoperative. **C and D,** Female, preoperative and postoperative. *(Courtesy Brian W. Davies, MD.)*

move into position. If intravenous conscious sedation (IVCS) or general anesthesia is used, the patient will be very groggy and need to be positioned by the team. The patient is not moved until the anesthesia provider states it is safe to begin the positioning process. IV lines and airway maintenance are prime considerations in the patient's physiologic stability.

A safety belt is placed over the patient's thighs and secured to the OR bed. The belt should be loose enough to allow the passage of several fingers underneath and tight enough to prevent flexure of the large group of leg muscles. The safety belt should be visible by the team at all times before and after the procedure. If additional blankets are added over the patient, it is advisable to replace the strap over top of the blankets. If the extra blankets are placed over the safety strap, the strap is not visible to the team and it is difficult to verify its security before and after the application of drapes. The patient's arms should be secured by wrist straps or tucked in at the sides of the patient with the draw sheet. The sheet is wrapped over the arms and secured under the patient, not tucked in under the mattress. Tucking the sheet under the mattress causes pressure from the weight of the

patient and the mattress. Patients receiving local anesthetic procedures may become apprehensive if their hands are "tied down." Some patients are more cooperative if they are permitted to rest their hands loosely on armboards or in their lap.

The final resting position of the patient will be designated according to the type of procedure performed. The surgeon and anesthesiologist give final approval of the surgical position. Modifications based on each patient's needs and physiology should be individually addressed. Considerations for circulatory and respiratory support are important. Prevention of musculoskeletal or neurologic injuries is accomplished by using positioning devices. The use of foam and gel-filled pads prevents pressure to body parts. Table 5-1 lists several areas of potential patient injury caused by positioning. Figure 5-11 shows pediatric positions, padding, and security straps. Table extensions should be used as needed, and care should be taken to use appropriate tables with designated weight limits. Consult manufacturer's recommendations concerning safe weight limits. After the patient is draped, care is taken to avoid placing instrumentation on the patient's body.

Table 5-1 **Potential Patient Injury Caused by Positioning**

Five Basic Positions	Potential Patient Injury	Prevention
Supine	Pressure to posterior buttocks, sacrum, genitalia, back of head, heels, elbows	Padding with gel-filled cushions, sheep skin, egg-crate, air mattress, donut
	Neurovascular injury caused by hyperextension or hyperflexion of a joint	Arms whould not be hyperextended beyond 90 degrees
Prone	Pressure to anterior face and forehead, endotracheal tube injury, eyes, ears, breasts, genitalia, knees, dorsum of foot	Padding with gel-filled cushions, sheep skin, egg-crate, air mattress, donut
		Observe for chest excursion; use chest rolls
	Shoulder dislocation	Caution is needed for circumduction of arm for armboard placement
Lateral	Pressure to lateral face and eye, medial knees, and lateral ankle; neck displacement, shoulder nerve injury	Padding with gel-filled cushions, sheep skin, foam, egg-crate, air mattress, donut
Sitting	Pressure to posterior buttocks, sacrum, genitalia, head, heels, elbows	Padding with gel-filled cushions, sheep skin, foam, egg-crate, air mattress, donut
Lithotomy	Pressure to posterior buttocks, sacrum, genitalia, back of head, heels, elbows	Padding with gel-filled cushions, sheep skin, foam, egg-crate, air mattress, donut
	Neurovascular injury to legs, ankles, feet	Padded stirrups, correct anatomic position without hyperflexion or hyperadduction of joints
	Crush injury to hands from table gatch	Observe hand when raising or lowering end of table

SKIN MARKING AND PREPARATION
Skin Marking

Precision incision lines are necessary for most plastic and reconstructive procedures. Prime consideration is given to the exterior appearance of the wound as well as the underlying restructuring. Most incisions follow natural tension lines of the skin and are concealed by folds or hair patterns. Predrawing or outlining the intended surgical knife blade pattern is part of the planning process.

Methods of marking the surgical site commonly include measuring anatomic structures with a tape measure, calipers, or schematic before the antiseptic skin prep. Areas such as the face, nose, and ears may be compared with a photographic template. Commercially packaged and sterilized skin-marking pens are available in a variety of tip widths and ink colors (Fig. 5-12). Some plastic surgeons prefer to use bottled dyes like methylene blue, indigo carmine, and brilliant green. These dyes can be applied with a sharpened stylus or the wooden end of a cotton-tipped applicator. Larger incisions may be overscored with the tip of a sterile needle, breaking the skin surface after the patient is anesthetized.

For larger markings on torso surfaces, the conscious patient will be asked to stand during the outlining process (Fig. 5-13). Procedures such as liposuction, abdominoplasty, and mastopexy require the skin to be pendulous for accurate measurement. The terrain of the skin would be shifted if the patient is marked in a recumbent position (Fig. 5-14). Adequate privacy and room warmth should be provided for the comfort and security of the patient.

Skin Preparation

The patient's skin prep may consist of hair removal and cleansing with an approved antimicrobial solution. Extremely hairy surfaces may be heavily contaminated with microorganisms. Hair follicles and oil ducts contain many resident flora that can cause complications in wound healing. Methods of hair removal include clipping, shaving, and depilatory chemicals. Clipping and shaving can cause cuts in the skin surface. Depilatories can cause chemical irritation and edema of the skin and mucous membranes and should not be used near the eyes or genitalia. Scalp hair can be clipped before shaving. Studies have shown that there is no appreciable increase in wound infection when conservative shaving procedures are used compared with radical shaves. The least amount of hair is removed as possible. The eyebrows are not shaved because they may not grow back evenly. Hair removal should take place as close to the time of the procedure as possible.

Cleansing the skin before the procedure may include prewashing with a degreasing agent to remove surface oils. Cotton-tipped swabs dipped in antimicrobial antiseptic should be used to clean the umbilicus. Foreign substances such as glass, cinders, or dirt imbedded in a traumatic wound must be thoroughly cleansed from the site. Soft synthetic brushes may be needed to dislodge the debris.

The surgical site is squared off with absorbent towels and prepped in a circular motion from the incision site outward to the periphery. Gloves are worn during the prep to prevent the introduction of additional microorganisms to the area. Care is taken to prevent pooling of solutions. Sterile cotton

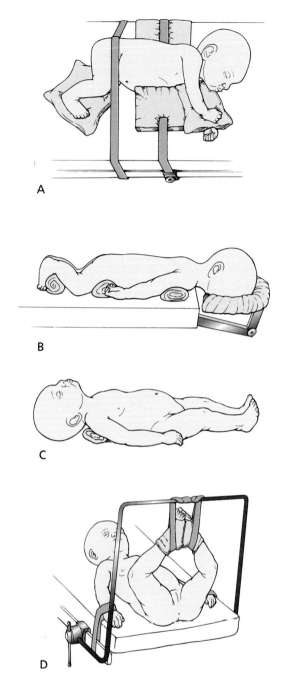

Fig. 5-11 Examples of pediatric patient positions.

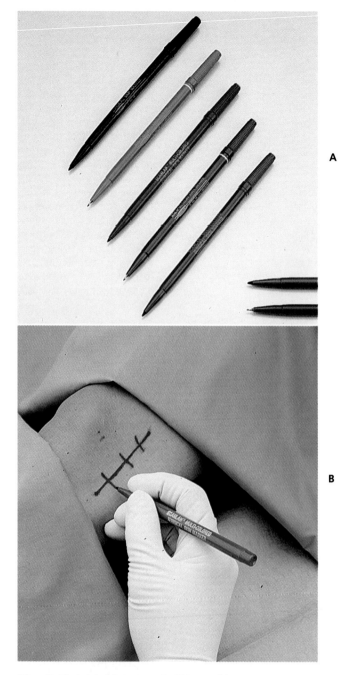

Fig. 5-12 A, Marking pens. **B,** Skin marking. *(Courtesy Scanlon, International, St Paul, Minnesota.)*

balls can be used to occlude the ear canals for facial preps. Tissue injury may occur if the patient's skin is kept in prolonged contact with chemical antiseptics. Table 5-2 lists commonly used antimicrobial skin preparation agents. Care is taken to avoid scrubbing off the measured markings made for incision sites. Prep solutions should not be heated because they can lose effectiveness if the concentration is altered by evaporation. In addition, the patient may suffer burns to the skin from over-heated solution. Consult the manufacturer's recommendations.

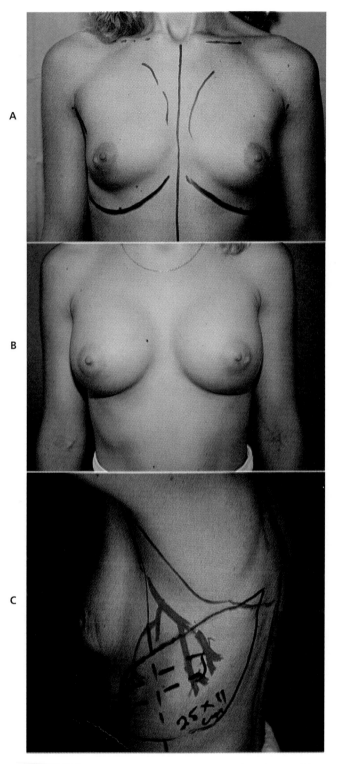

Fig. 5-13 Marking for augmentation. **A,** Preoperative. Simple color marking to outline area of undermining for placement of implants. **B,** Postoperative. **C,** Examples of multicolor skin marking to identify vascular structures of a flap. *(Courtesy Brian W. Davies, MD.)*

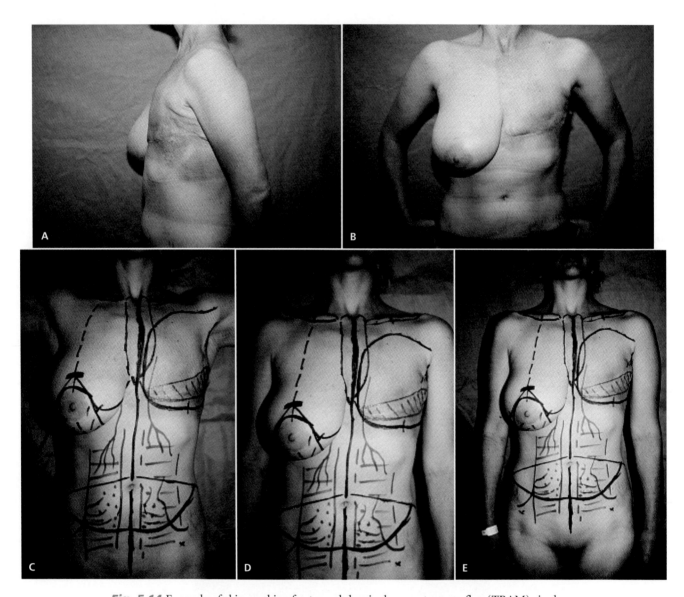

Fig. 5-14 Example of skin marking for transabdominal myocutaneous flap (TRAM) single pedicle for left breast reconstruction and right breast mastopexy. **A and B,** Preliminary photos for premarking to evaluate extent of scar and potential for reconstruction. **C,** Process of marking while standing with arms raised. **D and E,** Final markings while standing with arms down. *(Courtesy Brian W. Davies, MD.)*

Table 5-2 **Antimicrobial Skin Preparation Solutions**

Solution	Antimicrobial Action	Notes
Ethyl alcohol	Gram-positive and gram-negative bacteria, fungi, viruses, tuberculosis (TB)	Flammable; vapors; drying to skin; degreasing agent
Iodophor	Gram-positive and gram-negative bacteria, fungi, viruses, TB	May have enhanced action when combined with alcohol; inactivated in presence of biologic matter; may cause reaction in iodine-sensitive person
Chlorhexidine gluconate	Gram-positive and gram-negative bacteria, viruses	Not good for TB or fungi; ototoxic; avoid use on mucus membranes; can damage eyes; has sustained action for several hours postapplication
Chloroxylenol	Gram-positive bacteria	Not effective against other microorganisms
Hexachlorophene	Gram-positive bacteria	Not effective against other microorganisms; neurotoxic; avoid use on broken skin
Triclosan	Broad-spectrum	Cumulative action; safe for use around face and eyes

Bibliography

Anderson LG, Leroux CL: Routine surgery, routine patients? never, *Plast Surg Nurs* 16(1):41, 1996.

Association of Operating Room Nurses: *Standards, recommended practices, and guidelines,* Denver, 1997, AORN.

American Society of Plastic and Reconstructive Surgical Nurses: *Core curriculum for plastic and reconstructive surgical nursing,* ed 2, Pitman, NJ, 1996, ASPRSN.

Atkinson LJ, Fortunato NM: *Berry and Kohn's operating room technique,* ed 8, St Louis, 1996, Mosby.

Cehaich K: Preparing the pediatric patient for surgery, *Plast Surg Nurs* 14(2):105, 1994.

Grunert BK, Maksud DP: Psychological adjustment to hand injuries: nursing management, *Plast Surg Nurs* 13(2):72, 1993.

Hart D: The psychological outcome of breast reconstruction, *Plast Surg Nurs* 16(3):167, 1996.

Holden P: Psychosocial factors affecting a child's capacity to cope with surgery and recovery, *Semin Periop Nurs* 4(2):75, 1995.

Maksud DP, Anderson RC: Psychological dimensions of aesthetic surgery: essentials for nurses, *Plast Surg Nurs* 15(3):137, 1995.

McCain LA: A woman's psychological response and adjustment to the breast cancer diagnosis, *Plast Surg Nurs* 13(2):77, 1993.

McEwen D: Intraoperative positioning of surgical patients, *AORN J* 63(6):1059, 1996.

Moser S: Social service collaboration: meeting the patient's psychosocial needs, *Plast Surg Nurs* 13(2):84, 1993.

Murphy L: Preoperative skin preparation of patients, *Plast Surg Nurs* 13(2):101, 1993.

Pruzinsky T: Psychological factors in cosmetic plastic surgery: recent developments in patient care, *Plast Surg Nurs* 13(2):64, 1993.

Roth RA: *Perioperative nursing core curriculum,* Philadelphia, 1995, WB Saunders.

Spencer KW: Significance of the breast to the individual and society, *Plast Surg Nurs* 16(3):131, 1996.

6 Understanding Skin and Wound Management

Cells are the smallest functional units. Individually, cells throughout the body differ in structure and contain various work structures called *organelles*. Each type of organelle performs a different task, such as generating energy, manipulating protein, digestion, excretion, and genetic replication. As the fundamental unit of life, each cell has a specialized role.

Collections of cells performing specific unified tasks are referred to as *tissue*. Similar types of tissues that are grouped together to perform a collective function are the basic structural components of organs. A group of organs that work together in concerted effort is a system. Skin, for example, is referred to as the integumentary system because it is comprised of many tissues, organs, and structures that work together to perform particular functions (Fig. 6-1).

Variances in tissue types, location, structure, and function influence healing and remodeling. Body surfaces, such as the dermal cover, subsurface layers, and bony framework, are critical elements in plastic and reconstructive surgery. Each body surface, whether superficial or deep, is subject to alteration, restoration, or neostructure. Most of the body is the working realm of the plastic and reconstructive team with few exceptions, such as the eyeball, brain, spinal cord, and other major organ systems.

Success or failure of a plastic or reconstructive procedure depends on the skill of the surgical team, but the patient's healing is contingent on his or her tissue properties. The team measures the success of the procedure objectively for form and function. The patient measures success or failure by subjectively assessing superficial aspects for beauty and scar size.

TISSUE STRUCTURE AND FUNCTION

Tissue structure varies according to location in the body and function. The four main histologic types of tissue are shown in Table 6-1. Tissue can be categorized by texture ranging from very soft and loose to hard and compact. Although minimal tissue handling is optimal, necessary handling of tissue layers is based on the cellular design and mechanism of healing. For example, tissue with fine cellular layers, such as mucous membrane, is manipulated with fine forceps and sutured with fine absorbable material. Using crushing clamps and heavy-gauge, nonabsorbable suture would significantly interfere with healing.

Surface Layers

The skin is a multilayered, multifunctional body cover. As the largest and heaviest organ of the body, assessment of the skin is one of the best measurements of generalized wellness. Functionally, the skin, when intact, is multipurpose as shown in Table 6-2.

The two main skin layers are the epidermis and the dermis. Thickness of the skin and its layers is determined by location. Skin thickness of combined epidermis and dermis ranges from 4 mm on the back to 1.5 mm of scalp.

Epidermis (cuticle or scarf skin)

The epidermis is the outermost layer of the skin. It is organized into five levels of stratified squamous epithelium and contains no organs, nerve endings, or blood vessels. It renews itself every 15 to 30 days according to the body surface area, age of the individual, and generalized condition. The basic anatomy and physiology of epidermal layers are as follows:

- Strata corneum: 20 to 30 layers of flattened, nonnucleated, keratinized cells filled with sclerotic protein forming the surface of the skin. Accounts for 75% of the epidermal thickness. Cells are shed from this level. Referred to as the *horny layer*. Thinner in hairy, thin-skinned areas.
- Strata lucidum: Composed of flattened eosinophilic cells. More apparent in thicker-skinned areas. Organelles and nuclei are absent. Thinner and less developed in hairy, thin-skinned areas.
- Strata granulosum: Flattened, polygonal cells laden with basophilic granules arranged in three to five layers create a penetration-resistant, cementlike protein. Mitotic activity in this level creates cells for renewal of epidermal layers. Thinner and less developed in hairy, thin-skinned areas.
- Strata spinosum: Mitotic activity in this level takes place at the junction of the basal, referred to as the malpighian layer, creating cells for renewal of epidermal layers. Nucleated cuboidal and polygonal prickle cells are bound together on the surface by protein filaments (tonofibrils). These filaments may minimize the effects of abrasion. Thicker-skinned areas have tougher filaments.
- Stratum basale (strata germinativum): A single cell layer that overlies the junction of the epidermis and dermis. Intense mitosis in this layer in combination with the basal and the spinosum causes epidermal regeneration. As cells are generated, they migrate upward toward the surface. Melanocytes, located between basal cells and in hair follicles, create melanin that causes skin pigmentation. Melanin enters and accumulates in keratocytes causing superficial skintone color and ultraviolet protection. Exposure to sunlight causes darkening of existing melanin and accelerated generation of new melanin.

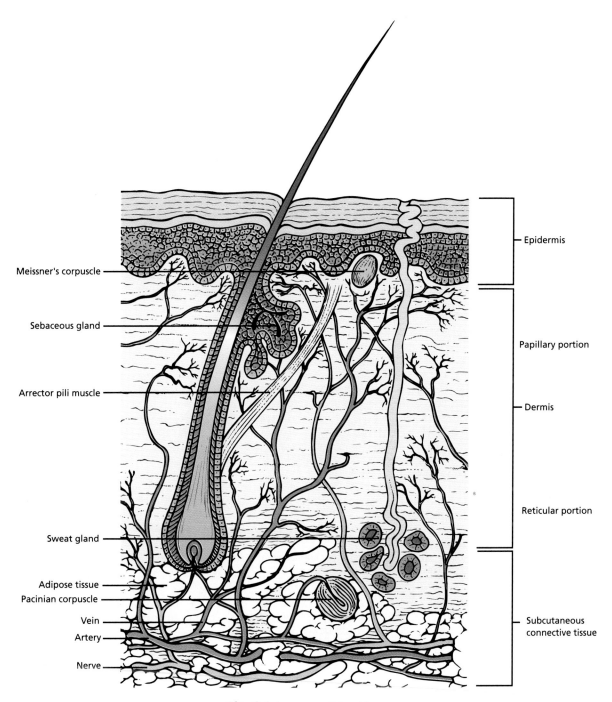

Meissner's corpuscle

Sebaceous gland

Arrector pili muscle

Sweat gland

Adipose tissue

Pacinian corpuscle

Vein

Artery

Nerve

Epidermis

Papillary portion

Dermis

Reticular portion

Subcutaneous
connective tissue

Fig. 6-1 Anatomy of the skin.

Table 6-1 **Four Basic Histologic Tissue Types**

HISTOLOGIC TISSUE TYPE	DESCRIPTION	IMPLICATIONS TO PLASTIC AND RECONSTRUCTIVE TEAM
EPITHELIAL TISSUE		
A. Types		
1. Simple	Single layer of cells (endothelium) that lines the blood vessels, heart, and lymphatics	Delicate tissue that is easily damaged by rough handling
2. Stratified	Several layers of cells that form the skin, gastrointestinal tract, genitourinary (GU) tract, reproductive tract, oropharynx; lines area that serve as a passage; reduces friction with mucus; can convert into keratin	Superficial layer of body cover; surface modifications are performed here; forms hair and nails
3. Transitional	Combination of simple and stratified layers found in ureters and bladder	Encountered during GU reconstruction and neoconstruction
B. Cellular surface structure		
1. Squamous	Flat	
2. Columnar	Tall, cylindrical	
3. Cuboidal	Square-shaped	
CONNECTIVE TISSUE		
A. Fluid	Blood, lymph, chyle, cerebrospinal fluid, synovium vitreous and aqueous, and mucinous material	Care with body substance isolation and provision of hemostasis
B. Fibrous		
1. Areolar	Loose network forming the frame for subcuticular tissue.	Reorganized during liposuction and fat transplantation procedures
2. Adipose	Fat that fills the loose network; visible in fetus at 14 weeks' gestation; not found in eyelid, penis, scrotum, labia minorum, cranium, and lung tissue	
3. Reticular	Forms firmer framework for organs and vessels	
C. Supportive		
1. Cartilage	Avascular, no lymphatics or nerves	Structural integrity is altered during rhinoplasty and otoplasty; cartilage may be used as graft material; radical neck reconstruction may involve tracheal rings or laryngectomy for multidisciplinary treatment
a. Hyaline	Translucent, articular, and rubs against other articular surface; forms the epiphyseal line in long bone, portions of the nose, and tracheal rings	
b. Costal elastic	Becomes fibrous with age; found in ribs, nose, trachea, and larynx	
c. White fibrocartilage	Forms circular menisci in joints and between vertebrae	
d. Yellow elastic	Found in auricle of ear, eustachian tubes, and epiglottis	
2. Erectile	Found in corpus cavernosa, clitoris, and nose	
D. Hard	Bony surfaces covered with periosteum except at articulations and cartilaginous areas of circulatory insertion points	Reconstruction requires framework of underlying bone or graft material; autologous bone may be harvested from graft site for neoconstruction; donor bone may be used as transplant material
1. Cancellous bone	Spaces are filled with red marrow; erythroblasts and smaller vessels	
2. Compact bone	Hollow center filled with yellow marrow (higher fat content) and larger vessels	
MUSCLE TISSUE		
A. Visceral	Smooth, involuntary muscle; hollow organs, vessels, glands, areola, scrotum, iris of eye	Skeletal muscle may be used to replace bulk lost to debridement; vascularized flaps replace radical tissue excisions
B. Skeletal	Cylindrical, striated, voluntary cells	
C. Cardiac	Branching cells, nonnucleated, less fibrous connective tissue	
NERVE TISSUE		
A. Types		
1. Neuron	Cells generate and conduct nerve impulses; has multiple cytoplasmic fibers on one side (dendrites) and a single myelinated extension from the other side (axon)	Nerves may be injured during any procedure
2. Neuroglia	Insulate and support neurons in central nervous system	
B. Classification by activity type		
1. Afferent	Sensory	
2. Efferent	Motor	

Table 6-2 **Functional Physiology of the Skin**

Skin Functions	Examples
Protection	Waterproof barrier; pigmentation guards against ultraviolet rays of the sun; diminished impact and friction injury; can expand to accommodate subsurface enlargement such as edema or pregnancy
Regulation	Maintains constant internal environment; works in concert with temperature controls; evaporation and absorption control
Regeneration	Reconstructs own structure
Absorption	Minimal intake of chemical substances; can be beneficial or harmful
Communication	Tactile sense delivers information about environment
Excretion/ secretion	Serves as exit point for some metabolic waste; physiologic lubricant
Vitamin D production	Sunlight exposure causes generation of fat-soluble vitamin D for calcium absorption
Sense of self-esteem	Subjective sense of well-being and acceptance when body surface conforms to perceived norms
Health indicator	Objective assessment of color, temperature, texture, hydration, topography, tactile response, odor, and comparison with accepted norms for age, sex, and race provides generalized health information

Each epithelial layer consists of keratin-producing (keratinocytes) cells. Keratin is modified into functional components such as hair and fingernails on select body surfaces. Over-activity of the spinosum and basal levels can increase epidermal thickness in normally thin areas causing psoriasis. The cell renewal rate in psoriasis is approximately 7 days instead of the normal 15 to 30 days.

Dermis

The dermis, also known as *corium* or *cutis vera*, is composed of papillary and reticular layers of flexible connective tissue. Superficially, the dermis has an irregular surface of papillae that interdigitate with the strata basale of the epidermal layers. This peglike interlacing is more dense in areas of the body that are under constant tension or pressure, which in turn reinforces the sturdiness of the surface. These papillary vascular projections are referred to as *rete*. The papillary layer comprises 20% of the dermal thickness and is connected to the underside of the basale by a reticular network referred to as the *lamina reticularis*. This complex forms the basement membrane. The dermal structure as a whole is a loose, areolar connective tissue that contains pain and touch receptors, blood vessels, and lymphatics. Macrophages and mast cells are abundant in the meshwork. A protein and polysaccharide compound produces a macromolecule that has a large capacity for holding water. The dermis is a key element in wound repair and tissue healing.

From fetal life to adulthood, collagen fibers thicken and collagen synthesis decreases. In old age, elastin diminishes and the skin looses its suppleness. Pathologic skin and ligament conditions of lost elasticity and faulty collagen fibril processing include cutis laxa and Ehlers-Danlos syndrome.

The dermis contains a rich blood and lymph supply. In some areas, arterial and venous communication is direct without utilizing a capillary mechanism. Arteriovenous shunts allow for thermoregulation and blood pressure control. Capillary networks are located in the papillary layer to nourish the epidermis. Effector innervation of the dermis is derived from postganglionic fibers of the sympathetic ganglia of the paravertebral chain. Affector innervation is a superficial dermal network of free nerve endings, hair follicles, and encapsulated sensory organs, such as Meissner's and Pacini's corpuscles.

Below the dermis is a looser, fatty layer, the panniculus adiposus, which is referred to as the *subcutaneous layer*. Beneath the subcutaneous tissue is a vestigial layer of striated muscle referred to as the *panniculus carnosus*. The looseness of this structure allows for movement of the skin over supporting musculature. In males, the distribution is through the nape of the neck, deltoids, triceps, abdomen, lumbosacral region, and buttocks. In females, the fatty layer extends through the breasts, abdomen, buttocks, epitrochanteric area, and anterior thighs.

Each area of epidermal-dermal-adipose layering (integument) overlies fascial sheeting in various arrangements specific to corresponding musculature. The fascial layer is a fibrous-areolar tissue that supports the superficial skin layers and encases the muscle. This fibrous sheet covers the body's musculature throughout superficial and deep bundles. Adipose cells occupy areolar spaces rendering it soft and pliable, permitting vessels, nerves, and lymphatics to penetrate its course. The superficial fascia is directly below the integument and is the point to which injection of local anesthetic should extend for the best effect. Sensory nerve fibers run through this area, and anesthetic is easily absorbed.

The deep fascia is tough and less pliable. Encasing the muscles, the deep fascia runs the length of the bundle and terminates in strong, fibrous tendons that attach to bones beneath the periosteum. Incisions or tears greater than 10 mm are sutured meticulously to prevent herniation of underlying structures.

Accessory Appendages to the Skin

Modifications in the epidermal layer cause varying degrees of keratin deposition. Thickness and durability are functionally related to location of keratiniztion. Hair, for example, is modified keratin fibers. It is designed to be flexible and serves to protect and warm specific areas where it grows. Nails are more compact, translucent keratin. They are useful for the protection of each distal phalanx. Under normal circumstances, nails are achromatic.

Other skin appendages include glands, blood vessels, and sensory organs. Glands arise in the dermis, and some exit the body through ducts that penetrate the epidermis. Other glands empty into the superior segment of hair follicles.

Hair Follicles

Hair follicles are invaginations of epidermal epithelium that terminate in the dermal layers in hair bulbs. The bulb is encircled with a capillary bed to nourish the entirety of the follicular structure. Loss of this blood supply results in death of the follicle. A specialized sheath of connective tissue encircles the follicle in the dermal layer. Small bundles of smooth muscle cells, referred to as *arrector pilli,* form attachments to the surrounding connective tissue in a diagonal fashion. As arrector pilli contract, the shaft of the hair is straightened to an upright position. This contraction causes the superficial skin to dimple and pucker, creating "goose bumps" (cutis anserina).

Straighter hair is stronger and more cylindrical on cross section. Curly hair is weaker and more flattened or ovoid on cross section. The diameter and length-potential of hair is proportionate to its location on the body. Scalp hair grows to indefinite lengths. Eyelid hairs are fine and do not grow past the end of the follicle. Eyelashes grow a specific length and stop. Beards grow continuously. Pubic hair is usually coarse and thick to provide greater protection and padding in a vulnerable area.

The character of hair, such as color, texture, and volume, depends on age, sex, race, and location on the body. Hair color is caused by melanocytes near the hair root that enter the medulary and cortical cells of the hair shaft.

Hair growth patterns alternate between activity cycles lasting several years and rest periods lasting up to 3 months. Some growth patterns are age-dependent and are triggered by sexual maturation. Scalp, face, and pubic hair growth is dependent on hormonal activity of the adrenal and thyroid glands and the gonads. Mitotic activity of hair follicles is directly influenced by androgens, which are male hormones. Hair-bearing surfaces are found everywhere on the body except on the soles, palms, lips, glans penis, clitoris, and labia minora. Early hair follicles are visible around the eyes and scalp during the ninth fetal week. Hair cutting or shaving does not affect the hair regrowth rate. Clipped eyelashes usually grow back to their normal length. Shaving eyebrows, however, may cause irregular regrowth and is not advised.

Nails (ungues)

The dorsal tip of each phalanx is tipped with a plate of specialized, keratinized cells. Proximally, the nail root is covered by stratum corneum referred to as the *eponychium,* or cuticle (Fig. 6-2). A sheet of hard keratin, known as the *nail plate,* rests on a bed of epidermis (nail bed). Nail bed layers are continuous with other surfaces of the digit with the exception of stratum corneum, which is actually continuous with the nail plate. The nail matrix is deep in the nail root and generates cells that move distally over the nail bed to form the nail plate. The white, crescent-shaped area at the base of the nail plate is the lunula, which is framed by a ridge of skin (cuticle). The peripheral blood supply may be assessed through the translucent nail plate but should not be the sole determinant of oxygenation of the patient. Nails are chemically similar to the surface epidermis.

Glandular structures and ducts

Sebaceous and suderiferous glands are found within the dermal layers of the skin. Sebaceous glands are referred to as *holocrine glands* because the oily secretion, sebum, also carries cellular debris. Holocrine glands are small, sacculated structures that contain acini cells that proliferate and produce rounded cells full of fat globules. The cells swell and burst, discharging fatty material and cell remnants into several passages that merge into a single duct. This duct empties into a hair follicle or on nonhairy areas directly onto the surface of the skin. Interruption of sebum flow is responsible for acne. Testosterone controls this cycle in males, and ovarian and adrenal androgens exert influence in the female. Sebum is a lubricant with minor antibacterial and antifungal properties. It also forms part of the vernix caseosa that covers the fetus. The palms and soles lack sebaceous glands, but they are numerous on the scalp and face and around natural body orifices. The largest (meibomian glands) are located on the eyelids.

Eccrine and apocrine glands are suderiferous glands. Eccrine glands are widely distributed over the entire surface of the body and are responsible for producing 700 to 900 grams of sweat per 24 hours. These simple structures are coiled, tubular glands consisting of a secretory component embedded in the dermis with a funnel-shaped exit path (pore) leading directly to the skin's surface. Secretions from these glands are clear and watery, produced in association with physical activity, and serve to cool the body's surface by evaporation. The presence of catabolites in sweat demonstrates that eccrine glands serve also as excretory mechanisms. These glands are most numerous on the palms, soles, and forehead.

Apocrine glands are located only in the axillary, perineal, and areolar areas in combination with eccrine glands. Apocrine glands are larger than eccrine glands and are embedded in subcutaneous tissue. These glands secrete a viscous fluid and have ducts that open into hair follicles. Initially, the secretion is odorless, but quickly develops an odor caused by bacterial decomposition. These glands secrete in response to stress or excitement. In animals, apocrine and sebaceous glands are thought to release

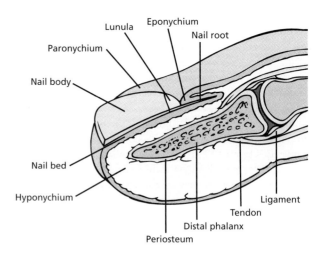

Fig. 6-2 Saggital view of distal fingertip including nail and nail bed.

pheromones, which are hormones thought to cause sexual attraction. Modified apocrine glands are found in the ear canals and secrete cerumen (earwax). Breasts also are modified apocrine glands. Suderiferous glands are found on every area except the lips, nipples, and glans penis.

Circulation of the epidermis and the dermis

Arterial vessels form two separate plexuses. One is located between the papillary and reticular layers, and the other is located between the dermis and the subcutaneous tissue. Each dermal papilla (rete) has one ascending artery and one descending vein. Two separate venous plexuses compliment the arterial network. A third venous plexus passes centrally through the dermis. The vascular structure of the skin is far more complex than that needed for tissue nourishment. The circulation also serves as a thermoregulatory apparatus.

Lymphatic vessels arise from interconnecting cell spaces in the dermal papillae. The lymphatic vessels are the thickness of a single endothelial cell layer and have a proportionately large lumen. They serve to carry debris and cellular proteins from the extravascular compartment of the dermis. The lymphatic circulation forms two plexuses that follow the structure of the arterial plexuses, superficially and deep. The plexuses drain into the lymph nodes.

Innervation of the epidermis and dermis

Many afferent nerve fibers terminate in the face and extremities. Few terminate in the back. The cutaneous nerves contain axons with cell bodies arising from the dorsal root ganglia. Main trunks enter subcutaneous tissue and branch out into webs of nervous fibers in the dermis in a horizontal plane. Some fibers ascend, following the pathway created by blood vessels. Many terminate in the superficial dermal layers and basement membrane, but few extend and terminate in the epidermis. Nerve endings are either encapsulated or free fibers. Encapsulated endings are usually myelinated and located in the dermis and superficial dermal layers. Peripheral free nerve endings that terminate beyond the dermis are unmyelinated fibers.

Skin type distinctions

The two basic types of skin are glabrous (smooth) skin and hairy skin. Glabrous skin is found on the palms and soles. The surface is marked by ridges and sulci arranged in unique configurations referred to as *dermatographics*, or *fingerprints*. These ridges first appear in the fingertips during the thirteenth week of fetal life. The glabrous epidermal layer is very thick. Eccrine glands are present in the dermal layer, but a marked absence of hair follicles and holocrine glands is characteristic of this tissue. Sensory end-organs are encapsulated.

Hairy, thin skin has hair follicles, eccrine glands, and holocrine glands. Apocrine glands are found in the axilla and groin. Sensory structures are not encapsulated.

Langer's Lines

The skin is very mobile and has a great capacity for stretching. The pregnant woman's abdomen expands greatly to accommodate her fetus. Often, the enlargement results in dermal tears referred to as stretch marks. Initially, they appear red *(striae gravidarum)*, but soon fade to white *(linea albicantes)*. Striae usually cross natural skin tension lines in a perpendicular manner.

In 1861, Carl von Langer (1819-1887), an Austrian anatomist, found that natural lines in the skin are caused by static and dynamic tension. Static forces intrinsic to the layers of the skin cause any wound to gape. Elastic and collagen fibers oriented parallel to the skin create a natural tension, giving the skin its firmness (Fig. 6-3, *A-C*). Dynamic forces work in the same direction as muscle pull. These lines are most visible while changing facial expressions (Fig. 6-3, *D*). A wound that crosses perpendicular to these natural lines of tension will have a widened scar. Intentional incisions should follow the natural creases and folds for the best cosmetic effect. An understanding of the mechanics of skin anatomy and physiology is essential for optimal outcomes of plastic and reconstructive surgery.

Subsurface Structural Layers

Under the epidermal and dermal surface layers is a framework of cartilage and bone. Structural modifications often include remodeling subsurface layers. Some reconstructive procedures involve grafting autologous cartilaginous and bony mass from one area to another area of the body. Donor bone is also used to fill defects and stabilize and remodel the structural framework.

Cartilage and bone have distinct anatomic and physiologic properties. Cartilage is found at the ends of long bones between bony articulations and is a tough connective tissue. It is an actively regenerating surface with a high elastin and collagen content, yet it is avascular. Nourishment to cartilage is from capillaries in the perichondrial covering. Mobile articular surfaces have no perichondrium because nourishment is derived from synovial fluid. Cartilage is not innervated and has no lymphatic circulation. (See Table 6-1 for the different types of cartilaginous connective tissues.) The growth site (epiphyseal line) in long bones is cartilaginous tissue that is invested with osteoblasts (precursor bone cells) and hardens into bone to generate length (endochondral bone formation). At maturity, the growth site hardens completely and stops growing in length. Flat bones are an exception to this process, not having a preliminary cartilage mass to remodel. They regenerate by directly producing osteoblasts in the periosteum and resorbing old bone in the marrow cavity (intramembranous bone formation).

Bone is a hard connective tissue. Compact bone is dense and smooth, whereas cancellous bone is softer and more latticelike. Structurally, bone is composed of minerals, such as calcium, phosphorus, potassium, copper, magnesium, sodium, and sulfur. The internal cavity contains marrow from which blood cells are derived (hematopoiesis). Long bones are compact with yellow, fatty marrow. They increase in length at cartilaginous epiphyseal lines. Flat bone and long bone ends are internally cancellous containing red marrow. Bone is covered with periosteum except at articulations and cartilaginous areas. Periosteum adheres to bony surfaces and conducts insertion points of vessels, nerves, and lymphatic vessels.

Bone strength and remodeling involve balanced stress points. Absence of weight bearing causes bone to demineralize. Donor bone serves as an organic space holder during healing. Osteoblasts cause demineralization leaving a trabecular network

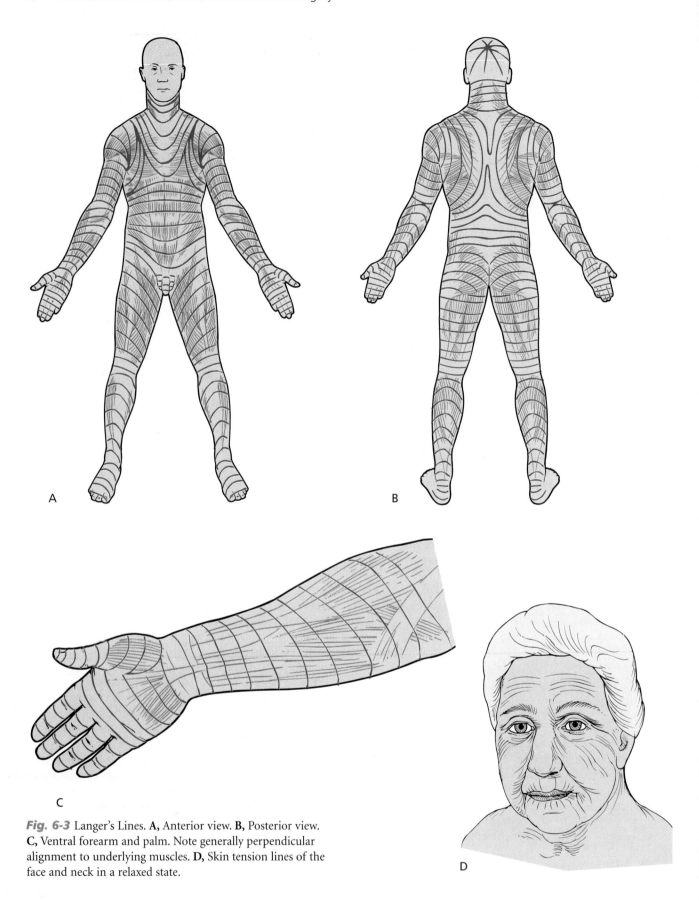

Fig. 6-3 Langer's Lines. **A,** Anterior view. **B,** Posterior view.
C, Ventral forearm and palm. Note generally perpendicular
alignment to underlying muscles. **D,** Skin tension lines of the
face and neck in a relaxed state.

for natural osteoblastic recalcification. Once the process is complete, the transplanted bone is indistinguishable from naturally occurring bone.

CONSIDERATIONS AND TECHNIQUES IN WOUND MANAGEMENT

Wound Healing Processes

Wound repair can only happen in the presence of intact circulation and living tissue. The inflammatory process is a natural body defense that involves autologous tissue and cellular changes activated in response to a stimulus. The purpose of inflammation is to protect and effect repair to damaged tissue and remove debris, such as dead cells or microorganisms. The severity of tissue injury will dictate the level of inflammatory response. Immunocompromised patients have decreased immune response because of altered white blood cell function.

Localized injuries that cause a separation of tissue layers stimulate moderate inflammation, which allows for healing. Burns or frank tissue destruction may interfere with inflammatory response because circulatory mechanisms have been damaged. Reparative cells cannot be delivered to the site of injury.

In comparison, generalized systemic assault, such as sepsis or anaphylaxis, generates a total body inflammatory response and is a potential life-threatening event. Cardinal signs of local and systemic inflammatory responses are described in Table 6-3.

Localized inflammatory response

During the first few hours after tissue is injured or a wound is created, a coagulum consisting of thrombus and a cellular exudate (polymorphonuclear leukocytes, lymphocytes, and macrophages) coats and fills the area (agglutination). The thrombus contains a network of fibrin that aids in hemostasis, epithelialization, and fibroblast migration. A solid cover is created by dehydration of the coagulum. The polymorphonuclear cells marginate and line the area. Within 2 days, macrophages predominate the wound. Capillary endothelial buds cannulate the area, increasing vascularization to the site. During this phase, the endothelium has a rapid replication period. The main localized inflammatory response remains in effect for approximately 5 days.

Epidermal wound resurfacing

Epidermal healing is activated before dermal healing. Within a few hours of tissue disruption, epidermal cells begin to migrate from the edges and line the walls of the wound (epithelialization) under the newly forming clot. It is not known if the

migrating cells are derived from undifferentiated epithelial cells, stem cells of the basal layer, or keratinocytes. Mitotic activity causes the migrating cells to increase in number within the first 24 to 48 hours as the epidermis thickens. Epithelialization in a well-approximated wound closed by primary intention can be completed in 24 hours.

Mechanisms of wound healing

Wound healing is directly related to whether the wound is closed and the timing and mechanism of the closure.

Primary intention. In primary intention, the epidermal edges are clean and are approximated by suture, staples, or adhesive devices (Fig. 6-4). Key components for closure by primary intention are (1) the quality of blood supply to the margins is sufficient and (2) no infection or contaminants are in the wound. Although these criteria are met, the strength of the healed wound depends on the deep dermal and subcutaneous tissues. Meticulous hemostasis supports adequate remodeling of deeper layers. A "golden time period" for closure by primary intention is affected by mechanism of injury, anatomic location, and potential for contamination. If wound edges look questionable after the prep, then an alternate closure method should be used. Some sources indicate that 6 to 8 hours is reasonably safe for closure of wounds on most body surfaces, such as arms, legs, and superficial chest or back. The hand or foot should be closed within 3 hours because of risk for contamination (Fig. 6-5). Closure of facial wounds may be delayed as long as 24 hours under clean circumstances.

Secondary intention. In secondary intention, the wound is not closed. Healing takes place from the base of the wound by the formation of granulation tissue if a good dermal base has been preserved. Collagen is deposited, and the wound naturally diminishes in size by significant degrees of contracture. The inflammatory exudate and blood dry to form a scab, creating a barrier to external infection. Dried scab and crusty material on the surface of a wound prevent epidermal migration across the injury, delaying reepithelialization. Wounds that are kept moist epithelialize faster because the new tissue remains soft and pliable. Skin grafting can be done later for a more aesthetic appearance. Concave surfaces can have a reasonable cosmetic result depending on the color match of the graft (Fig. 6-6).

Tertiary intention (delayed primary closure). In tertiary intention, the wound is debrided, irrigated, packed, and left open. Granulation tissue forms, and the wound edges are brought together 4 to 6 days after the injury. This is the method of choice for contaminated, traumatic wounds (Fig. 6-7).

Influences on Wound Healing

Age of patient

The condition of tissue is often age-related. Epidermal-dermal planes shift with age caused by decreased vascularity of aging. Decreased tensile strength allows tissue to tear and break down easily in response to suturing. The wound has low resistance to suture tension and should be reinforced with wound closure tape strips. Very young patients may heal much better because their tissues are healthier.

Table 6-3 **Cardinal Signs of Inflammatory Response**

LOCALIZED	SYSTEMIC
Redness	Flushed, erythema
Swelling	Generalized edema
Pain	Somatic pain
Sensation of heat	Fever
Altered function	Dizziness, weakness

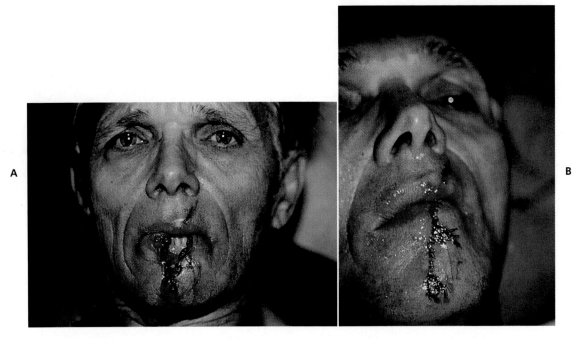

Fig. 6-4 Tramatic wound closure by primary intention **A,** Before. **B,** After. *(Courtesy Brian W. Davies, MD.)*

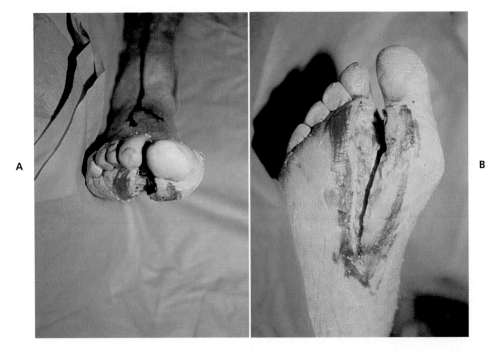

Fig. 6-5 Wounds of foot have a higher incidence of infection. Careful debridement and primary closure are performed within a few hours of injury. *(Courtesy Brian W. Davies, MD.)*

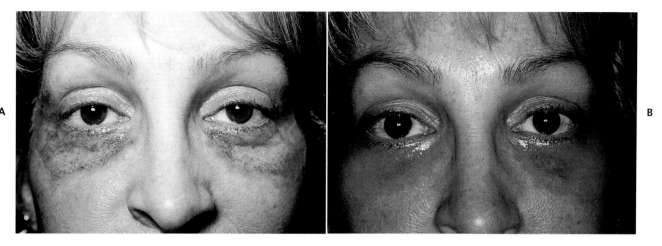

Fig. 6-6 Secondary intention after CO_2 laser resurfacing around female patient's eyes. *(Courtesy Brian W. Davies, MD.)*

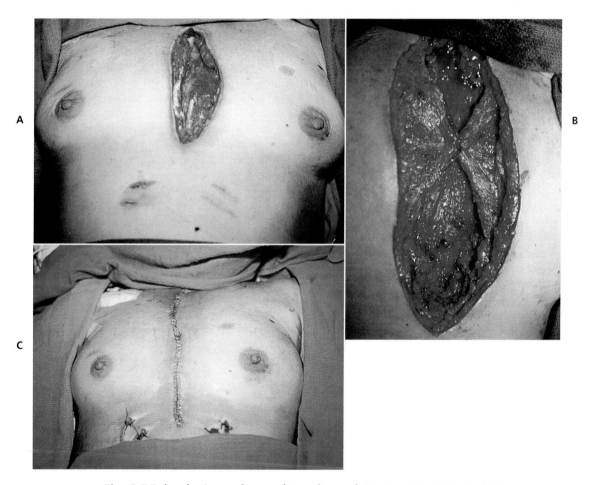

Fig. 6-7 Delayed primary closure of sternal wound. *(Courtesy Brian W. Davies, MD.)*

Condition of integument before injury

Healthy tissue has a better chance of optimal healing. Frail, damaged tissue is systemically impaired and takes longer to heal with less desirable results. Radiated tissue is an example.

General health

Physiology and psychologic state of being play a large role in wound healing. Lifestyle is a potential predictor of outcome. Potential for injury or exposure to harmful elements predispose the patient to poor wound healing. Studies have shown a connection between the mind and body. Depression can delay healing. A patient who is socioeconomically unable to afford proper supplies, nutrition, and health care is prone to an undesirable outcome. Cognitive impairment can predispose the patient to unintentional self-harm. Cultural or folk remedies may also cause harm. An underlying illness such as cancer can affect wound healing.

Nutritional status

Altered nutrition, either more than required or less than required, places the patient at high risk for poor wound healing. Alcoholics, even those who appear to be appropriate for height and weight, are usually nutritionally depleted. Adequate vitamin and mineral intake facilitates tissue repair and cellular level healing. Fluid balance is critical.

Mobility

Generalized inactivity predisposes the patient to alteration of all major organ systems, including the integument. Patients who remain bedfast become easily weakened and are at risk for reinjury caused by falls during syncopal episodes.

Wound condition

Origin, shape, depth, size, and location of the wound influence how well it heals. Oily or pigmented skin generates more scar tissue than fair skin. Hypertrophic scar tissue remains within the border of the wound. Keloid scar tissue extends beyond wound margins. Foreign body reaction can impair healing processes. Dead space or hematoma provides a breeding ground for microorganisms. Infection prevents tissue remodeling. The use of a drain may affect wound healing serving as a portal for infection.

Cardiopulmonary status

Oxygenation is dependent on heart and lung function. Prolonged periods of hypoxia, anemia, and/or peripheral vascular disease decrease the body's ability to perfuse tissue.

Endocrine status

Dysfunctions such as diabetes, adrenalopathy, and immunodeficiency alter the patterns of healing by interfering with cellular metabolism, catabolism, and anabolism.

Procedural considerations

The type of surgery performed; skin preparation; duration of procedure; tissue handling techniques; and hemostatic, closure, and dressing methods directly affect wound healing. Glove powder can cause starch granulomas. Dressings play a role in healing.

Chemical effects

Prolonged use of medications, such as steroids, anticoagulants, antibiotics, antiinflammatories, colchicine, and antineoplastics, alter the body's ability to use natural forces for healing. Corticosteroids, for example, inhibit collagen fiber synthesis and accelerate degradation of tissue. Neovascularization and epithelialization are delayed. The dermis thins, leaving the tissue less trauma resistant. Caffeine and nicotine alter circulatory status and can cause delayed healing.

Hemostasis

Prevention of blood loss, pooling, and accumulation in the wound provides an optimal environment for wound healing. Mechanical, chemical, and thermal methods of hemostasis are most frequently used.

Mechanical hemostasis. Direct pressure is the first-line hemostatic approach, such as with pressure dressings. Hemostats, ties, and clips are commonly used as well. Blind clamping of bleeding vessels is discouraged because nerves and tendons may be damaged. Bone wax provides pressure over bleeding bony surfaces, but excess can cause a foreign body reaction. Tourniquets over limbs and digits can provide a bloodless field. Tissue expanders can suppress bleeding from the inside out.

Chemical hemostasis *Gelatin sponges* can be applied dry or moistened in sterile saline with thrombin or epinephrine added. The sponge, if left in the wound, will liquefy in 2 to 5 days. When left in the wound, care is taken to avoid overpacking the area. The sponge can absorb many times its own weight and cause compression injury to surrounding vessels and nerves.

Thrombin solution directly clots the fibrinogen in blood. It is used for small bleeding and oozing points. Thrombin should not be permitted to enter open vessels.

Microfibrillar collagen initiates natural coagulation mechanisms and stimulates platelets to aggregate. Collagen is of bovine origin and available in sheet or fiber form. Excess fiber in the wound can cause adhesions.

Cellulose is impregnated into gauze or cotton. It is absorbed by the body in 2 to 7 days. It is not used with thrombin or left in the body near the spinal cord, nerves, or bone fractures.

Fibrin glue is useful for hemostasis of venous oozing. It is mixed and applied at the time of use.

Epinephrine is commonly mixed with local anesthetics to promote vasoconstriction. It is not used for procedures involving digits, ears, the tip of the nose, or the penis. Patients with peripheral vascular disease are at risk for tissue sloughing if vasoconstrictive agents are used.

Thermal hemostasis. Thermal hemostasis can be established by extreme heat or cold application to the area. Common methods of providing thermal heat hemostasis include electrocautery, photocoagulation with a laser, and an argon beam coagulator. Tissue-sparing application involves prevention of charring. Devitalized cells cannot repair themselves. Excess charred debris creates a media for infectious processes. Cold hemostasis is generated by cryoprobes and iced solutions.

Types of Wounds

A wound is an intentional or unintentional interruption of tissue integrity. Intentional wounds are made under controlled conditions in a deliberate pattern. The potential for contamination is kept at a minimum, and closure is selected according to the type of healing required for the wound integrity of the body part. Tissue regeneration is reasonably predictable, and scarring is within acceptable parameters. Strength of the healed wound permits a return to function after a prescribed period of time.

Wound Categories

Wounds are categorized according to anatomic site, origin, level of contamination, depth, tissue loss, and potential for repair. The anatomic site is important because location on the body influences the rate of healing and the risk for infection. Wounds on the face and neck have less potential for infection than a wound of the foot or hand (Fig. 6-8). Incisions in a nonmobile anatomic site heal with less disruption than wounds across a joint or a prominent body part. Flexible areas tend to have more scar contracture.

Wound origin can help predict the viability of tissue in situ for healing. Devitalized, avascular tissue does not perfuse and cannot heal. Cleanly incised edges may indicate a better blood supply for tissue repair. Trapped particulate matter, chemicals, dirt, and other foreign substances prevent wound healing. Deep wounds have dermal tissue loss and may extend into the superficial fascia, muscle, or bone.

Wounds are classified according to the potential for infection. The risk for infection increases while the wound is open to the environment. Additional infection risk factors include the presence of drains, contaminants, and known infectious process. Wounds are not classified until completely closed at the end of the procedure. The purpose of the classification system is to predict and possibly prevent potential infections. This cannot be known until all events surrounding wound manipulation are known, which is at the end of the procedure. Wound classification is described in Box 6-1.

Restoration of tissue continuity is important for optimal wound repair. Staples, sutures, tape strips, specialized dressings, and hemostatic agents and/or devices are used to approximate wound edges or bridge gaps left by tissue loss.

Surgical wounds

Surgical wounds are created under controlled circumstances, and if linear, they have clean edges. Approximation is easier and performed with little difficulty. Placement of the wound is selected by the surgeon according to the type of procedure, anatomic site, and need for visualization of the working environment. An incision can be placed according to skin tension lines for minimal scarring. Examples of surgically created wounds include incision, punctures for drains, occlusion banding, and chemical resurfacing.

Traumatic wounds

Traumatic wounds are unintentional, random interruptions in tissue integrity (Fig. 6-9). Tissue is at risk for devascularization, progressive injury involving other body systems, loss of function, and impaired neurovascular activity. Gunshot, stab, and slice wounds have little tissue damage other than the point of contact unless underlying structures are involved. Many can be closed by primary closure with low incidence of infection. Sometimes a small scar will result.

Box 6-1 **Wound Classification**

CLEAN WOUND (Potential Infection Rate: 1% to 5%)
Wound created under optimal sterile conditions
Primary closure, wound usually not drained; some closed systems are used
Sterile technique not breached during surgical procedure
No inflammation present
Natural body orifice not entered

CLEAN-CONTAMINATED WOUND (Potential Infection Rate: 8% to 11%)
Primary closure, wound drained
No inflammation or infection
Minor break in technique occurred
Natural body orifice entered under controlled conditions without spillage or microbiologic contamination (genitourinary, gastrointestinal, oropharyngeal, respiratory)

CONTAMINATED WOUND (Potiential Infection Rate: 15% to 20%)
Open fresh traumatic wound of less than 4 hours' duration
Acute, nonpurulent inflammation
Major break in technique occurred
Gross spillage and/or contamination from gastrointestinal tract
Genitourinary or biliary tracts with infected urine or bile

DIRTY AND INFECTED WOUND (Potential Infection Rate: 27% TO 40%)
Old traumatic wound of over 4 hours' duration from dirty source or with retained necrotic tissue, foreign body, or fecal contamination
Organisms present in surgical field before procedure
Existing clinical infection with or without purulence or incision to drain abscess
Perforated viscus

Tension wounds. Tension wounds are created by blunt, ripping forces. The edges are often ragged and uneven. The force causes a triangular tear that leaves devascularized tissue on at least two sides of the flap. The only blood supply comes from where the flap is still attached to the point of contact. Vascularity is preserved or the delicate flap will be lost. The tissue degrades quickly, and despite precision handling, a large scar results.

Triangular closure involves placing the initial suture at the apex of the flap and cautiously approximating and everting the edges. The knots are tied away from the devascularized side of the flap. Great care is exercised to avoid strangulating the tissue. The sequence of suture placement may make a difference. Using less suture and reinforcing tissue approximation with tape wound closure strips may prevent overhandling of delicate repairs. Tension wounds frequently happen over thin-skinned areas, such as the shin or bridge of the nose. Penile zipper injuries are tension wounds.

Compression wounds. Compression wounds include injuries caused by industrial machinery, motorcycle, or motor-vehicle accidents. The tissue is crushed and ripped, causing

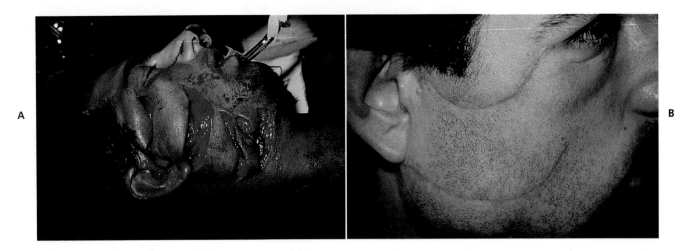

Fig. 6-8 **A,** This male patient encountered a boat propeller while swimming. **B,** Careful debridement and primary closure improve the chance for good results. *(Courtesy Brian W. Davies, MD.)*

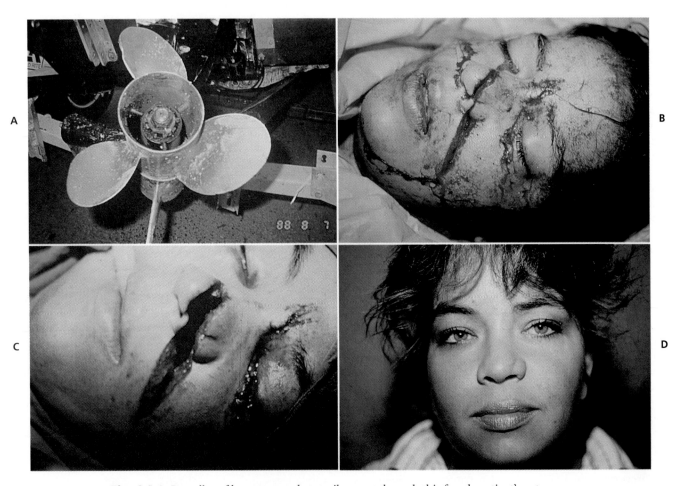

Fig. 6-9 **A,** Propeller of boat mounted on trailer went through this female patient's automobile windshield. **B-D,** Traumatic wound repair and progressive reconstruction produces good results. *(Courtesy Brian W. Davies, MD.)*

ragged surfaces down to the superficial fascia. Large portions of tissue are devascularized and deinnervated. Some may extend into bone and other organ systems. Debridement and irrigation under pressure may be needed to prepare the tissue for healing by secondary intention. The goal of treatment is to prepare the tissue for granulation from the wound base up.

Repair of compression wounds may need a multistage, multidisciplinary plan of care. Punch press or wringer-roller type injuries usually cause degloving of skin, crushed or fractured bone, neurovascular compromise, and other disfigurement.

Burn wounds. Burn wounds are classified by how deeply the tissue is affected. The full effect of the injury may not be realized until days later when devitalized tissue sloughs off. Secondary burn wounds can occur in response to exothermic reactions to plaster casting materials that have been applied with warm water.

Injection wounds. Injection wounds are caused by paint guns or other mechanized, pressurized devices. This type of wound is usually deep, with tissue necrosis appearing later as a secondary effect.

Puncture wounds. Animal or human bites leave an irregular surface defect. The potential for infection is high. Treatment will vary according to the type of bite and the anatomic site of injury. Animals with sharp, pointed teeth can perforate joint spaces and major vessels. Infants bitten around the head and face are at risk for cranial perforation through sutures and fontanels. Many deep punctures may not be irrigated. Large herbivores, such as cows and horses, cause serious crush-injury not conducive to debridement. Generally, the larger the defect, the less prone to infection. Small, deep punctures frequently become infected because of trapped microorganisms.

Incidental wounds

Incidental wounds are caused by pressure, such as decubitus ulcers over a bony prominence. Poor positioning can cause pressure in areas such as the posterior occiput, ear, heel, elbow, sacrum, and scapulae. These wounds are a form of compression wounds but have developed over a period of time. The primary force is devascularization that causes tissue sloughing. Wound healing is unpredictable and may require prolonged phases of treatment including skin grafts. Most incidental wounds cannot be closed by primary intention.

Complications of Wound Healing

Complications alter wound healing in some individuals. Types of common complications include the following:

Hemorrhage

Blood can pool forming a hematoma. Circulation is interrupted, which provides a breeding ground for infection (Fig. 6-10).

Infection

Abscess formation in solid tissue can tunnel through to other areas of the body. Patients with diabetes and malnutrition are at high risk.

Abnormal scar formation

Adhesions. Filmy bands of scar tissue form that bind organs together. Some can impair function of a part. Many require surgical release to restore function.

Keloid. Over-sized, darkened, gnarly scars that overextend the borders of the wound are common in dark-skinned individuals. These are commonly found on the ears, chest, extremities, and lower abdomen (Fig. 6-11). Treatments include corticosteroid injection, compressive dressings, surgical excision, and radiation therapy.

Hypertrophic scar. Spread scars are common over joints and stress points. They are sometimes confused with keloids because they are red. Hypertrophic scars do not extend over the border of the wound and often improve without intervention in time. Steroids can be used.

Contractures. Scars can form that decrease range of motion and function of a joint or body part. Other areas include tissues surrounding implants. Muscles and nerves shorten. Disuse atrophy can result.

Neuroma. Nerve endings can become encased in scar tissue. A painful mass is palpable.

Granuloma. A foreign body is encased in scar tissue.

Nonhealing wounds

Chronic friction and altered blood supply lead to nonhealing wounds referred to as ulcers. Debridement followed by delayed primary closure is usually the treatment of choice.

Mechanical wounds. Friction from clothing, dressings, casting material, or other irritant prevent healing by disrupting the granulation process.

Chemical wounds. Environmental wastes or acidic body secretions, such as pancreatic and gastric enzymes, cause lysis of tissue.

Stasis ulcers. Occluded venous circulation causes aseptic necrosis of tissue. The extremity may appear reddened and swollen, and it may feel warm to touch.

Ischemic ulcers. Occluded arterial circulation causes avascular necrosis and hypoxic tissue injury. The extremity may appear pale, grey, or bluish, and it feels cool to touch.

Disruptions of wounds

Hernia. Subsurface layers separate leaving the skin intact. A bulge is felt over the surface of the area. Organs may protrude into the bulge. It can be a previous surgical site.

Dehiscence. Superficial wound edges separate 5 to 8 days after the operation. This may signal an infectious process, and any exudate should be cultured.

Evisceration. Edges open to the deepest layer with internal organs visible or extruding through the wound.

Fistula. This is an abnormal tunnel or passage between two organs.

Sinus tract. This is an abnormal tunnel or passage leading from the inside to the external surface of the body

WOUND CLOSURE MATERIALS

The first sutures were probably made of linen. Historic writings dating back to 2000 BC refer to strings and animal tendons for ligating and suturing. *The Samhita,* an eastern Indian text written between 600 and 1000 BC by Sushruta, refers to horsehair, cotton, strips of leather, and fibers from tree bark used as wound closure material. Galen (130-200 AD) used twisted strands of animal gut or silk for primary closure of wounds. The term *catgut* is derived from the original term, *kitgut,* which was sheep intestines used in ancient Arabic fiddle strings. Surgical gut suture material is still made from sheep or beef intestine. Synthetic polymer sutures have modernized wound closure, but natural silk and surgical gut continue to be widely used.

Sutures

Sutures are placed in tissue using a sterile technique. Uniform tensile strength is the measurement of tension or pull that a strand of suture can withstand before it breaks when knotted. Tensile strength is proportionate to the diameter of the strand.

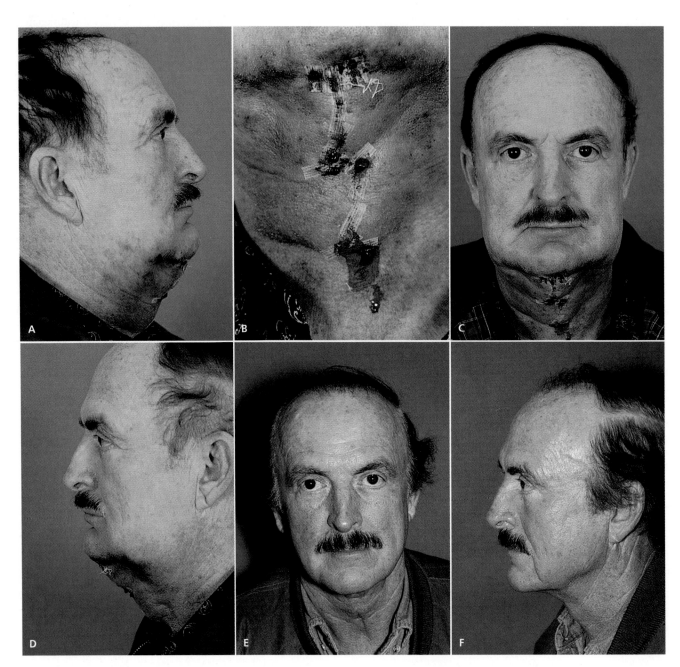

Fig. 6-10 **A and B,** Postoperative hematoma after excision of excess anterior neck skin. **C and D,** Postoperative healing of anterior neck hematoma. **E and F,** Remote postoperative wound healing of anterior neck hematoma. *(Courtesy Brian W. Davies, MD.)*

Smaller diameters of suture are less traumatic during suturing and leave less knotted bulk to promote tissue reaction. Suture sizes range from heavy 7 to very fine 11-0; ranges vary according to type of composition. Absorbable and nonabsorbable materials are used. Some are natural, and others are synthetic.

Absorbable sterile sutures are prepared from animal collagen tissue or from synthetic polymer. They are absorbed by the body but may be treated to delay or enhance the absorption rate. Nonabsorbable sterile sutures are fibers of natural or synthetic material that are not absorbed. The retained suture material becomes encapsulated, remaining in tissue for prolonged periods of time without causing a harmful reaction.

Monofilament and multifilament suture strands are commercially available. Monofilament suture is a single strand, and multifilament suture is made of multiple strands spun or braided together. The choice of which type and construction of suture material to use depends on the biologic effects of the material in the body, such as absorption potential or inertness. Wound size and location are considerations when favorable cosmetic results are desired. Infected or contaminated wounds can be the source of a fistula or a sinus formation along a suture tract, especially if braided suture is used. Coarse suture can cause a "rope-burn" friction effect as it passes through tissue. Monofilament suture is less traumatic.

Suturing techniques, such as continuous or interrupted stitches, are used according to tissue strength, suture type, condition of the wound, and cosmetic result desired. The key to wound closure is approximation, not strangulation of tissue edges. Strangulation inhibits blood flow causing devitalization of tissue. Knots are tied loosely so the edges are everted slightly but in approximation with each other (Fig. 6-12).

Needles

Eyed needles made of bone were used until the Renaissance. Straight and curved steel needles became popular in the 1800s. Progressively, surgeons have modified needle design throughout the centuries. Permanently attached needle-suture material (swaged-on) developed in 1928 simplified surgical wound closure technique.

The body of the needle is available in many gauges and sizes. Available degrees of curvature allow for many combinations of thickness, length, and angulation of the needle shaft. Configuration of the needle can range from straight to 5/8 circle curvature. The needle point is sharpened into specific configurations for specific types of tissue. Various tips include taper point, cutting edge, and blunt-tipped. Taper point atraumatic needles are conical without a cutting edge along its shaft. They enter tissue by pushing it aside. Cutting needles are sharpened into two or three opposing ridges along the distal portion of the shaft for ease of tissue penetration. They split through layers by slicing a small hole for passage of the suture.

Staples

Skin edges are everted with a tissue forceps, and a single staple is applied with each squeeze of the handgrip. Skin staples are removed 5 to 7 days after the operation. As the wound heals, the skin flattens out to form an even surface with an excellent cosmetic result.

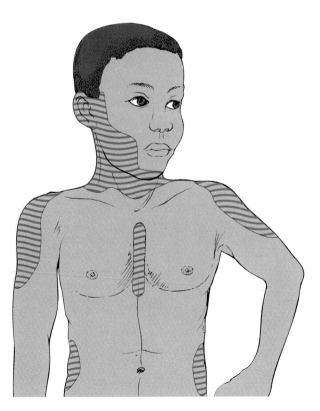

Fig. 6-11 Common keloid distribution.

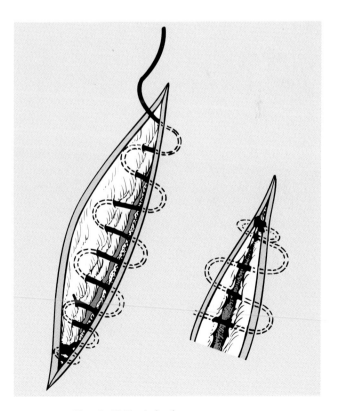

Fig. 6-12 Buried subcutaneous suture.

Wound Closure Tape Strips

Adhesive-backed strips of microporous nylon (Proxi-strip) or polypropylene (Steri-strip) or rayon acetate are placed at 1/8-inch intervals across the incision line. They are used for primary closure skin edges of superficial lacerations or in conjunction with skin sutures or staples to support the wound during healing. They are sometimes used as reinforcement after suture or staple removal.

Skin edges should be clean and dry or prepared with a tacky substance, such as tincture of benzoin. A forcep should be used to apply the strip because tissue adherent to gloved fingers may render the adhesive strip nonadherent.

Wound Dressing

Studies have shown that a moist environment promotes epithelial migration. Dressings serve as a temporary cover in a functional capacity. Important aspects of dressings include achieving hemostasis, creating appropriate pressure to prevent edema, absorption of excess fluids, and support for healing structure. Other dressing considerations are provision of moist physiologic environment, prevention of contamination, and ease of removal. Dressing modalities differ according to the type of procedure and surgeon preference. See Table 6-4 for an overview of wound care materials.

Table 6-4 **Wound Care Materials**

Dressing Material	Composition and Properties	Indications for Use	Advantages	Disadvantages	Notes
Alginate	Originates from brown seaweed; highly absorbent; becomes a gel when exposed to exudate creating a moist environment	Used for infected and noninfected wounds with moderate to heavy drainage; some are used for tunneling wounds	Can absorb 20 times its own weight in fluid; rehydrates wound and facilitates debridement; requires secondary dressing cover	Contraindicated for use with light exudate or dry eschar; can promote bacterial growth if used with occlusive dressing cover; not used with third-degree burns	Packaged as ropelike fibers or pad; do not use with alkaline solutions; packaged sterile; remains in place 2 to 4 days
Composite	Composed of two or more moisture-enhancing materials in combination with absorbent material	Used for partial or full-thickness wounds with moderate to heavy exudate; can also be used over fresh granulation or necrotic tissue	Facilitates debridement and allows for moisture/vapor exchange; safe for use over healthy or infected tissue; easy to apply and remove	Should be placed in area with border of healthy intact tissue for anchoring; should not be used for light exudate; may cause excess moisture loss; can become very adherent	Check manufacturer's recommendations about use with adjunct topical medications
Exudate absorber	Added to wound surface to eliminate dead space and absorb exudate; minimizes odors	Used for full-thickness wounds with moderate to heavy exudate; can be used with necrotic wounds; some can be used as lining material before packing and surface dressing	Can absorb five times its own weight in fluid; rehydrates wound and facilitates debridement; requires secondary dressing cover	Contraindicated for use with light exudate or dry eschar	Supplied in bottles or packets; clean wound and irrigate before use; fill the wound cavity to eliminate dead space and line the defect
Foam	Semipermeable, either hydrophilic or hydrophobic	Creates a moist environment and affords thermal insulation	Nonadherent; repels contaminants and is easy to apply and remove; absorbs light to moderate exudate; can be used with compression dressings; requires secondary dressing cover	Not used for dry wounds; can cause maceration of adjacent skin	Some erythema or itching may occur during the first 24-hours; not used with occlusive dressings; change more frequently if exudate is heavy

Table 6-4 **Wound Care Materials—cont'd**

Dressing Material	Composition and Properties	Indications for Use	Advantages	Disadvantages	Notes
Gauze	Composed of woven or nonwoven materials; can be impregnated; used as primary or secondary dressing; can be natural or synthetic material; nonocclusive	Used for wound protection, wicking, and absorption; can be used wet or dry; packaged in rolls, pads, or strips	Moderately absorbent; less expensive to use and can be used in combination with other material; can be used as packing	Need to be changed frequently; can leak or strike through; can dry out causing injury to healing tissue	If applied wet and allowed to dry, gauze can be used as debridement agent; may be saturated with oils, iodophor, bismuth, petroleum jelly, scarlet red
Hydrocolloid	Occlusive, adhesive wafer; the contact layer may differ in composition; creates a moist environment; supplied in packets, tubes (paste), oral discs, and wafer; can be cut to fit	Clean wounds will granulate and necrotic wounds will debride autolytically	Impermeable to contaminants; self-adhesive and can remain in place for 3 to 5 days without tissue damage; slight to moderate absorption	Not used with heavy exudate, sinus tracts, or infection; not intended for full-thickness wounds exposing bone; unable to visualize the wound; occlusive properties inhibit air-exchange; can injure fragile tissue at wound edges	Safe to use under compression devices and wraps; can be used at ostomy sites or areas affected by incontinence
Hydrogel	Water or glycerin-based gel, gauze, or sheet dressing that has high moisture content; supplied in tubes, packets, spray, liquid	Used for partial and full-thickness wounds; good for burns, necrosis, and radiated tissue	Very soothing; can rehydrate dried tissues; used to fill dead space and facilitate debridement	Not used for absorption of exudate because of inherent moisture content; can dry out easily; not a bacterial barrier; may be difficult to secure to wound	Keep covered after application to prevent evaporation of the gel
Transparent film	Adhesive, semi-permeable membrane; bacterial and water barrier; permeable to oxygen	Waterproof, but permeable to air and moisture vapors; bacterial barrier	Promotes a moist environment for new granulation and autolysis of necrotic tissue	Not used for infected wounds; periphery of wound needs to be intact to apply the film; may be hard to apply	Used for superficial and partial-thickness wounds with minimal exudate
Skin sealant	Barrier film applied in liquid form that dries to form a plasticlike barrier coating; supplied in liquid form and individual wipettes	Used on intact skin surrounding a wound, ostomy site, or over a surgical incision closed by primary intention	Waterproof barrier	Can sting raw skin when applied; has alcohol base to cause drying by evaporation	Some have vapors may be harmful to inhale as product evaporates

Bibliography

American Society of Plastic and Reconstructive Surgical Nurses: *Core curriculum for plastic and reconstructive surgery,* ed 2, Pitman, New Jersey, 1996, ASPRSN.

Atkinson LJ, Fortunato NM: *Berry and Kohni's operating room technique,* ed 8, St Louis, 1996, Mosby.

Bennett RG: *Fundamentals of cutaneous surgery,* St Louis, 1988, Mosby.

Cawson RA, et al: *Pathology: the mechanism of disease,* ed 2, St Louis, 1989, Mosby.

McCance KL, Huether SE: *Pathophysiology: the biologic basis for disease in adults and children,* ed 2, St Louis, 1994, Mosby.

Monacada GA: The healing wound: clinical management, *Plast Surg Nurs* 12(2):56, 1992.

Osak MP: Nutrition and wound healing, *Plast Surg Nurs* 13(1):29, 1993.

Rook A et al: *Textbook of dermatology,* ed 4, Oxford, England, 1988, Blackwell Scientific.

Rothrock JC: *The RN first assistant: an expanded perioperative role,* ed 2, Philadelphia, 1993, JB Lippincott.

Trott A: *Wounds and lacerations: emergency care and closure,* St Louis, 1991, Mosby.

Wound closure manual, Somerville, NJ, 1994, Ethicon.

7 Surface Modifications

Patient concerns about outward appearance are frequently treatable with surface modification. The epidermis and dermis can be peeled, excised, sanded, bleached, and/or tinted. The results can be dramatic, despite the simplicity involved with the change. More complex procedures involving external tissue transfers can improve function as well as form.

CHEMEXFOLIATION (CHEMICAL PEELS)

Chemical peels are topical agents used to minimize or remove superficial skin irregularities, such as acne scars, fine wrinkles, and hyperpigmentation (Box 7-1). Tissues are destroyed by the chemexfoliant causing new tissue to regenerate. The best results are attained in fair-skinned individuals with minimal sun damage and shallow surface scars.

Patients at risk for perioral herpetic lesions should be treated prophylactically with acyclovir 400 to 1000 mg po for 24 hours before the operation, continuing treatment for at least 2 to 10 days after the operation. Dosage and duration are individualized per patient need. This treatment is also used with other resurfacing procedures, including laser, that may involve the vermilion border. Herpetic outbreaks are painful and can take several weeks to completely heal. The lesions can extend the full length of the resurfaced area (see Fig. 5-7).

Additional preoperative preparation for chemexfoliation may include use of bleaching cream or gel. The patient will be instructed to avoid sun exposure, electrolysis, depilatories, waxing, abrasive cleansing, and Retin-A. On the day of a chemical peel, males are instructed to avoid shaving.

Preoperative skin preparation is performed by washing the surface with antimicrobial soap and rinsing with clear water. Skin oil and grease are removed with alcohol or acetone. Ether can be used to augment the depth of a trichloroacetic acid (TCA) peel.

Dermal collagen and elastic tissue increase after a peel. Connective tissue can increase 0.2 to 0.3 millimeters in the subepidermal layer. Melanin decreases in the epidermis. Full-face chemexfoliation should not be performed within 3 months of full raised-flap rhytidectomy. Injury to the flap may result.

Retin-A

Tretinoin cream (Retin-A) is a vitamin A derivative used to stimulate collagen synthesis at the cellular level. It is indicated for use in fine wrinkles and irregular pigmentation of the face over a period of several months. It is commonly used as a pretreatment for dermabrasion and other types of chemical peels. Tretinoin has skin-lightening properties.

Trichloroacetic Acid

TCA is not systemically absorbed and has little or no effect on any major organ system. It is considered safe for use in the presence of liver or cardiac disease. TCA is indicated for use in deeper wrinkles, scarring from acne, and sun-damaged areas. Preoperative skin treatments include bleaches, retinoids, and/or alpha hydroxy acid (AHA). Supplemental estrogen is withheld for several weeks before the operation to help minimize the potential for postoperative hyperpigmentation.

TCA solution is applied in concentrations of 20% to 50% strength proportional to the depth of desired chemexfoliation. The skin will look frosted within 10 to 20 seconds after application. Pinker tones indicate lighter peel, whereas whiter frost indicates a deeper peel. Areas other than the face require lower concentrations to avoid scarring. When using topical anesthetic gel consisting of lidocaine 2.5% and prilocaine 3.5%, the concentration of TCA should not exceed 30% because the anesthetic gel enhances the depth of the peel.

The preparation is removed between 1 and 5 minutes after application. The skin can be rinsed with water. The dermal serum neutralizes the solution. The skin will appear red, and the patient will feel a burning sensation. Soothing ice packs provide comfort and decrease edema. TCA applications may be repeated

TRETINOIN CREAM

(Retin-A: 0.05% to 0.1% concentration)
Works at the cellular level to produce new collagen.
Results are apparent if used longer than 6 months. May be
used as pretreatment for dermabrasion or laser resurfacing. Is sometimes used in combination with hydroquinone.
Can cause dryness, photosensitivity, and skin sensitivity. No
anesthesia is used.

ALPHA HYDROXY ACID (AHA)

mini peel: 30% to 75% solution)
Natural acid found in foods. Used weekly for 2 to 6
months, then every two to three treatments twice per year.
Continued application by patient at home of 5% to 10%
cream twice per day after initial treatment. No anesthesia
is used.

TRICHLOROACETIC ACID (TCA)

(20% to 50% solution)
Should be used with caution in darker-skinned patients.
Preoperative skin preparation with Retin-A 0.05% or AHA
is performed by the patient for 2 weeks before initial peel.
Topical bleaching agent may be included. Face may appear
ruddy as a result. No anesthesia is used.

PHENOL (CARBOLIC ACID)

(Baker-Gordon solution: 3 ml 88% phenol, 2 ml H_2O, 8
gtts liquid soap, 3 gtts croton oil)
Skin appears white after application. Layered strips of fabric,
tape, or paper can be applied over the chemexfoliant for 24
to 48 hours to deepen the results. When the tape is
removed, the skin is dusted with antimicrobial thymol to
encourage crusting. Intravenous conscious sedation and
physiologic monitoring by anesthesia provider is performed.

several times over a period of several months to attain the desired
effect. After the operation, sun exposure must be avoided. Crusts
will form over the peeled area and these must remain undisturbed
by picking or excess facial movement. Facial cleansing with a mild
cleanser followed by hydrocortisone cream is recommended for
the best results. Bacterial infection may occur for which systemic
antibiotics are prescribed. Hypertrophic scars may require an
intralesional injection of steroids and compression.

Alpha Hydroxy Acid

AHA is derived from fruit, milk, and sugar acids. Stronger concentrations used by physicians to rejuvenate skin act by epider-
molysis and detachment of keratocytes. Lesser concentrations
used by consumers in facial rinses, makeup bases, and moisturiz-
ers act by preventing corneocyte cohesion and stratum corneum
thickening. AHA does not have the side effects associated with
other peel products. Some individuals experience some redness
and minimal stinging. The best results are attained by fair-
skinned patients with minimal rhytid formation. Darker-skinned
patients may experience hyperpigmentation and streaking.

AHA is applied starting at the forehead and working down
the face in sections. The solution is left in place for 2 to 3 minutes. The concentration and duration of application are determined by the surgeon in response to the desired effect. The
skin appears erythematous in response to the peel. Subsequent
peels may be left in place for up to 6 minutes. Petroleum jelly is
applied around areas such as the eyes, nares, and lip edges to
prevent accumulation. After the timed period is completed, the
AHA is sponged off using a 1% sodium bicarbonate solution.
Cool water is used to complete the rinse, and the face is patted
dry. Hydrocortisone 0.5% cream is used to minimize swelling.
Postoperative instructions include continued avoidance of sun
exposure and irritants. Gentle cleansing twice per day and
moisturization with a non-AHA product are recommended.

Phenol

Phenol is used for chemexfoliation of moderate to severe sun
damage. Hyperpigmentation is permanently lightened, therefore darker-skinned individuals are not good candidates for
phenol use. Areas peeled by phenol will appear whiter and shiny
after healing is complete.

The average penetration through the epidermis and the dermis
is 0.3 to 0.6 mm. The depth of chemexfoliation is greater with
lower concentrations of phenol. High concentrations coagulate
protein, blocking the depth of penetration. Phenol is absorbed
systemically, detoxified by the liver, and excreted in the urine.

The patient will be heavily sedated and should be monitored
during the procedure for cardiac (especially atrial) dysrhythmia. Full face peels may precipitate a cardiac event. The phenol
peel limited to small areas over increments of 15 to 20 minutes
may reduce the risk of cardiac problems. The face is divided
into six segments for application to minimize the amount of
chemical absorption (Fig. 7-1, *A and B*). The total application
process may take more than one hour. The skin surface will
frost over very quickly. The patient will sense an intense burning sensation. Occlusive skin surface taping after full face phenol peels can enhance the depth of penetration (Fig. 7-1, *C and
D*). Petroleum jelly or A&D ointment can be applied as a mask
over the face instead of taping.

The skin is rinsed with tap water after removal of the mask
(Fig. 7-1, *E*). A&D ointment is applied daily after mild cleansing
until reepithelialization is complete. The pigmented layer will be
permanently changed. Sunscreen is required because the patient
will have no pigment-mediated sun protection in peeled areas.

Nursing Care of the Patient During
a Chemical Peel

Chemical peels are administered by the physician with caution.
Routine peels are usually uncomplicated, but it is advisable to
monitor the patient for changes in vital signs or cardiac rhythm.
Monitoring should be done by an anesthesia provider or a qualified perioperative registered nurse

Before administering a peel, the skin is washed with soap and
water followed by a degreasing agent. Cotton-tipped applicators
or soft brushes are used to swab on the solution. Application to the
face should extend into the hair and vermilion lines to avoid
streaks and demarcation patterns. Care is taken to not allow the
solution to enter the eyes or ears. Severe damage may result.

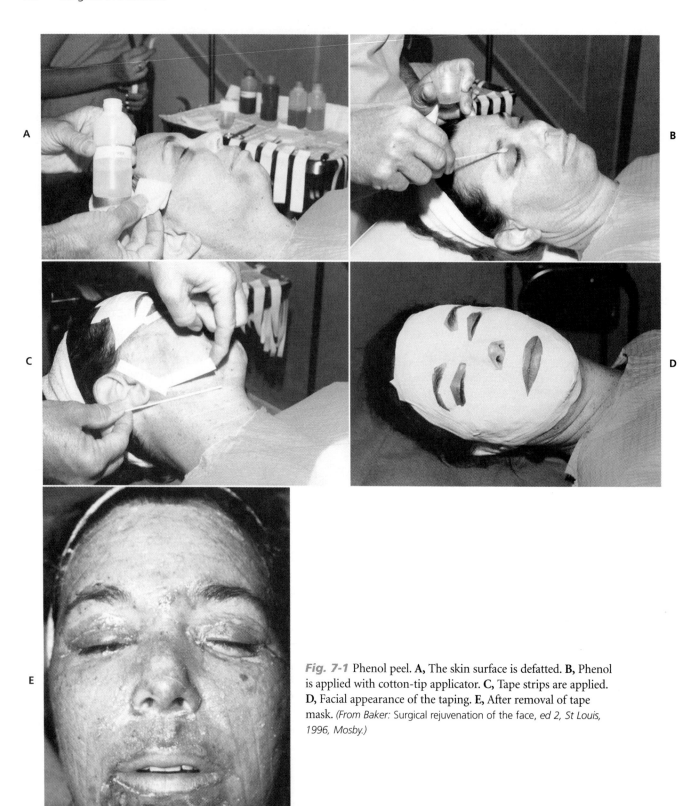

Fig. 7-1 Phenol peel. **A,** The skin surface is defatted. **B,** Phenol is applied with cotton-tip applicator. **C,** Tape strips are applied. **D,** Facial appearance of the taping. **E,** After removal of tape mask. *(From Baker:* Surgical rejuvenation of the face, *ed 2, St Louis, 1996, Mosby.)*

The patient may feel stinging and burning for 24 hours after the procedure. The skin appears to have a second-degree burn when the tape is removed. The skin will be edematous and will develop a crusty surface. Cleansing with water is gently done followed by application of a soothing ointment. As the crusts fall away over a period of 2 to 3 weeks, the skin will look reddened. This will last approximately 10 to 12 weeks. The patient should be cautioned about sun exposure for at least 6 months. Sunscreen with sun protection factor (SPF) 15 or higher is very important. The sun can cause hyperpigmentation (Boxes 7-2 and 7-3).

DERMABRASION

Scarring caused by acne vulgaris or other conditions such as rhytids cause the skin surface to appear gnarled and uneven. Skin surfaces with roughened terrain appear coarse and unaesthetic. A dermabrader is a hand-held device used to mechanically even the layers of dermal tissue (Fig. 7-2).

Nursing Care of the Patient During Dermabrasion

The patient is placed under general anesthesia or administered local anesthesia with intravenous conscious sedation (IVCS). The skin is thoroughly cleansed of oils and dirt. Topical ethyl chloride may be applied to freeze the skin into a firm working surface. Other methods include tumescent injections in the face consisting of sterile normal saline with lidocaine, bicarbonate, and epinephrine added. Topical application of eutectic mixture of local anesthetics (EMLA), which is a local anesthetic cream, enhances pain relief. The tumescence provides a firm working surface without the use of cholorofluorocarbons. Use of a wire brush instead of a mechanized dermabrader decreases the amount of aerosol.

Mechanical smoothing of the firmed surface is performed with wire brushes, abrasive discs, diamond bur, and other "sanding" appliances. During the procedure, the field becomes very bloody and aerosol-laden. The surgical team should wear personal protective attire, such as eyewear and side shields. A full face shield is advised. Larger contours can be shaved down with a scalpel before proceeding with the dermabrasion process. Pin-point burs can be used for small discolored areas, such as traumatic tattoos.

The surface is denuded leaving a raw weeping wound that heals smoothly. The newly healed area will appear pinker and will heal lighter than the surrounding tissue. Pores may appear more prominent. Wound care is similar to the healing of a graft donor site. The wound is allowed to heal by secondary intention over a period of several weeks.

PHOTOTHERMOLYSIS (LASER RESURFACING)

Photothermolysis can be performed for fine lines and wrinkles, pigmented areas, sun-damaged skin, and shallow scars. Tattoo removal is discussed later in this chapter. Preoperative skin preparation begins 3 to 6 weeks before the procedure. Topical application of Retin-A, bleaches, alpha hydroxy acids, or dexamethasone cream conditions the skin for treatment, reducing actinically injured cells and suppressing melanocytes. Patients

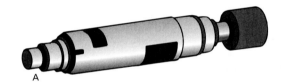

A

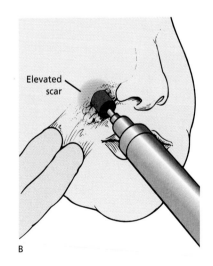

Elevated scar

B

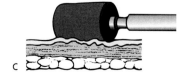

C

Fig. 7-2 Dermabrasion.

Box 7-2 **Contraindications of a Chemical Peel**

Severe sun damage
Radiated tissue
Active personal herpes simplex I
Scleroderma
Dark skin tones
Asian skin
Oily skin

Box 7-3 **Complications of a Chemical Peel**

Full-thickness skin loss
Hypertrophic scarring
Infection
Irregular skin tones
Persistent redness of skin
Milia
Pruritis

with a history of perioral herpetic outbreaks are pretreated with acyclovir or a comparable antiviral agent. This regimen continues for several days after the operation (Box 7-4).

Laser procedures can be performed using local, regional, or general anesthesia. Topical anesthesia, such as 2.5% lidocaine and 2.5% prilocaine cream (EMLA), is not highly effective. Vasoconstrictors added to the local anesthetic agent can diminish the absorption of laser light. Many types of laser are used, but argon, carbon dioxide (CO_2), and Candella lasers (tunable dye) are most commonly used (Table 7-1). Laser variations include Q-switching and pulsed applications. Patient selection ensures success of the procedure.

The argon laser is useful for vascular lesions, port-wine stains, and strawberry hemangiomas. Some tattoos can be revised or removed by this method. Most treated lesions will lighten between 50% to 80%.

Box 7-4 Contraindications for Laser Resurfacing of Skin

Active perioral herpetic lesions
Accutane therapy 6 to 12 months before the operation
Unbleached, dark skin
Scleroderma
Radiation therapy

Table 7-1 **Examples of Lasers Used for Skin Surface Modifications**

Type of Laser	Spectrum of Light	Notes
Argon	Blue-green	Used for treatment of superficial vascular lesions, pigmented areas and some inflammatory lesions; absorbed by hemoglobin
CO_2	Infrared	Has a red aiming beam to make the invisible infrared laser visible; absorbed by water
Tunable dye (Candela)	Yellow	Used to treat port-wine stains and vascular ectasis; very selective vascular destruction; absorbed by pigmented tissues
KTP:YAG	Green	Used to treat tattoos, vascular lesions, and pigmented lesions; good for removal of black, yellow, or blue colors; works well for dark-skinned patients; articulated arm
Alexandrite	Red	Used to treat tattoos, particularly blue, black, and green; not good for orange or yellow; fiberoptic: flexible arm

KTP:YAG: Potassium titanyl phosphate:yttrium aluminum garnet.

The pulsed CO_2 laser is delivered by an articulated arm and is delivered through a handpiece. It is a precise cutting tool for debulking lesions and as a dermal layer (Fig. 7-3). The CO_2 laser also can be used with a microscope. Each light pass with the CO_2 laser removes a surface layer of approximately 100 microns. The CO_2 laser is absorbed by water. The field remains bloodless and combines positive results of both chemexfoliation and dermabrasion (Fig. 7-4). The skin surface landmarks are visible, and the level of tissue can be determined easily. Deep rhytids may be retreated 2 or 3 months after the operation. Milia and pruritis are not uncommon after the procedure.

The Candela laser is highly selective in vascular destruction and minimizes associated scarring and epidermal texture changes. The active media is yttrium aluminum garnet (YAG), alexandrite, argon, or krypton. The Candela Company has developed a skin-cooling device that minimizes the thermal effect of the laser without decreasing the effectiveness of the laser. Use of this device increases the amount of possible laser power used and may reduce the number of treatments needed to effectively remove a skin defect by 30%.

Nursing Care of the Patient During Laser Resurfacing Procedures

The areas to be resurfaced are marked with a skin marker. As the laser light is passed over the skin, the lased tissue is wiped away with a moist sponge. Areas of thicker collagen will be lased several times. Yellowing of the tissue indicates denaturation of protein.

After treatment, cool packs are applied to decrease swelling. The wounds are cleansed with vinegar solution (1 teaspoon vinegar:1 pint water), and bacitracin without zinc, petroleum jelly, or Preparation H is applied to encourage epithelialization and prevent infection (Fig. 7-5). Dressing materials, such as occlusive semipermeable saturated mesh gauze, may be used. Healing usually takes place in 2 weeks with resultant erythema clearing over an additional 6 months.

Laser safety

Appropriate eye protection of the correct optical density is necessary for all personnel, including the patient, during laser therapy. Corneal eye shields may be used for additional patient protection. The color of the lens of the glasses or goggles is not an indicator of protection. Each type of laser has different precautions and safety requirements (Fig. 7-6). Failure to provide safe conditions may cause irreversible damage to nontargeted tissues, including the skin and eyes. Drapes and some endotracheal tubes may be an ignition source if exposed to laser light. Fire-prevention protocol and emergency procedures should be established by each facility. Warning signs and proper protective eyewear are placed outside the OR door during laser use in case additional personnel must enter the room during the procedure.

Only appropriately trained and credentialed individuals should be allowed to work with or operate lasers. Laser plume (smoke) may carry mutagenic viral material and is hazardous. A smoke evacuation system is recommended because plume is moist and can accumulate in regular suction apparatus.

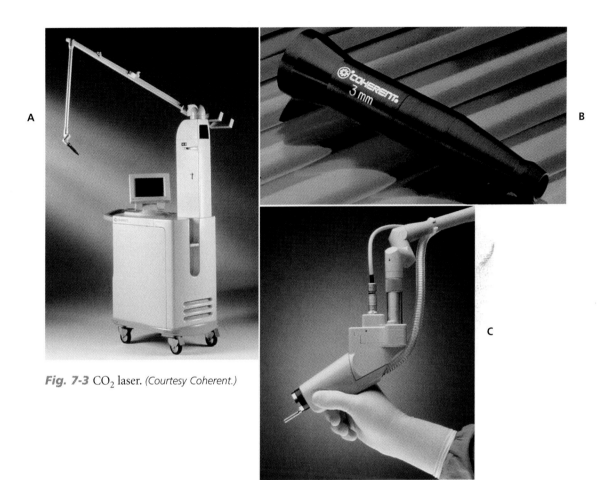

Fig. 7-3 CO_2 laser. *(Courtesy Coherent.)*

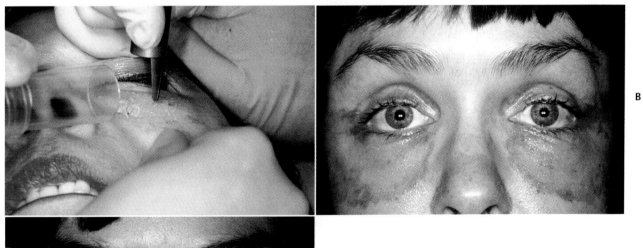

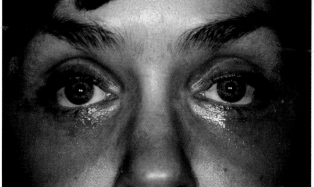

Fig. 7-4 CO_2 laser resurfacing around female patient's eyes. **A,** Intraoperative. **B,** Two days postoperative. **C,** One week postoperative. *(Courtesy Brian W. Davies, MD.)*

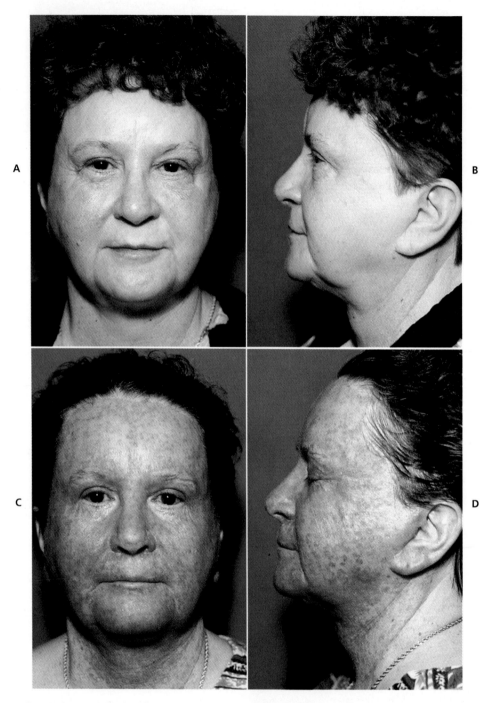

Fig. 7-5 Laser resurfacing of face. **A and B,** Preoperative skin condition. **C and D,** If postoperative skin care regimen is not followed, postoperative candida infections can result. *(Courtesy Brian W. Davies, MD.)*

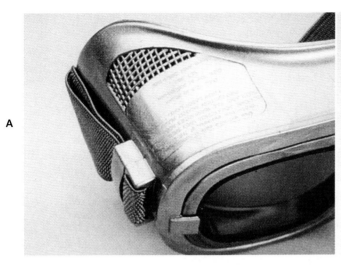 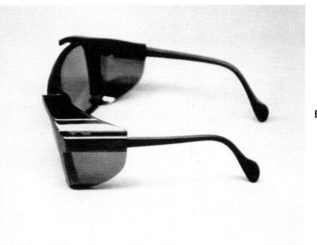

Fig. 7-6 Goggles (**A**) or glasses (**B**) with side shields of the appropriate optical density are worn by personnel working in the presence of lasers. *(From Ball:* Endoscopic surgery, *St Louis, 1997, Mosby.)*

OTHER AESTHETIC SKIN MODIFICATIONS

Resurfacing also includes lightening, tinting, and restoration after treatment of pathologic conditions such as hypertrophic scars or excisional biopsies.

Bleaches

Phenolic preparations and nonphenolic derivatives are skin-lightening agents. Phenolic compounds include hydroquinone and hydroquinone-combination preparations. Nonphenolics include tretinoin and azelaic acid.

Hydroquinone 4%, a phenolic preparation in a moisturizing cream for dry skin or a gel for oily skin, is a bleaching agent used once or twice per day to lighten epidermal hyperpigmentation and irregular skin tones. Commercial preparations may also contain glycolic acid for exfoliation, SPF 19 sunscreen, and/or sunblock. Tinted formulas are available to blend into skin tones. Formulations without sun protection are used at night when sun exposure is not a risk. Separate sunblock may be applied if used during the day. Skin patch testing should be done to assess sensitivity to the product. Slight redness is not abnormal, but frank edema, vesicles, and widespread inflammatory response are considered a sensitivity or allergic reaction. Safety during pregnancy and breast feeding has not been established. Skin absorption studies have not been performed. Only small areas are treated at a time.

Skin bleach is frequently used for 2 weeks preoperatively to prepare the skin for dermabrasion or laser resurfacing. Sometimes it is used if the physician determines that the patient may develop postoperative hyperpigmentation. Kojic acid is also used for the same treatment if hydroquinone is irritating to the skin. Retin-A (tretinoin) is sometimes used in combination as a lightener.

Generalized skin lightening for conditions such as cholasma, freckles, melasma, or age spots can be accomplished with skin bleach. The bleaching process is stopped if the area treated shows no response to treatment after 2 months. When the desired level of lightening is attained, avoidance of sun exposure is critical. The sun stimulates melanotic activity, nullifying the effects of the bleaching agent. Sunblocks and screens should be applied before any sunlight exposure and should be continued indefinitely.

DERMAPIGMENTATION (TATTOOING)

Dermapigmentation, also known as tattooing, can be intentionally permanent (professional or amateur) or accidental (traumatic). Intentional permanent tattoos are commonly created as symbols of personal identity, for decoration, or for cosmetic or restorative purposes.

Professional, Permanent Tattoos

Under local or topical anesthesia, professionally applied tattoos in a medical environment are injected very evenly at the same level of tissue by penetrating needles. Most of the application devices are mechanized with preset depth guides to 3 mm for most tissue and 1.5 mm for eyelids. The pigment is deposited in the superficial dermal and papillary layers by angled and straight needles. Eyelid injection is angled between the lash follicles and does not penetrate the tarsal plate or muscular layers. Care is taken to avoid damaging the lash follicle or permanent lash loss may occur.

The colors can be very deep and bright or subtle. The pigment is composed of carbon, copper, iron, cobalt, chromium, and titanium. Personnel who apply this pigmentation should be aware that extreme amounts of these metallic pigments may cause artifacts that interfere with some nuclear scans, such as computerized tomography (CT) scans and magnetic resonance imaging (MRI). Medical-grade tattoo pigments are commercially prepared and sterilized in a suspension of water and glycerin in an alcohol base. The alcohol evaporates during the sterilization process.

Professional tattoos applied in a medical environment are used to cosmetically enhance lip lines, eyebrows, and eyelash lines. Other purposes include restoration of the nipple/areola complex and camouflage of irregularly pigmented tissues and scars (Fig. 7-7).

Nonmedical Tattoos

No regulatory mechanism is in place to control the source or compilation of tattoo pigments found in other tattooing environments, such as tattoo parlors. Many artists who perform decorative tattooing are highly trained and talented. They commonly use commercially prepared pigments and equipment. Some use customized blends. Many are aware of the importance of sterility and the risks associated with bloodborne disease. The use of mechanized equipment allows the pigment to be deposited evenly in the dermis in a manner similar to medical-grade application.

Amateur tattoos are not as complex. They are commonly injected by the bearer at varying layers of tissue using varying types of available pigment, usually an ink. The application is not performed uniformly or under sterile conditions and may

tend to fade as the person's body ages. These are usually found in young people who have impulsively administered the mark as a sign of affiliation with a group or gang. Sometimes they are applied as a sign of affection for another individual. As the bearer matures, the primary affiliation may change, causing the person to seek removal. Fortunately, amateur tattoos are usually less difficult to remove than professionally applied tattoos.

Tattoos applied during World War II in concentration camps were applied in a similar manner to amateur styles. The single-hued pigmentation was placed in varying layers and can be removed by conventional methods. Many individuals bearing the tattoos of the holocaust decline removal in remembrance. Sensitivity to this preference and rationale is important.

Traumatic tattoos occur through industrial injection machines, motorcycle and bicycle injury, explosions, and other chemically mediated skin accidents. The pigmentation is usually deep, often beyond the first layer of dermis. Careful removal

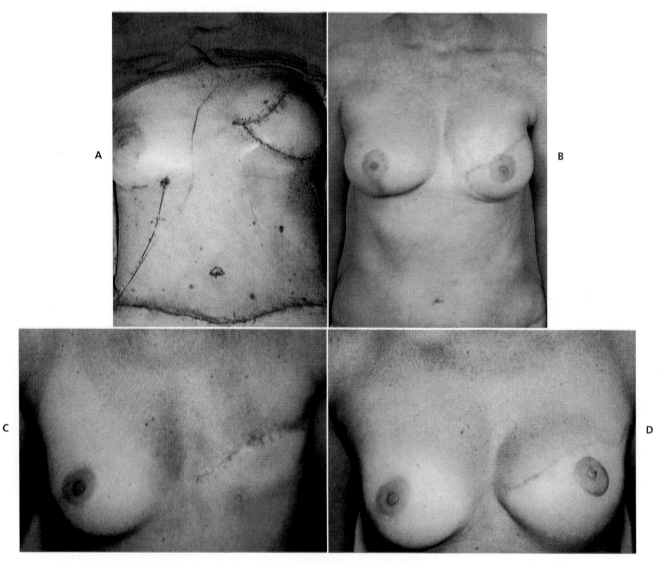

Fig. 7-7 Left breast reconstruction with nipple tattoo. **A and C,** Prior to tattooing. **B and D,** After tattooing. *(Courtesy Brian W. Davies, MD.)*

of road dirt, chemicals, and foreign material from deep tissue helps prevent traumatic tattooing. Some wounds require multiple debridement sessions as the foreign material migrates toward the surface. Occasionally, the foreign material is encapsulated and forms a granulomatous mass. Many of these lesions can be removed by lasers, dermabrasion, excision, and skin grafting. Scarring is common.

Removal of a Tattoo

When the bearer no longer feels the desire to wear a permanent tattoo, he or she may seek removal. More than one method may need to be employed to remove them. A combination of spectrums from multiple laser types may be used for between six to ten treatments to remove the tattoo (Table 7-2). Patient education should include the knowledge of risks and benefits of removal, especially the potential for multiple procedures and potential complications.

The composition and hue of the tattoo pigment determine the method of removal. White, pink, flesh-toned, and red pigments may darken or turn black if exposed to Q-switched or pulsed lasers. Base components of these shades are often ferric oxide, a form of iron (a rusty shade). This chemical converts by chemical reaction to ferrous oxide, also a form of iron (black), when exposed to laser light. The mechanism of this change involves a form of oxidation and is not clearly understood. Some titanium mixtures also turn black when exposed to laser light, although it appears white when first applied by the cosmetician.

Many tattoo pigments contain mercury, cobalt, and chromium. Tattoo pigment is intracellular when left undisturbed. Laser light causes the cell to rupture sending the debris into the extracellular tissue. Dissemination of these chemicals into the tissues can precipitate a cell-mediated sensitivity reaction up to and including allergic anaphylaxis. Each subsequent laser treatment can release more of the substance into the system causing sensitivity to a pigment substance increasing the threat of potential allergic reaction.

Laser treatments for tattoo removal are scheduled 6 to 8 weeks apart. Some fading of the treated area continues between treatments. The patient is instructed to avoid sun exposure and to wear a strong sunscreen or a sun block.

Table 7-2 **Laser Spectrums Used in Multi-Colored Tattoo Removal**

Color of Tattoo	Range of Laser (nm)	Spectral Range of Laser
Red	505-560	Green
Orange	500-525	Green
Yellow	450-510	Blue-green
Green	630-730	Red
Blue-green	400-450	Blue-violet
	505-560	Green
Blue	670-730	Red
Purple	550-640	Green-yellow-orange-red
Black/gray	600-800	Red

Patients, who have an excision of malignant melanoma in a tattooed limb can have unusual gross pathologic tissue appearance. Pigment can migrate from the tattoo to regional lymph nodes giving a darkened appearance to gross observation. The nodes are then differentially diagnosed. Microscopically, the histology looks normal, and mass spectrometry reveals the presence of metallic pigment if the visual changes were caused by tattoo dyes.

Basic Skin Care

There are no substitutes for essential skin care. Twice-daily cleansing, exfoliation, and moisturization provide superficial benefits to the skin (Fig. 7-8). An adequate diet rich in vitamins A, C, E, and B complex supplies cellular-level benefit to skin structure. Eight to ten glasses of water per day are necessary for proper hydration of tissues.

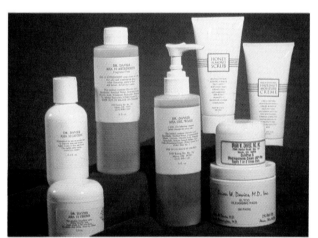

A

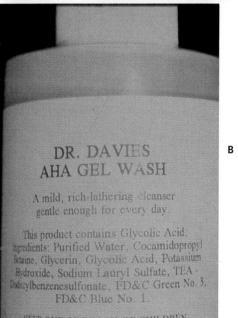

B

Fig. 7-8 A, Basic skin care as prescribed by Dr. Davies. **B,** Alpha hydroxy acid is a major component of many skin care products. *(Courtesy Brian W. Davies, MD.)*

Table 7-3 **Skin Lesions**

SKIN LESIONS	APPEARANCE	INCIDENCE	NOTES
BENIGN			
Keratoacanthoma	Round, smooth dome with central crater filled with keratin	Sun-exposed areas of body; ages 60 years and older	Arises from a hair follicle; can resolve spontaneously; need biopsy to rule out squamous cell carcinoma (SCC)
Keratosis	Rough, red-brown, scaly patches	Found on skin areas exposed to the sun	Can convert into SCC
Moles (nevi)	Clusters of pigmented or nonpigmented cells; flat or raised above the surface	Common in most humans from birth	Continuous irritation can cause changes leading to precancerous condition
MALIGNANT			
Basal cell carcinoma	Pearly or ivory bump with small blood vessels or sore that will not heal; becomes a central depression with rolled edge; ulcerates	Most common form; found on face, neck, nose upper trunk, and ears	Does not metastasize; spreads locally and changes the structure of normal skin; slow growth without lymphatic or vascular invasion; may be familial
Squamous cell carcinoma	Warty growth, pink nodule, or sore that will not heal; Two types: in situ and invasive	Common in sunnier locales, particularly closer to the equator; upper face, ears, and hands	It can metastasize; treatment of metastasis is not very effective; usually middle-age or elderly patient; spreads quickly
Malignant melanoma	Can develop in a preexisting mole; jagged edges with multi-color hue; usually black, and/or blue	Late teen years and older; anywhere on the body; associated with infrequent acute sun damage	One of the most deadly forms of cancer; can spread to lymph nodes and major organs; may be familial; often a single lesion

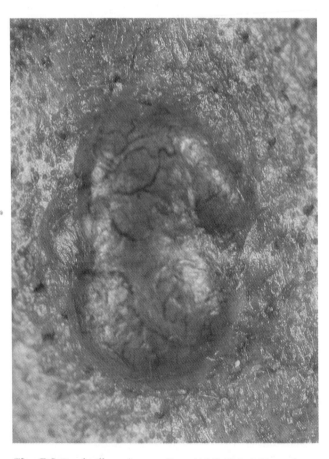

Fig. 7-9 Basal cell carcinoma. *(From Habif: Clinical dermatology, ed 3, St Louis, 1996, Mosby.)*

Exposure to Ultraviolet Rays (UVA and UVB)

Prevention of overexposure to natural or artificial ultraviolet rays is important. Use of sunscreen SPF 15 or above, a wide brimmed hat, and avoidance of sun exposure during the hours of 10:00 AM to 3:00 PM are suggested to minimize the risk of skin cancer and other skin lesions. Medications such as antibiotics, diuretics, hypoglycemics, and antiinflammatories increase sensitivity to the sun. Patients using Retin-A or AHA also are at increased risk for sun damage to the skin.

A history of severe sunburn with blistering increases the risk of skin cancer later in life. People with fair skin and hair are at the greatest risk. Preseasoning skin in a tanning bed gives no protection from subsequent sun exposure. Tanning beds are also a source of harmful rays. Cosmetic manufacturers include preparations of sunscreen in many foundation and cover cream products.

DIAGNOSTICS AND TREATMENTS OF SKIN LESIONS AND NEOPLASMS

Photodamage and exposure to chemicals such as arsenic, coal tar, creosote, pitch, and radium are common causes of abnormal skin lesions (Table 7-3).

Malignant Skin Lesions

Basal cell carcinoma

Basal cell carcinoma (BCC) is the most common form of skin cancer (Fig. 7-9). Fortunately, it grows slowly and rarely

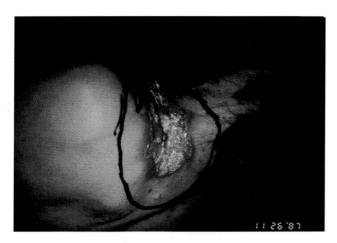

Fig. 7-10 Advanced basal cell carcinoma. *(Courtesy Brian W. Davies, MD.)*

Box 7-5 **Four Primary Types of Basal Cell Carcinomas**

NODULAR
Raised nodular lesions with pearly borders; telangiectatic vessels around edges and surface; some are pigmented and may resemble melanomas; at 1 cm in size, the center ulcerates; this is referred to as a *rodent ulcer;* can cause tissue destruction in area; infiltrative types commonly recur; variations include adenoid and infiltrative

SUPERFICIAL
Flat, erythematous macular lesion; grows into an ulcerated scaly patch with a pearly border; found on the trunk and extremities

MORPHEALIKE
Indurated plaque found on people with keloids or other fibrous disease such as Dupuytren's contracture; the borders are not easily defined with the naked eye; can recur often after excision

INVERTED
Pitlike crater without ulceration; cells invade the dermis and subcutaneous tissue without obvious surface growth; the morphology appears like a nodular-type growth pattern, but infiltrative qualities are present

metastasizes. The average rate of growth for all types is 1 centimeter per year for the first 2 years. After the first 2 years, the rate will vary according to type (Fig. 7-10). Histologic studies are done to determine which type of BCC is present. Before beginning treatment, a biopsy is essential. Specimens should be handled with care to prevent a wrong diagnosis. The treatment will be planned according to the type of cell described by the pathologist.

The BCC lesion appears most commonly on sun-exposed surfaces. Fair-skinned people are at the highest risk. Other factors include previous radiation therapy and arsenic ingestion. Extremely rare varieties may have genetic links. There are four basic types of BCC (Box 7-5). Variants of common nodular BCC structures are also described as adenoid and infiltrative. These types require frozen section on biopsy and very clear marginal excision because they are very aggressive. Recurrent BCC in excised tissue is even harder to cure. Recurrent BCC can occur anywhere from 1 week to 10 years after removal and looks like a cystic, macular, papular, or scaly lesion near the site of previous excision. The recurrence rate increases with each time the lesion is excised and recurs. In some individuals, tumor cells continually arise in newly formed scar tissue.

An unusual form of BCC has some qualities of both BCC and squamous cell carcinoma (SCC). It is known as metatypical BCC or basosquamous cell carcinoma. It may in fact be a form of small cell SCC rather than BCC. It is difficult to differentiate this type of cell from BCC or SCC. If treated as a simple BCC, the prognosis becomes grim if in fact it is SCC, which is more deadly. This is the most aggressive form of skin cancer and may metastasize (Fig. 7-11).

Squamous cell carcinoma

SCC is the second most common skin and mucous membrane cancer (Fig. 7-12). This malignancy is more common after the age of 60 years and is found on the ears, hands, and upper face. Most lesions on the ears are SCC rather than BCC. Males have a higher incidence than females. Rare SCC on scalp, legs, and trunk is more commonly found in females. Patients who have immunosupression therapy for an organ transplant often develop SCC. Arsenic or chemical exposure to tars is an influence in some individuals.

The average patient waits 1.2 years before seeking medical intervention. The SCC lesion grows in response to sun exposure or mercury vapor light sources. Light-skinned individuals and albinos are vulnerable. Patients with darker complexions rarely develop SCC.

SCC is classified as in situ, or invasive, and grows twice as fast as BCC. Histologically, SCC cell types are classified as well differentiated, moderately well differentiated, and poorly differentiated. Invasive SCC cells may display no adhesion, and they may break off and metastasize more easily. It rarely arises from the skin de novo but begins as a scaly pre-malignant macule or papule that becomes nodular. It usually ulcerates causing the border to indurate. A crust forms over the top. It can travel along a perineural pathway and spread proximally to other structures. It can also take a lymphatic route. SCC is also known to occur on mucous membrane where metastasis is more likely. Lesions of the ear can spread more easily than lesions on other sites. Undifferentiated cell types have nearly a 100% metastasis rate.

Follow-up care for SCC includes reexamination every 3 months for the first year after the operation and every 6 months for the next 4 years. SCCs may recur or metastasize within 3 years after initial treatment (Box 7-6).

Malignant melanoma

Malignant melanoma is the most deadly type of skin cancer (Fig. 7-13). It arises de novo or from preexisting lesions from

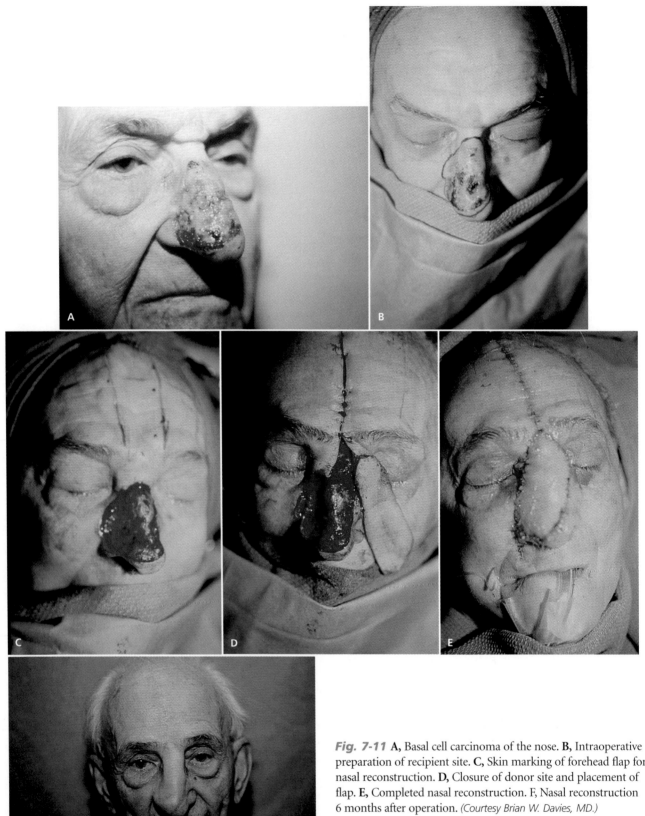

Fig. 7-11 **A,** Basal cell carcinoma of the nose. **B,** Intraoperative preparation of recipient site. **C,** Skin marking of forehead flap for nasal reconstruction. **D,** Closure of donor site and placement of flap. **E,** Completed nasal reconstruction. F, Nasal reconstruction 6 months after operation. *(Courtesy Brian W. Davies, MD.)*

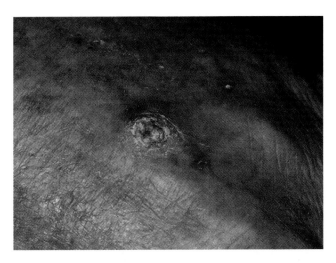

Fig. 7-12 Squamous cell carcinoma. *(From Habif:* Clinical dermatology, *ed 3, St Louis, 1996, Mosby.)*

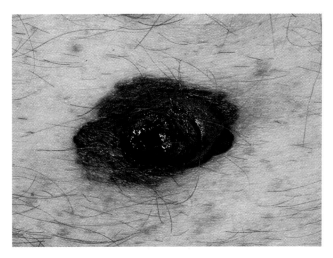

Fig. 7-13 Melanoma. *(From Habif:* Clinical dermatology, *ed 3, St Louis, 1996, Mosby.)*

Box 7-6 **Factors Influencing Failure to Cure Cutaneous Squamous Cell Carcinoma**

Size > 3 cm
Duration > 1 year
Poorly defined cells
Neural invasion
Location on either mucous membrane or ear
Location in scar tissue
Location in previously rediated tissue
History of previous SCC treatment

Box 7-7 **Prognostic Variables in Malignant Melanoma**

AGE
Females: Between 40 and 50 years of age
Males: Between 50 and 60 years of age

SEX
Females: A higher incidence with better prognosis; thinner less invasive lesions
Males: Older males have worse prognosis

ANATOMIC LOCATION
Females: More on lower extremities
Males: More on trunk
Best prognosis for either is on the extremities or the head and neck

SIZE OF LESION
Lesion size is difficult to estimate on gross examination because of irregular border;
< 3 cm has approximately 49% 5-year survival rate;
> 3 cm has approximately 9% 5-year survival rate;
Small pigmented macules and/or papules nearby may be regional, lymphatic, metastatic emboli and not direct extensions; depth of invasion and thickness are directly related to severity (Clark's levels)

ULCERATION
Is usually a poor prognosis, and often indicates a larger, traumatized tumor

---

melanotic cells. Approximately 1 in 250 people will develop this cancer in his or her lifetime. Fair-skinned individuals are at particular risk. People with red hair have a higher incidence. Familial forms are an autosomal dominant trait. Prognosis depends on many variables (Box 7-7). Earlier detection has improved survival, although surgical treatments are relatively the same as they have been for several years.

In evaluating a patient for potential melanoma lesions, the acronym ABCD is used. A is asymmetry, B is border irregularity, C is color (black-brown-red-blue mix), and D is diameter of 6 mm or more. The thickness and depth of invasion are difficult to ascertain without more invasive testing. A wide and deep excisional removal of the lesion for biopsy is usually performed. A margin of 3 to 5 cm in continuity of the lymph node drainage and depth to the deep fascia is excised. Patients at risk may need a lymph node dissection. The degree of severity is microscopically diagnosed using Clark's melanoma microstaging criteria (Fig. 7-14). This is based on the degree of dermal invasion by the melanoma.

The hormones of pregnancy can trigger an existing mole or nevi to convert to a melanoma. During a normal pregnancy, a woman may normally develop hyperpigmentation in various areas of the body. This is caused by estrogen, progesterone, and melanin-stimulating hormone. The lesion is evaluated the same as if the patient was not pregnant. If delivery is eminent, the excision may be delayed until the baby is born. The patient is instructed that oral contraceptives and subsequent pregnancies

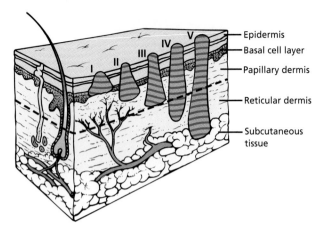

Fig. 7-14 Clark's microstaging criteria.

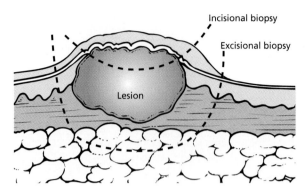

Fig. 7-15 Incisional and excisional biopsy.

Table 7-4 **Four Types of Malignant Melanoma**

TYPES	NOTES
Superficial spreading melanoma	70% of melanoma in Caucasians; grows in width before deep invasion; legs of females and upper back of both sexes
Primary nodular melanoma	12% of melanoma in Caucasians; commonly deeply invasive and ulcerated
Lentigo malignant melanoma	5% of melanoma in Caucasians; head, neck, and dorsum of hands
Acral lentiginus melanoma	8% of melanoma in Caucasians; forms in glabrous skin of palms or soles, distal extremities, ungual areas; accounts for 60% of malignant lesions in dark-skinned individuals

need to be avoided for the next 2 years at a minimum. The risk of recurrence is high during the first 2 years after delivery.

Follow-up is critical. All patients should be examined every 3 months for the first year after the operation and should be scheduled for additional follow-up according to the diameter (Breslow's classification) and depth (Clark's staging levels) of the excised lesion from that point on. Patients with lesions less than 0.76 mm in diameter (Clark's level II) should be examined yearly after the first year. If the lesion is 0.76 mm to 1.49 mm in diameter (early Clark's level III), the patient should be examined every 6 months from that point on. Chest x-ray examination and liver function tests are done for all patients at 6- to 12-month intervals. Patients with melanomas larger in diameter than 1.50 mm and deeper than 4.0 mm should be referred to an oncologic center for definitive treatment.

Surveillance is necessary for the remainder of the patient's life. Melanomas often recur or metastasize within 5 years of diagnosis. Melanoma has a poor 5-year survival rate, especially if the lesion exceeds 3.65 mm in depth. Statistically, survival rates are improving up to 69% at 10 years with early diagnosis

and treatment. The patient will need continual examinations for at least 10 years after the operation (Table 7-4).

Excisional Biopsy

Excisional biopsy is indicated for lesions less than 1.5 cm in diameter. The margin should be 2 mm of clear skin in the elliptical circumferential periphery of the lesion. Marking the orientation of the lesion is important for the pathologist. The entire lesion and palpable tissue mass are removed.

Incisional Biopsy

Incisional biopsy is indicated when the amount of skin to be removed is in a critical location of the body. This may be performed if the lesion is large and requires the removal of much skin. A scalpel can be used, but a punch is a better choice for a full-thickness core specimen. Only part of the lesion is removed (Fig. 7-15).

Mohs' Microsurgery and Tissue Mapping

Mohs' surgery is a specialized method of serial, excisional biopsy in uniform tangential layers and mapping tissue borders and layers. The freshly excised tissue is carefully oriented to the wound and mapped by location. The pathologist examines the tissue at all margins including depth and width. Stains, such as haematoxylin, eosin, and select immunoflourescents, are used to determine the histologic indicators of diagnosis. This technique is used most often for nonmelanotic lesions such as SCC and BCC. Mohs' histographic surgery is useful for treating recurrent or recessed skin cancer in a scarred or radiated area. The tangential sections create a deep defect that requires secondary revision at a later date (Fig. 7-16).

TREATMENT OF SKIN SURFACE DEFECTS

Skin surface defects, such as tissue loss by trauma or therapeutic excision, are interventionally closed or allowed to heal by natural physiologic methods. Treatment decisions are made based on the initial cause of the defect, amount of tissue loss, degree of contamination, blood supply, tissue viability, and location of the defect. Wounds closed by primary intention normally have the lowest level of microbial load and need no topical antiinflammatory or antibacterial creams or ointments. Some of these agents can cause interruption of the natural fibrin seal that forms over the closed wound.

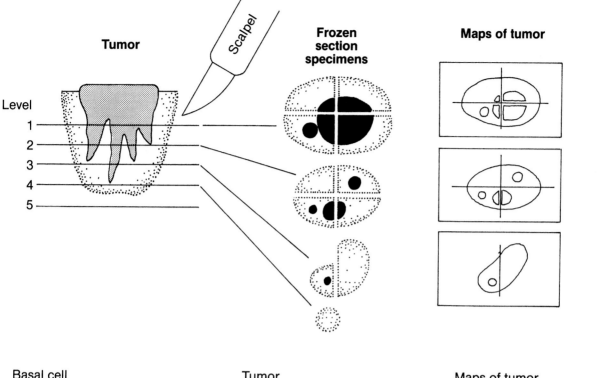

Basal cell
    carcinoma with
    fingerlike
    projections of
    tumor in the
    dermis

Tumor
    sliced with
    scalpel and
    cut into
    quadrants before
    frozen section;
    dark areas
    represent tumor

Maps of tumor
    location drawn
    from frozen
    section specimens,
    indicating areas of remaining
    tumor that must be removed

Fig. 7-16 Microscipically guided excision of cutaneous tumors—Mohs' micrographic surgery. *(From Habif:* Clinical dermatology, *ed 3, St Louis, 1996, Mosby.)*

Desiccation

Curettage and desiccation are used to remove lesions from the skin. Curettings should be sent for histologic confirmation of cell type. Desiccation destroys cells and renders the tissue histologically indistinct. The disruption of the tissue makes it difficult to determine if the entire lesion has been removed, and the lesion can reappear. Desiccation is performed with electrocautery or laser. Plume from a thermodesiccation device is considered biohazardous and should be evacuated from the surgical field with a filtered smoke evacuation device. Patients having desiccation of warts or lesions under local anesthesia should also be given a mask to wear to prevent inhalation of the airborne particulate. A mask, gloves, and eye protection should be worn when changing the filter on the smoke evacuator.

Topical Chemotherapy

5FU (fluorouracil) can be used topically to destroy select lesions at the cellular level by interfering with deoxyribonucleic acid (DNA) synthesis. This drug causes an inflammatory reaction that may play a part in tumor destruction. Only small, superficial BCCs can realize a cure. The drug is applied in a cream twice per day for 4 to 6 weeks. Some inflammation will occur at the site that is treated with topical steroids. This method gives good aesthetic results if used for the correct type of lesion and is reasonably priced. For patients with a history of hypertrophic scars and irregular pigmentation, this may be the treatment of choice. Deeper tissue lesions treated by 5FU cream may give the appearance of resolving, but in fact may be delving deeper into the tissues. This can cause delayed treatment and result in extensive tissue damage.

Radiation Treatment

Radiation may be used to treat some skin conditions. Unfortunately, years after radiation treatment for conditions such as acne, the patient may develop SCC at the site. Cure rates for BCC are between 87% to 94%. After treatment, the highest recurrence rate is around the nose and scalp. Ulcerated lesions caused by radiation often appear.

Radiation treatment is contraindicated for patients under 40 years of age, because they commonly develop postradiation sequelae, such as radiodermatitis and radiation-induced skin cancer.

Cryotherapy

Few studies have been performed to test the efficacy of cryosurgery, although it has been used for more than 20 years. Studies have shown a 95% cure rate for primary BCC and an 89% cure rate for recurrent basal cell lesions. Other lesions are not widely reported in the literature. Cryotherapy has no specific dose requirements but is placed in contact with target tissue for a timed therapeutic effect. Other specialties such as gynecology have used this method for many years to treat premalignant or chronic conditions.

Cryotherapy is delivered by topical application of a freezing chemical or other instrumentation. A freezing chemical can be applied topically to augment other procedures, such as dermabrasion. It has been applied to the skin in studies as a pretreatment for laser therapy with varying degrees of success. Liquid nitrogen is delivered via cryoprobe to a specific lesion. In some respects, oddly-shaped lesions in hard-to-reach places may respond to cryotherapy better than to Mohs' microsurgery.

GRAFTS AND FLAPS

Transposition, mobilization, shifting, and movement of biologic tissue are complex mainstays of plastic and reconstructive surgical procedures that utilize grafts and flaps (Fig. 7-17). The potential degree of graft or flap complexity depends on the patient, donor source, and wound conditions. The intent of tissue transfer will not be successful if any of these entities are omitted from the equation. Depending on the type of tissue and the donor source, placement of these biologic materials may be permanent or temporary (Box 7-8 and Box 7-9).

Skin Grafts

Skin grafts can be classified as split-thickness (partial-thickness) or full-thickness. These include the epidermis, dermis, and varying levels of subcutaneous tissues and structures (Fig. 7-18). A skin graft is the transfer of a segment of epidermis and dermis by separating it from its original blood supply (donor site) and placing it on a new location of the body (recipient site). The graft adheres to the new surface by attaching to a layer of natural fibrin glue that forms naturally over the wound bed. Nutrients to the newly placed graft are transferred by plasmatic diffusion through the fibrin base. The process of diffusion and subsequent perfusion of the graft is referred to as *take.* The graft

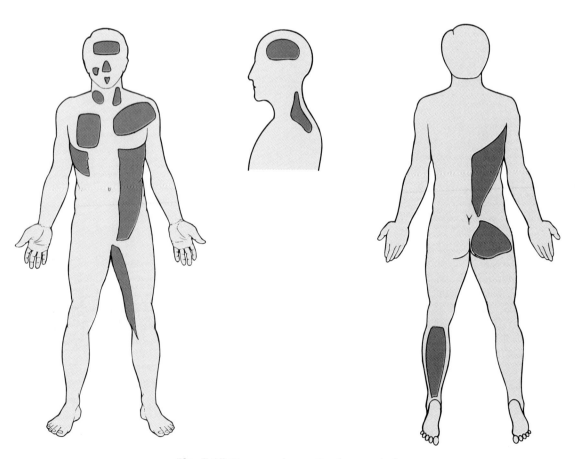

Fig. 7-17 Common donor sites for muscle flaps.

takes if the newly positioned tissue survives at the recipient site (Fig. 7-19). Favorable conditions for the take of a skin graft are described in Box 7-10. Thinner grafts take more readily because the diffusion has fewer layers to penetrate. Thicker grafts have higher metabolic needs because they have more dense tissue and accessory components.

The patient should be closely assessed for factors that could cause graft rejection. Hematoma can cause graft separation. Medications such as aspirin, anticoagulants, antiinflammatory agents, or vitamin E should be discontinued at least 14 days before the surgical procedure to minimize the possibility of bleeding. Hypertension also contributes to the possibility of postoperative hematoma. The risk of hematoma is greatest within the first 10 to 12 hours after the operation.

The neovascular blood supply to the graft is established by the vertical migratory insertion of vessels from the wound bed and the spread of endothelial cells originating in the old vessels of the transferred tissue. This process is referred to as inosculation. Thicker grafts can realign cut vessel surfaces on the underside of the graft with the migration of vessels in the wound by the same endothelialization process.

Graft procurement pain can be deceased by topical application of EMLA to intact skin 1 to 5 hours before surgery. EMLA should not be used as a postoperative analgesic because it is not a sterile preparation. Gloves should be worn for the application process. After application, an occlusive dressing is placed over the intended surgical site. The product should be kept out of areas of broken skin. It also may be harmful to eyes and mucous membranes of the ears. Chlorhexidine nullifies EMLA effectiveness and should not be used for skin prep. Minimal amounts of the drug become absorbed into the systemic circulation. Additional local infiltration anesthesia can be used to augment analgesia.

Split-thickness skin grafts

A graft less than full-thickness of the skin is referred to as split- or partial-thickness skin graft. Categorization is based on the level of thickness and the constituents of the procured skin segment and is not an absolute measurement. The intrinsic site of procurement can vary in thickness; therefore the depth and constituents of the tissue will differ. Tissue taken from the eyelid varies greatly from tissue taken from the thigh.

Epidermal grafts. Early grafts consisted of autologous epidermal shavings placed in the recipient site. The result was negligible structure, no pigmentation, and wide scar contracture. This process progressed to spatially multiplying the cells in a culture medium to cover larger surfaces. This is lifesaving in burn wound management. The area heals in a lighter shade than surrounding tissue.

Thin grafts. This form of skin graft includes the epidermis, portions of papillary dermis, and most, but not all, of the basal cell layer of the donor site. This graft takes quickly because it requires minimal nourishment to remain viable. This enables its use over less vascularized areas. There are no hair follicles or glands. Scar contracture is wide. Most of the main skin constituents remain at the donor site allowing rapid healing by secondary intention. The same area can be used as a donor site again. This is useful for burn patients because multiple donor sites may be hard to find.

Box 7-8 Classification of Grafts by the Source of Donor Tissue

AUTOLOGOUS GRAFT
Transfer of tissue from one site to another site on the same person

ISOGRAFT
Transfer of tissue from one genetically identical person to another

ALLOGRAFT
Transfer of tissue between the same species

XENOGRAFT
Transfer of tissue between two different species

Box 7-9 Biologic Tissues Used for Temporary and/or Permanent Transfer

Epidermis
Dermis
Adipose tissue
Mucous membranes
Fascia
Tendons
Nerves
Bone

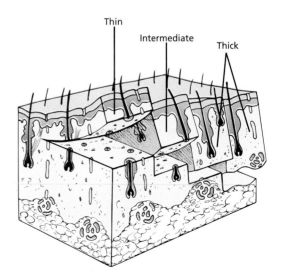

Fig. 7-18 Free skin grafts.

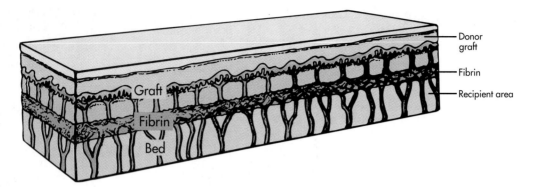

Fig. 7-19 The process of take of a free skin graft.

Moderately thick grafts. This form of skin graft includes the epidermis, the full basal layer, and the majority of the papillary dermis. The healed graft is hairless and dry because only portions of the glands and follicles are included. The site may feel itchy because of the dryness. The donor site heals reasonably well by secondary intention because residual epithelial elements remain. Pigmentation may vary in the healed recipient site and is often darker than the donor site. This graft provides durable and functional cover to the recipient site.

Thick grafts. This form of skin graft incorporates 70% to 80% of the thickness of the epidermis/dermis complex. This leaves a donor site of bare reticular dermis with visible subcutaneous surfaces. Meticulous wound care of the donor site is important because tissue slough could result in full-thickness tissue loss requiring intense treatment.

Take of thick grafts is more difficult because of the thickness of the donor graft and requires a well-prepared, viable recipient site for neovascularization. The healed result is more aesthetically pleasing because scar contracture is less than other split-thickness grafts, and the tissue is far more durable. This method is commonly used for hand and foot skin grafts.

Full-thickness skin grafts

Full-thickness skin grafts contain epidermis, dermis, and all constituents except adipose tissue. The condition of the recipient site is critical to the success of the graft take. The donor site results in a wound the same size and shape of the recipient site. The surgeon usually closes the donor site by primary intention. Optimal healing of the newly grafted sited results in close tissue match of color and consistency. The desired outcome is attained by an aesthetic appearance (Fig. 7-20).

Composite skin grafts

Skin grafts (epidermis/dermis complexes) that include other types of tissue, such as adipose, cartilage, and/or mucous membrane, are referred to as composite grafts. Composite grafts are usually small and limited to use in highly vascular areas of the body, such as hair-bearing surfaces, the nipple/areola complex, the nose, and the ears. The technique for this type of tissue transfer is tedious and requires careful approximation. More complex methods may include microvascular surgical technique. Neovascularization and inosculation are rapid and begin within hours of the graft. The donor site is closed by primary intention or allowed to close by secondary intention with the resultant scar contraction that follows.

Procurement of Skin Grafts

Dermatomes are cutting devices used to procure skin grafts of varying thicknesses. Original graft procurement devices consisted of various free-hand knives. Depth of donor tissue was dependent on the skill of the surgeon. The donor tissue was not always consistent in depth and width. Modification of the free-hand knife included placing an adjustable guard over the blade to guide the surgeon's incisional pass over the donor site (Fig. 7-21). Tangential excision is more precise with the guard in place (Box 7-11).

Drum dermatomes were invented in the early 1930s. The Padgett semicircular drum dermatome measures 4 by 8 inches on the surface and has an adjustable blade (Fig. 7-22). The Padgett blade is seated in an adjustable handle to control the

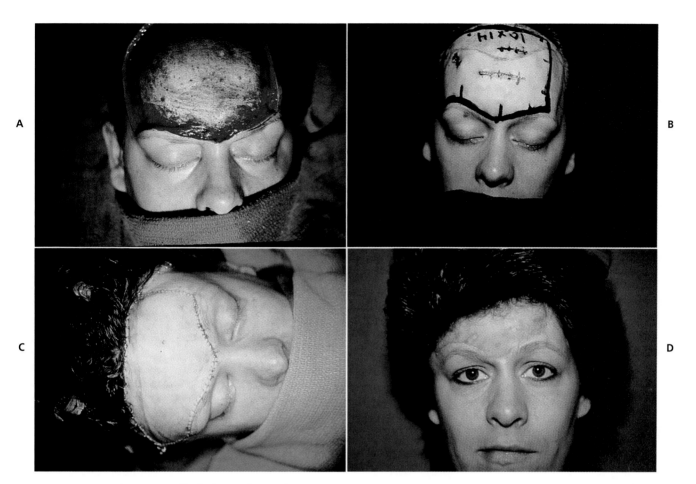

Fig. 7-20 Full -thickness skin graft. **A,** Intraoperative recipient site. **B,** Intraoperative graft planning. **C,** Completion of graft placement. **D,** Postoperative graft healing. *(Courtesy Brian W. Davies, MD.)*

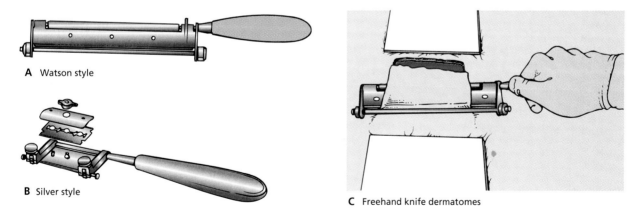

A Watson style

B Silver style

C Freehand knife dermatomes

Fig. 7-21 Free-hand knife dermatomes.

depth of procurement. The Reese drum dermatome controls the depth by placing shims. Glue, or most recently double-sticky tape, is placed on the drum before taking the graft.

Powered dermatomes are driven by pressured air or electricity (Fig. 7-23). The power causes the blade to oscillate. The Brown dermatome is commonly used to take uniform grafts of unlimited length from smooth surfaces. Irregular contours can be evened out by injection of sterile saline or mixtures of lidocaine with a vasoconstrictor into subcutaneous tissue. This helps eliminate bumpy terrain and minimizes blood loss at the same time.

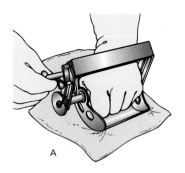
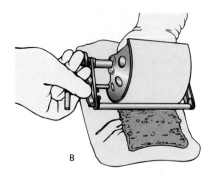
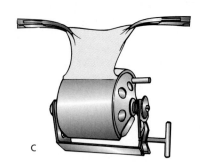

Fig. 7-22 Drum dermatome.

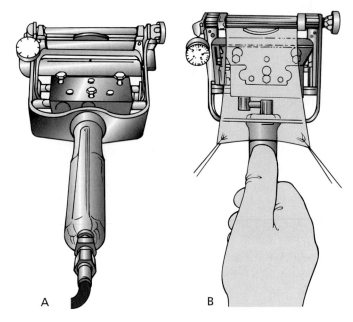

Fig. 7-23 Powered Brown dermatome.

Box 7-11 **Free-hand Graft Knives**

Blair
Humby
  ■ Braithwaite
  ■ Watson
  ■ Bodenham
  ■ Cobbett
Weck
Goulian
Ferris-Smith

The surface cover potential of a donor graft can be increased in size by meshing. The donor tissue is passed through a machine, and tiny symmetrical slits are cut, allowing expansion of the graft in a meshlike manner (Fig. 7-24). Older meshers use a carrier slide to secure the skin during meshing. Newer models have eliminated the use of a carrier. After placement of the meshed graft over the recipient site, fibrin from the recipient bed accumulates in the open meshwork of the donor graft causing optimal conditions for reepithelialization. Healed mesh grafts often have a cobblestone appearance.

Care of the donor site includes pain management, protection from infection, and maintenance of moisturization. Topical application of antimicrobials can assist in retaining moisture that encourages reepithelialization. The formation of a scab can serve as a biologic method of retaining moisture at the site of healing. Common antimicrobial and moisturizing dressings include Xeroform gauze and gauze saturated with Scarlet Red. Stimulation of epithelial layers is desired. Pain is more commonly associated with the donor site than the recipient site.

Care of the recipient site includes maintaining graft positioning until fibrin adherence has occurred. The duration varies according to location and thickness of the graft. The donor graft can be meshed to conform more easily to the contours of an irregular wound. Excess pressure from dressings can impair circulation and prevent neovascularization. The wound edges are treated the same as any other primarily closed wound. Collections of serous fluid should not be milked or squeezed from the grafted recipient wound. This would cause disruption of the adherent surfaces and stop neovascularization. Serous fluid can be aspirated with a sterile needle and syringe, and the dressing can be readjusted for even coverage, taking care not to shift the grafted tissue.

Graft coverage of an irregular surface, particularly a concave surface, may need a bolus dressing acting like a stent. The gauze is evenly placed over the newly grafted site and tied in position with suture ends (Fig. 7-25). Placement is secured with even pressure over the entire grafted surface. Great care is exercised when changing this dressing. Two pairs of forceps should be used; one to stabilize the graft in place and the other to slowly lift off the dressing. This is done very cautiously to prevent peeling the graft from the wound if adherent to the surface of the graft.

Tissue Flaps

A tissue flap maintains a connection with its original blood supply. The direction of the incision lines is directly related to the direction of the blood supply. A flap is dissected free on one or more sides with at least one side remaining attached to its origin (Fig. 7-26). The vascular and innervated attachment is referred to as a pedicle (foothold). Exceptions include a flap that is dissected free of the remaining connection and reattached elsewhere (referred to as a *free flap*). One side of the free flap is anastomosed microscopically to a new blood supply at its new location.

Postoperative flap monitoring

Blood flow in the flap is monitored during preparation and after transfer. One method involves the IV instillation of fluorescein. Within 5 to 10 minutes the drug perfuses to the capillary level and is visible in the tissues under a Wood's lamp. Doppler use may be indicated to check blood flow in larger vessels. The two most common causes of flap failure are loss of arterial blood flow and venous congestion. Tension on the flap by edema can compromise the viability of the arterial blood supply. The patient is instructed to avoid smoking because it compromises the flap by causing vasoconstriction.

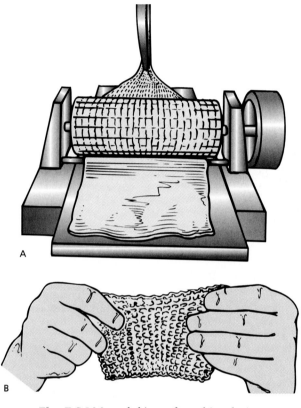

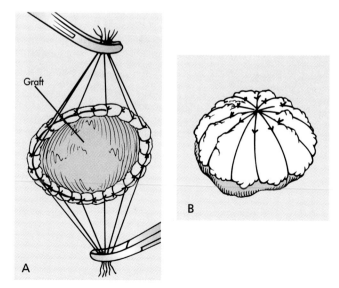

Fig. 7-24 Manual skin graft meshing device.

Fig. 7-25 The skin graft is tied in place and covered with a Bolster dressing.

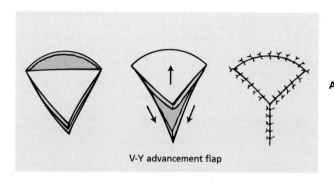

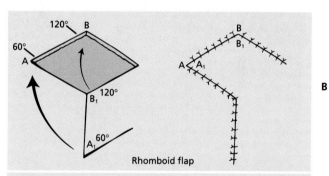

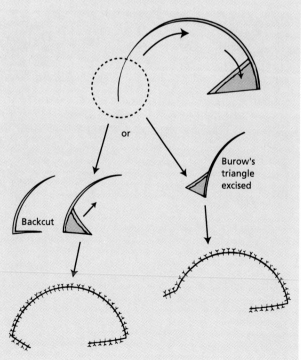

Fig. 7-26 **A,** V-Y advancement flap. **B,** Rhomboid flap. **C,** Rotation flap: two methods of closure.

Flaps are created to reverse the direction of the lines of tension on an existing scar, such as in Z-plasty and related incisional configurations. Hypertrophic scars and keloids have poor aesthetic properties and cause flexibility problems in the overlying skin. Although no scar can be removed completely, the appearance can be improved by reversing the direction of tension on the skin and debulking hypertrophic tissue. Initial treatment consists of steroid injections and compression garments. When these methods prove unsuccessful, function can be partially or almost fully restored with surgical revision. Most insurance providers will not reimburse for aesthetic procedures but will usually cover restoration of function. Scar revision has the benefits of both form and function. Final results of scar revision may not be apparent for at least 1 year after the operation.

Types of flaps

Rotation flap. This semicircular flap is designed to cover soft-tissue defects in an immediately adjacent recipient site. The recipient site is looser tissue than the donor flap (Figs. 7-27 and 7-28). The donor site may be difficult to close and may require skin grafting. The base of the flap in the direction away from the rotation may have a dog-ear defect (Fig. 7-29). Excising a Burow's triangle may compromise the blood supply and should be performed with extreme caution.

Advancement flap. This flap is undermined on two, three, or four sides and brought forward to cover a close recipient site. The shape of the advancement flap determines whether the donor defect can be closed by primary intention. The remaining underside attachment is neurovascularly intact. Examples include the V-Y flap (see Fig. 7-26, *A*) and the bipedicle flap.

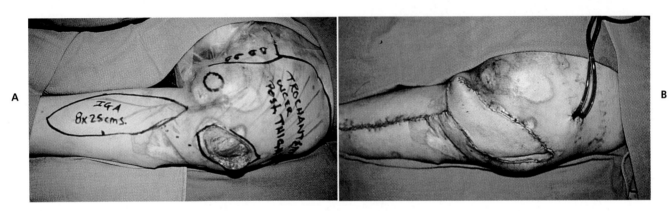

Fig. 7-27 A, Rotational flap from posterior thigh for pressure sore. **B,** Completed rotation flap. Note placement of drains. *(Courtesy Brian W. Davies, MD.)*

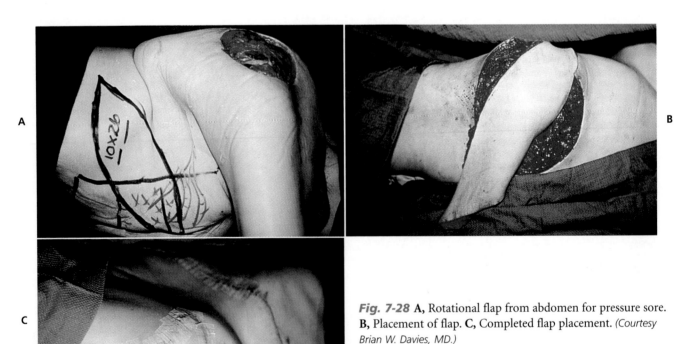

Fig. 7-28 A, Rotational flap from abdomen for pressure sore. **B,** Placement of flap. **C,** Completed flap placement. *(Courtesy Brian W. Davies, MD.)*

Pedicle flap. This mobilized, flexible flap is attached to a neurovascularly intact stalk. It can be tunneled or rotated to a distant recipient area with minimal risk to the pedicle. Orientation of the pedicle is important to avoid crimping the nerves and vessels in the stalk. This flap can be used to cover defects left from large tissue losses.

Island flap. This flap has a vascular pedicle that is raised completely from its bed and transferred to its resting location through a tunnel beneath the skin. The donor site is closed through primary intention. A transabdominal myocutaneous (TRAM) flap is a form of island flap discussed in Chapter 10 in reference to breast reconstruction (Fig. 7-30).

Transposition flap. This flap is designed to move or interposition tissue over or under normal tissue. This may be done to release scar tissue and lengthen the linear distance of tension lines. The direction and appearance of the wound is changed dramatically. Examples include Z-plasty, W-plasty, and rhomboid.

Myocutaneous and fasciocutaneous flaps

Survival of a muscular flap depends on the integrity of the vascular pedicle or the microvascular attachment (Table 7-5). Muscular function changes at the donor site and is not restored at the recipient site. The cutaneous surface may not be transferred with the flap. When transferred without the skin, the bulk of the muscle fills the recipient defect and can have a superficial skin graft at a later time. Some shrinkage may be evident if the innervation is disturbed.

Advantages of muscle flaps over skin flaps include a richer blood supply and higher resistance to bacterial invasion. There is less dead space when the body of muscle bulk fills the recipient defect. Blood vessels are larger in muscle tissue making microvascular anastomosis easier. Some muscles may retain function when the neurovascular stalk is intact upon transfer (Fig. 7-31).

Postoperative flap monitoring

Drains are used for 24 hours after the operation. Dressings are noncompressive and allow for drainage from the wound edges. Prevention of hematoma is critical to prevent separation of the flap from the donor bed. The flap is observed for color and capillary refill. Temperature and texture are monitored. A Doppler is useful for checking circulation in microvascular free flaps. Care is taken to not allow the patient to lie on the newly positioned flap. Innervation is not intact, and ischemic pain associated with poor flap perfusion may not be felt. The patient is taught to inspect the flap several times per day with a mirror.

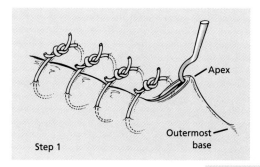

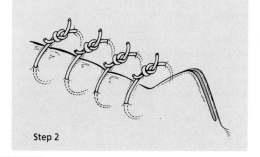

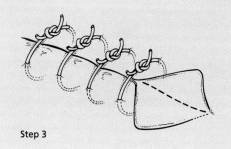

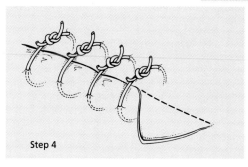

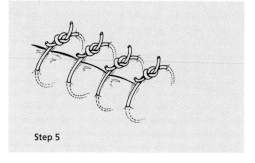

Fig. 7-29 Steps for straight dog-ear repair.

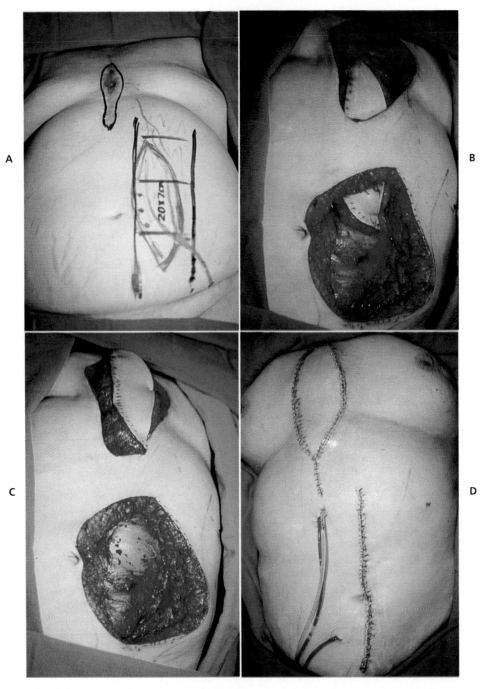

Fig. 7-30 **A,** Skin markings for abdominal myocutaneous island flap to cover a sternal defect. Note debridement lines around the sternal wound. **B,** Passing the abdominal island flap under the skin to the sternal defect. **C,** Placement of myocutaneous flap over prepared sternal wound. **D,** Closed abdominal wound and completed island flap placement. Note drain placement to prevent seroma and hematoma at the site. *(Courtesy Brian W. Davies, MD.)*

Leech therapy

Arterial blood supply brings oxygenated blood to the site of a tissue flap or replanted part, such as a limbs, a digit, ears, or the penis, and conversely, deoxygenated blood can accumulate at the site compromising tissue viability. Venous return routes may be complex to reconstruct, and neovascular formations take 3 to 5 days to form. Venous congestion and obstruction are serious complications that pose the threat of ischemia. Pressure caused by venous accumulation can be relieved by medicinal leech therapy.

What is a leech? A leech is a greenish-brown, muscular, wormlike, amphibious scavenger (Fig. 7-32). The most commonly used leech in plastic and reconstructive surgery is the

Table 7-5 **Muscle Flaps**

TYPE	DESCRIPTION OF BLOOD SUPPLY	EXAMPLES
Type I	Singular blood supply to single muscle body; rotates well because blood supply is usually proximal	Gastrocnemius, tensor fascia latae
Type II	Dual blood supply (major and minor); most common type of muscle vascularization	Gracilis, soleus, and trapezius
Type III	Dual blood supply (both sources are major blood supplies and may enter the muscle parallel or from either end); may have two vascular pedicles in same muscular flap	Rectus abdominis
Type IV	Has multiple vascular insertion points; division of any portion causes destruction of the supplied segment of muscle; these are of limited value for muscle flap transfer	Sartorius
Type V	Has one major and multiple minor vascular insertions; very important source of muscle flaps	Latissimus dorsi, pectoralis major

Hirudo medicinalis. This breed has been used by medical practitioners since 200 BC to treat everything from gout to hematomas. Although it is a hermaphrodite, it mates with another leech and lays eggs in a protective cocoon. It measures 12 to 20 cm in length with a suction device on each end and has a Y-shaped jaw with 300 tiny teeth. The gut contains *Aeromonas hydrophilia,* a nonpathogenic, gram-negative microorganism that is essential for the well-being of the leech. This microorganism can potentially become pathogenic in rare circumstances and is sensitive to some antibiotics such as Augmentin. Consult recommendations of the supplier for specific information about antibiotic therapy.

The leech produces an anticoagulant (hirudin), a vasodilator, and a mild anesthetic in its saliva. Its bite is essentially painless because of the natural anesthetic and attachment to denervated tissue. It consumes approximately 5 ml of blood (five times its own weight), becomes engorged, and falls off. The anticoagulant effect causes the bite wound to ooze for 6 to 10 hours. Blood drainage from the bite can range from 50 to 150 ml in 48 hours.

This continuous flow from the bite wound relieves the pressure caused by venous congestion and possibly prevents infection of the site. Arterial supply to the part must be adequate to support this process.

Use of leeches. Leeches are obtained through pharmaceutical suppliers. They are specially bred and raised for medicinal use on a single patient. They are almost extinct in the wild. Leeches cost between $6 and $15 each. They arrive at the pharmacy in a nested container filled with sterile distilled water with a special chemical additive. They are stored at 5° to 7° C (42° to 45° F), and the specially prepared fluid is changed every other day. The leeches will perish if placed in chlorinated tap water or exposed to temperatures over 20° C (65° F). The inner chamber containing the leeches has tiny holes through which the special fluid preparation can pass and a locking lid. No more than 50 leeches are stored in a 1 liter container.

Carefully cleanse and rinse the patient's skin. Creams and medication may repel the leech. Make a small bleeding nick in the skin with a sterile needle. To apply the leech (wearing nonsterile

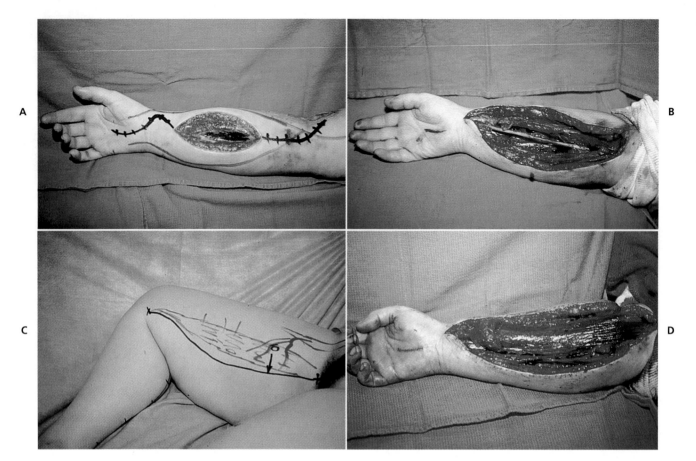

Fig. 7-31 Muscle free-flap. **A,** Right forearm skin markings to receive free-flap. **B,** Right arm prepared to receive gracillis muscle free flap. **C,** Marking on right thigh for procurement of gracillis muscle free-flap. **D,** Gracillis muscle free-flap in place in right forearm. *(Courtesy Brian W. Davies, MD.)*

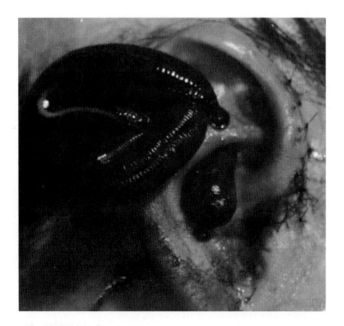

Fig. 7-32 Leech. *(Courtesy Leeches USA, Ltd, Westbury, New York.)*

gloves), extract the inner chamber allowing the fluid to drain into the outer canister. Carefully unlock the lid, remove the leech with forceps, and apply it on the intended site. A few drops of dextrose water placed over the desired site and covering the area with a tented gauze dressing or an opsite will prevent migration to an unwanted site. One or two leeches may be needed for a single finger. A large flap may need six or more to attain the desired result. According to need, leeches may be ordered by the physician for application every 2 to 5 hours until venous circulation is established.

After feeding, the leech may drop off the site or may need to be stunned with a cotton-tipped applicator dipped in 70% alcohol. When replacing a full leech with a hungry one, keep them at a distance from each other or the hungry animal will attach to the fed animal. Do not attempt to manually extract the leech because squeezing may force regurgitation of stomach contents that contain *Aeromonas hydrophilia* causing wound contamination. Some medication, including general anesthetics, may diminish its feeding habits. Tissue with poor arterial circulation repels the leech and may signal a failed surgical procedure.

If a leech is to be used again for the same patient, it can be forced to regurgitate by dipping it in 5% sodium chloride or "milking" its stomach contents out of its mouth. This is an unnecessary source of contamination for the caregiver because reused leeches do not feed well. Leeches only feed every 200 days, so keeping them around for reuse may not be practical. Used leeches are placed in 70% alcohol and disposed of as other biocontaminated or infectious waste. Leeches are never used between patients because they may transmit infections, such as hepatitis or human immunodeficiency virus (HIV). After treatment, unused leeches are returned to the pharmacy.

Nursing care considerations. Patients may find leeches repulsive and may not want to see the treated area during therapy. Patient and family education is important. Hematocrit and hemoglobin levels should be monitored closely because chemicals secreted by the leech can cause an anticoagulant effect and increase bleeding. Some patients can have a significant drop in these blood values after prolonged leech therapy.

BURNS

Critical issues for burn care and rehabilitation are primarily focused on resuscitation, prevention and management of sepsis, and the need for surgical intervention. Rehabilitation and cost containment are interwoven considerations. Initial burn management can determine the course of the patient's recovery. Rehabilitation is started the moment that treatment begins. The plan of care should reflect activities that integrate the preburn and postburn patient based on the physiologic and psychologic rehabilitation potential of the patient. Multidisciplinary caregivers include plastic and reconstructive surgeons, orthopedists, internists, infectious disease practitioners, nursing personnel, therapists, and many others.

Psychologic Considerations
Severe burns are devastating injuries. They can be horribly disfiguring to the body and incapacitating to physical motion. The memories of the burning event may cause psychologic problems, such as flashbacks and nightmares. Counselors and social workers are an important part of the burn care team.

From a perioperative standpoint, there are many factors involved in planning treatment and reconstruction procedures. Restoring form and function is a complex task. The first consideration is stabilization of the patient's condition followed by preservation of function. Form is important but cannot always be restored. The adult patient's preburn relationships, occupation, activities of daily living, and self-esteem will be forever changed.

The Pediatric Burn Patient
The pediatric patient has limited life experiences and minimal cognitive, emotional, social capabilities. He or she is dependent on others and is particularly vulnerable to influences that foster maladaptive behaviors. When hospitalized, he or she will commonly revert to immature coping mechanisms, such as regression or projection. Painful procedures will necessitate a controlled environment that enhances cooperation. Procedures such as

dressing changes, debridement, and grafting usually require general anesthesia. Consistency in approach to care will facilitate rehabilitation. Pediatric patients have not completed physiologic growth. Burn scars and contractures can alter expected growth patterns

Parents of burned children may impose blame on themselves. Family education should include the use and care of nonflammable, flame-retardant, or flame-resistant clothing and bedding. Fluffy dresses, petticoats, and tights can be easy targets for causing burns if not made of appropriate material. Some homemade Halloween and holiday costumes can fall into this category. These are often flammable or made of synthetics, such as nylon or polyester, that melt and adhere to skin when exposed to flame or high temperatures. Most fabrics treated for fire protection have special laundering instructions. Federal law regulates the fabrics used in the manufacture of children's clothing.

Assessment Of Burn Injury
Burn injury can be thermal, electrical, or chemical. Varying degrees of tissue damage occur, and the effect on multiple organ systems can complicate recovery.

Thermal
Thermal injury results from contact with open flame, hot liquids (scalds), or radiation. Rapid cooling with water can minimize the depth of the burn. Inhalation burns often accompany open flame burns. This is particularly true in children who have been playing with matches in a confined area, such as a closet. Complications also include massive edema of the respiratory tract and carbon monoxide (CO) poisoning from the smoke.

Scalds penetrate deeply and can be deceptive as to the extent of injury. Inhaled steam is not always clearly manifested. Several hours after the burn, the patient may experience respiratory distress caused by delayed tissue edema of the airway and/or lungs.

Electrical
Burns caused by electricity result from a current passing through the body to the ground. Associated flashes or flame may accompany the charge creating a secondary thermal wound. The severity of injury is determined by the duration of contact and the pathway of the current. Muscular components of organs in the direct path of the current undergo extreme contraction. Other traumatic injuries may be present. Cardiopulmonary arrest is common.

The superficial skin injury may be very small. It is not an indicator of the severity of the injury. As the current passes deeper through the tissue, it generates heat causing thermal coagulative necrosis.

Chemical
Chemical burns result from contact with or inhalation of acids, alkalis, or vesicants (blistering agents). They primarily destroy tissue by coagulating protein. Chemical burns are not primarily thermal burns, but a secondary exothermic reaction can occur with some chemicals, such as sulfuric acid or muriatic acid. Heat is created after contacting tissue and moist mucous membranes.

During treatment, all clothing is removed because chemical agent may be adherent. Brush off as much dry agent as possible, taking care not to create airborne dust that could be inhaled. Copious irrigation of the skin with water dilutes the effect of the chemical, even if it is activated by water.

The severity of the burn depends on the concentration of chemical, duration of contact, and the amount of tissue exposed. Some chemicals, especially alkaline varieties, continue to burn and destroy tissue for up to 72 hours. They cannot be neutralized. Some chemicals can be absorbed causing systemic toxicity.

Classification Of Burns

The severity of the tissue injury is determined by the cause and location of the burn. Understanding the types and severity of burns can be beneficial in the development of the plan of care (Fig. 7-33). Body size, age, and burn source will require modification in treatment modality. Perioperative care may include dressing changes under anesthesia, debridement, and possibly skin grafts or tissue flaps. Most severely burned patients will be long-term patients who undergo multiple procedures and treatments.

First-degree superficial burn

A first-degree superficial burn involves the outermost layer of the epidermis. Superficial erythema, dryness, and tissue damage occur without initial blistering. Some blisters may appear after 24 hours. The skin feels warm to the touch. The patient may experience fever and chills that is relieved by over-the-counter (OTC) antipyretics. Examples include sunburn and superficial scalds. Tissue healing is rapid, usually within 5 days.

Treatment. Cool, moist compresses or running water, OTC skin anesthetic spray, and gentle moisturizer with aloe. Top epidermal layers will peel. The skin may discolor or "tan" slightly.

Second-degree partial-thickness burn

A second-degree partial thickness burn involves all of the epidermis and varying depths of the dermis. This damage is characterized by cherry-redness, pain, blister formation, and a moist, mottled appearance. Some hair follicles and sebaceous glands may be damaged. Infection is a constant threat and can interfere with healing. Reepithelialization can take place if the epithelium is viable. Thick scars may form after healing occurs. Examples include scalds, flame-contact burns, and mild chemical burns. Patients with second-degree burns of 20% of the body surface area (BSA) (10% BSA if aged < 10 years or > 50 years) should be hospitalized. Any patient with second-degree burns of hands, feet, face, or perineum should be evaluated in a hospital setting for admission to the burn unit.

Treatment. Apply antimicrobial cream to a clean burn and cover with a transparent dressing. Contaminated wounds should be debrided and closed blisters left intact. Each time the dressing is changed the collagen build-up and eschar should be removed. Surgical or enzymatic debridement can be used to remove the buildup, exposing the newly granulating wound bed.

Wet dressings are applied and allowed to dry completely before removal. This is a form of mechanical debridement because the eschar sticks to the dried dressing gauze as it is removed. This can be very painful. Healing takes 21 to 28 days.

Scarring is common. If an infection occurs, the second-degree burn can convert to a full-thickness wound that requires a graft to heal.

Third-degree full-thickness burn

A third-degree full-thickness burn involves all of the epidermis, dermis, and subcutaneous tissue. It is characterized by a pearly-white, yellow, or charred appearance. There is little or no sensation in the area of a third-degree burn. The periphery of the burn extends into more viable tissue. These edges are usually second-degree burns and are very painful. This injury requires skin grafts in order for healing to take place. If left to slough, the area will appear denuded and can extend to the fascia. Hospitalization may be necessary if burns include hands, feet, face, or perineum. Many third-degree burns take months to heal and ultimately require grafts.

Treatment. Third-degree burn wounds will need escharotomy and enzymatic therapy in preparation for grafting. If the area of involvement is small enough, it can reepithelialize and ultimately close after a prolonged period of time.

Fourth-degree burn

A fourth-degree burn is the most devastating of all categories of burn injuries. Burn damage includes all skin layers and bone, tendon, muscle, blood vessels, and peripheral nerves. Necrotic muscle and bone are excised as soon as possible.

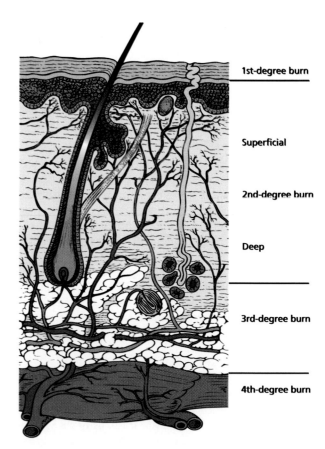

Fig. 7-33 Scheme of normal skin histology and the categorization of burn injury.

Treatment. A fourth-degree burn may require amputation if circulation cannot be reestablished with a flap. This type of burn is commonly found in electrical burn.

The total percentage of BSA that has been damaged by burns and the degree of that burn are calculated by using the Lund-Bowder chart (Fig. 7-34) or the Rule of Nines (adults) (Fig. 7-35). The percentage of burned surface area can be estimated by age, depth, and anatomic location of the burn. Pediatric body area is calculated by adult standards after the age of 15 years. Standardized estimates enable caregivers to plan for resuscitation and physiologic maintenance needs, particularly fluid replacement and nutrition.

Treatment of Burns

Treatment guidelines for the management of burns are based on preventing further injury. Many cells are initially injured but are still potentially viable and preserved if possible. Fluid-filled blisters may form over the surface. Burn blister fluid contains inflammatory mediators thought to be detrimental to microcirculation and could potentially damage localized microvascular structures. Rupturing the blister would remove the remaining natural barrier to infection of intact skin and is not indicated. The fluid can be aspirated at the edge with a needle and syringe leaving the blister epithelium intact.

Elevation and cooling are imperative since the intrinsic musculature of the hands, feet, and extremities cannot withstand ischemia. Surgical decompression by escharotomy, fasciotomy, and debridement may be indicated to release edematous tissues or tight eschar development, especially in circumferential burns. Splinting and positioning should be started as soon as possible after the injury to help preserve function, prevent contractures, and preserve as much neurologic function as possible. Gentle exercise may facilitate the resolution of edema and maintain joint mobility.

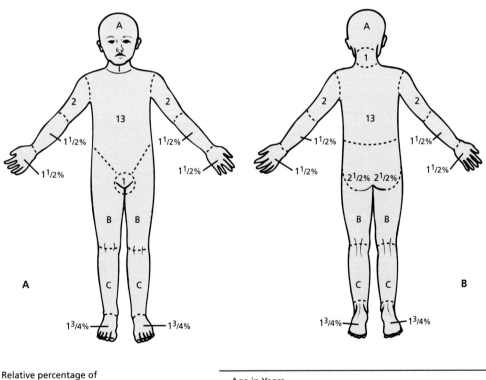

Relative percentage of areas affected by growth	Age in Years					
	0	1	5	10	15	Adult
A–1/2 of head	91/2	81/2	61/2	51/2	41/2	31/2
B–1/2 of one thigh	23/4	31/4	4	41/4	41/2	43/4
C–1/2 of one leg	21/2	21/2	23/4	3	31/4	31/2
Total percent burned		2° +		3°=		

Fig. 7-34 Lund-Browder chart to determine relative percentage of areas of burns on pediatric body. **A,** Anterior. **B,** Posterior.

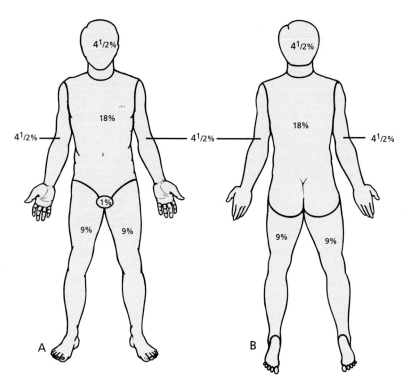

Fig. 7-35 Estimation of burn injury: rule of nines. **A,** Anterior. **B,** Posterior.

Biologic dressings

Biologic dressings are replaced every few days as determined by the physician until the burned area is ready for autologous skin grafting. These may be allografts from a living donor or cadaver, amniotic membranes, or a porcine xenograft. Synthetic skin has been used with some success. Biologic dressings help control infection, prevent loss of serum, decrease pain, stimulate epithelial formation, and promote the growth of granulation tissue.

Cadaver skin can be used as a temporary allograft over denuded areas. Cadaver skin is procured within 12 hours of death and can be refrigerated in culture media for 30 days. If frozen, the shelf life increases by several months. The skin is stored "unavailable for use" until biological testing for communicable diseases has returned negative. The skin is placed in an "available for use" status when all the tests have returned. Duration of allograft skin use is prolonged in immunosuppressed patients. Unfortunately, immunosuppression increases the patient's risk for infection.

Amniotic membranes have been used as a temporary allograft burn cover. This membrane is prepared by washing with a saline and penicillin solution. It is commercially processed and preserved. It has a shelf life of 1 week. It should not be used in penicillin-sensitive or allergic patients. The same biologic testing is done for this tissue as for cadaver skin. The amniotic sac is applied with its attached chorion against the burned surface. This dressing is changed every other day for 6 days. It appears to take, but this is only temporary.

Porcine tissue is used as an alternative temporary xenograft burn cover. It is commercially available and stores well. It does not appear to take and does not provide the same level of antibacterial protection as allograft materials.

Nonbiologic dressings

Dressings are changed frequently to control infection. Antimicrobial or chemotherapeutic agents are an important part of the dressing. The wound is cleansed of any old topical antimicrobial preparation before placing a dressing. Silvadene cream (silver sulfadiazine) is frequently used and is applied directly to the burned area to a depth of 1/16 inch, once or twice daily with a sterile gloved hand. A layer of fine mesh gauze is placed over next, followed by a soft, absorbent, fluffed gauze. Silvadene is not used for patients allergic to sulfa. A splint may be used and is held in place with an elastic bandage. Xeroform and Scarlet Red can be used over donor sites, partial-thickness burns, split-thickness grafts, and debrided wounds to promote epithelialization. Silvadene is not painful on application.

Sulfamylon 10% cream (mafenide acetate) penetrates eschar rapidly and is effective in reducing bacterial counts, especially on infected wounds. It is used in similar fashion to Silvadene cream, but absorption of Sulfamylon may result in metabolic acidosis. Acid-base balance is monitored by serum electrolyte values (particularly potassium levels > 5.5 mEq/L), urine pH < 4.5, and vital signs. Metabolic acidosis is characterized by deep, labored breathing because acidosis is a lack of oxygen at the cellular level. Patients with diabetes, sepsis, or shock are at particular risk. Sulfamylon causes a stinging sensation when applied. Some patients require analgesia for application of the cream. Other appropriate topical, antibacterial preparation is used if the patient is allergic to sulfa.

Nursing Considerations for Care of the Burn Patient

A patient presenting with obvious burn injury may also have additional trauma, such as fractures or hemorrhage that can complicate treatment. Injuries other than the burns are treated by level of severity. Tetanus toxoid is given prophylacticly. After stabilization of life-threatening conditions, the long process of burn treatment begins.

Initial care

Initial care and physiologic stabilization in the early hours after the burn are crucial. The first measure is to stop the burning process by removing clothing, jewelry, or anything in contact with the patient's skin. Airway maintenance is imperative, and assessment of the respiratory system is performed to discern any possible injury caused by inhalation of smoke, gases, or flame. Burns, char, black soot, singed nasal hair, blackened mucus, or excessive salivation may indicate serious oropharyngeal damage. Powderlike substances around the mouth and nose may indicate chemical inhalation. Wheezing and hoarseness may develop over a period of a few minutes or hours as the tissues of the airway become edematous. A tracheotomy tray should be immediately available. An assortment of endotracheal tubes (cuffed and uncuffed) and a laryngoscope may be needed. Severe cases may require a fiberoptic intubation either via the nasal or oral route.

CO poisoning may not be initially evident. Carboxy-hemaglobin occurs when the CO binds to hemoglobin and blocks oxygen transport. The patient will exhibit metabolic acidosis. Blood gas measurements of PO_2 are deceptive because oxygen is at normal tension because it cannot be unloaded. Cyanosis will not be present, and the characteristic cherry-red coloration may not be visible because of burned tissue. The CO content can significantly decrease within 2 hours with the patient breathing room air. Administering 100% oxygen can reverse this process within 20 minutes.

A nasogastric (NG) tube should be placed in severely burned patients to decompress the gastrointestinal tract. Respiratory distress may cause the patient to swallow air with excess salivation. He or she may develop an ileus. The NG tube can act as an esophageal stent and reduce the risk of vomiting and aspiration.

IV fluid replacement is established with a 16-gauge or larger IV catheter to support the intravascular compartment and maintain blood pressure. Ringer's lactate (crystalloid) is used to replace electrolytes and provide large volume expansion. Colloids such as albumin are given 24 hours after the injury to pull fluid back into the vascular space from the tissue. The IV access site should not be in the burned area if possible. A central line may be needed. Any patient with a 10% total BSA burn should receive fluid replacement therapy.

Burn shock

Renal function is dependent on blood pressure. Burn injuries cause massive fluid loss through evaporation, wound extravasation, and third spacing. Fluids leave the intravascular space at the site of injury over a period of 24 to 48 hours. This chemically-mediated systemic response is referred to as *burn shock* and happens throughout the body at the capillary level. Hypovolemic shock is a serious threat. Postburn edema is

expected. Patients at risk for inability to compensate for fluid shift because of physiologic illness include those with diabetes, cardiac problems, liver disease, gastrointestinal disorders, respiratory impairment, and renal disease.

Minimal renal function in the adult is urine production of 30 ml/hr. Children should have an output of 15ml/hr. Infants should produce 1 ml/kg/hr. A Foley catheter for continuous drainage is necessary. Burn shock subsides when the patient is able to maintain adequate urine production for 2 hours or more.

Burn cleansing is done as soon as possible, utilizing strict aseptic technique. Povodine iodine is a mild cleansing agent and is commonly used. Gentle debridement can be done at this time. Hair is removed from the site. The smell of burned hair may be disturbing to the patient. Shaving or clipping may be necessary.

Protective environment

A burn wound is easily contaminated before reepithelialization occurs. The environment should be designed to protect the wound from microbial invasion. Reverse isolation, laminar air flow, or a plastic isolator are examples of methods sometimes used to control the environment of the burn patient. Provide warmth because the burned patient loses body heat during fluid shifts. Hospital burn units generate levels of noise and disturbance that can cause sleep deprivation.

Pediatric considerations

Pediatric patients have thinner skin and greater surface area in proportion to body weight. Greater surface area loses more heat and fluid by evaporation. The metabolic rate is higher in children than in adults, even at a resting state. Urine output of very small pediatric patients from birth to 2 years of age may vary from hour to hour. Several hours of output should be evaluated in succession and compared with cardiac output.

Physiologic Approach To Postburn Reconstruction

Each area of the body has a specific pattern of care. Function of the burned part is the prime consideration followed by the aesthetics of form. The result of reconstruction will depend on the physiologic condition of the patient, quality and quantity of available autologous donor tissues, prevention of complications, and the skill of the restorative team.

Head and neck

Patients with sustained burns to the face fall into four categories of facial plastic surgery: emergent, urgent, essential, and desirable. Emergent procedures facilitate lifesaving measures, such as creating an airway after an oropharyngeal burn. Urgent procedures are performed during the acute phase to meet a need for immediate attention. These include a flap to cover exposed bone or cartilage, a graft to protect an exposed eye, or a release to allow the mouth to open for eating, access for anesthesia, or dental care.

Essential procedures restore function and aid with physical movement. Examples include release of contractures that impede movement, such as a neck release (Fig. 7-36) or an eyelid ectropian repair. Neck contracture causes facial distortion and is addressed as early as possible. When neck contractures are released, it sets the stage for further reconstruction.

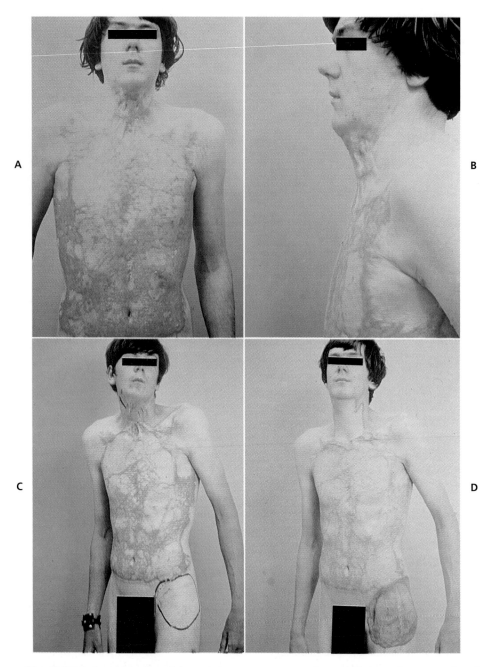

Fig. 7-36 A, Anterior view of thoracic burn contractures. **B,** Lateral view of contracted neck burn scar. Note limited extension of neck. **C,** Graft site marking on left anterior iliac crest for repair of anterior neck contracture. **D,** Healed graft site on left iliac crest and grafted anterior neck contracture. *(Courtesy Brian W. Davies, MD.)*

The eyelids are considered for early reconstruction because of their function and the aesthetic importance for the burn patient. Singed eyelashes should be trimmed away with small scissors coated with tobramycin or bacitracin ointment to prevent stray hairs from falling on to the conjunctiva. Full-thickness grafts or high-quality, thick split grafts can be used. Another area for early reconstructive consideration is the neck. Scalp wounds are allowed to heal with plans for the movement of hair-bearing flaps. Tissue expansion is used as needed.

Facial reconstruction consists of the cheek, nasolabial fold, lip, mouth, and the forehead. This is accomplished by using adjacent advancement flaps and skin grafts to replace tissue loss. The nasolabial fold is revised early before the scar has a chance to mature. The mouth and chin, however, benefit from a mature scar. Correction is done by means of splinting. Contoured areas are complex to restore. Mesh grafts heal in uneven pigment and texture (cobblestone), and although good for contoured areas, mesh grafts are not the graft of choice for facial restoration.

Damaged eyebrows and ears may be camouflaged by makeup and hair styling, especially for females. The ears are often restored last in a multistage otoplastic procedure. Missing ears can be fashioned from autologous rib cartilage covered by a local flap.

Desirable procedures include scar revision, resurfacing procedures, blending of irregular pigmentation, and other aesthetic modifications.

Upper extremities and hands

Treatment objectives of a burned arm and/or hand include functional aspects, such as fine pinch and power-grip in addition to appearance. Restoration to the workplace and self care are prime considerations.

Scar hypertrophy and contracture of the hand, elbow, and axilla complicate return to form and function. Prevent webbing between fingers by dressing each finger individually. Compression garments are commonly used in addition to standard burn tissue treatments. Physical therapy is progressively advanced as far as possible. The patient's physiologic condition and severity of the burn determine whether treatment is rendered on an outpatient basis or if hospitalization is necessary.

Anterior and posterior trunk

Burns of the trunk commonly present with upper and lower extremity burns. Trunk grafting is sometimes delayed causing the risk of contraction and hypertrophic scar development without creating any functional deformity. Burns to the anterior chest can create significant distortions to developing breasts. Debridement, especially around the nipple and areolar area, is done conservatively. Abnormal breast development or positioning can result from skin distortion caused by scar formation. Contractures across the thorax or in the axilla can cause breast tissue to shift medially or laterally. Contractures will need surgical release with breast reconstruction similar to procedures described in Chapter 10. Compression garments may decrease the formation of hypertrophic scar tissue.

Partial-thickness burns heal by reepithelialization in approximately 2 weeks after the injury in the absence of complications. A return to normal function is quick, and the aesthetic result is satisfactory.

Full-thickness injury is more extensive and necessitates early excision of damaged tissue. This procedure is usually accompanied by significant blood loss. The techniques used to control bleeding include hypotensive anesthesia, elevation of the legs during surgery, and the use of thrombin and epinephrine. Electrocautery is used sparingly (if at all) because it causes devitalized char and debris in the wound.

Perineum

Because of the bacterial environment and the many contours of this region, the treatment of perineal burns is both challenging and complicated. Superficial burns are treated with antimicrobial ointments. Larger burns, as with the female genitalia, are treated with the standard debridement of the full-thickness injury and skin grafting. For better contouring, mesh grafts are commonly used. Z-shaped incisions made into the scar tissue (referred to as *Z-plasty*) are used to lengthen contraction bands that may form.

Perineal reconstruction includes release of contractures, excision of hypertrophic scars, and/or resurfacing with grafts or local flaps. Complete external genitalia reconstruction, such as penile and/or scrotal and labial, may be necessary. Appearance and dysfunction are difficult obstacles to overcome. Reconstructive methods include tube pedicle flaps, or most recently, axial myocutaneous flaps. Fasciocutaneous free-flaps have had considerable success. Reconstruction of genitalia with flaps is performed after wound closure and scar maturation is complete. In the male patient, these flaps are designed to allow the placement of a penile prosthesis for erectile function and for the creation of a neourethra.

Lower extremities and feet

Aggressive management of burn wounds and the early physical management of scars has resulted in a lowered incidence of scar contractures and resulting deformities of the lower extremities. In the acute stage of the injury, elevation of the affected lower limb is important and is the best means of controlling edema. The treatment of the lower extremity is planned to regain or maintain unimpeded weight-bearing and ambulation. Early ambulation is encouraged, although judiciously controlled. Long-standing bed rest can cause complications, such as deep vein thrombosis and pneumonia. Circulatory status is greatly improved by ambulating, thus causing increased tissue perfusion, improved renal function, and more rapid clearing of burn shock edema.

The feet of the insensate patient, as found in diabetic neuropathy or spinal cord injury, are at high risk for burns. These patients delay seeking medical attention because they are often unaware of the injury because they lack pain sensation. Healing is prolonged because the wounds are commonly infected and the patient's circulatory status is impaired. Good management of the burned foot consists of careful cleansing, application of topical antibacterial dressing, and splinting to minimize scar formation of the toes and heel cord shortening.

Foot wound management is complicated by chronic pain, chronic instability of any soft-tissue coverage, ulceration of weightbearing or nonweightbearing areas, chronic osteomyelitis, contractures, gait abnormalities, and contour deformities.

Unyielding hypertrophic scars and contractures can cause secondary growth disturbances of the feet of children. Feet resurfaced with split-thickness skin grafts at an early age may require repeated releases and application of additional skin grafts until the child reaches maturity.

Misdiagnosis of the actual extent or depth of the burn injury can prolong the recovery period. Wounds that persist beyond 3 weeks should be debrided and grafted. Misdiagnosis of burn severity is sometimes complicated because the full extent of the wound may not be apparent for weeks or months after the initial burn. This can be adversely influenced by coexisting medical problems or other traumatic injuries.

Burn Complications

Hypertrophic scars

Hypertrophic scars result from the inflammatory responses caused by the release of polypeptide growth factors. These chemicals eventually lead to a thick deposition of a collagen and protein matrix at the site of injury. The result is a thickened scar over the length and width of the boundaries of the wound.

Controlling hypertrophic scars is challenging and often is beyond the control of the plastic reconstructive surgeon. Several techniques are used with some success. Pressure garments and silicone gel sheets have been reported to have produced favorable outcomes.

Contractures

Contractures are a common side effect of thermal burn injury. They can be prevented, or at least minimized, by an aggressive approach including early wound closure and physical scar management. While the burn scar tissue is immature, physical management with splints, casts (usually cylindrical), and elastic compression garment therapy can help preserve some function. The patient's mobility is monitored and increased frequently until the burn scar has stretched enough to allow maximum range of motion.

Decisions in the management of contractures are usually based on the age of the scar and the extent of the physical impairment. A contracture begins in the initial burn scar as it penetrates the dermal and subdermal layers. As the burn scar matures, the contracture advances into the deeper structures, including ligaments, tendons, and neurovascular structures. Contractures result in permanent shortening of tissue, which can only be released surgically. Methods such as flaps or Z-plasty are commonly used (Fig. 7-37).

The development of a lesion in a chronic, nonhealing scar is known as a Marjolin ulcer, first described by Marjolin in 1928 in a burn scar. SCC can arise in any chronic wound, such as venous stasis ulcers, chronic osteomyelitis, pilonidal sinus, and pressure sores. The majority of these ulcers occur in the lower extremity and have a high rate of regional metastasis. A biopsy and possibly a prophylactic nodal dissection are the initial treatments of choice.

Compartment compression syndrome

Edema caused by burn shock may cause compartment compression syndrome. The fascial covering of a part becomes snug and immobile against swelling tissue. Contracture bands interfere with circulation. This is commonly seen in circumferential deep burns. An escharotomy should be performed at the wound, but a compartment fasciotomy requiring anesthesia is usually necessary.

Bibliography

Anderson LL et al: Tattoo pigment mimicking metastatic malignant melanoma, *Dermatol Surg* 22(1):92,1996.

Anderson RR et al: Cosmetic ink darkening: a complication of Q-switched and pulsed-laser treatment, *Arch Dermatol* 129(8):1010,1993.

Armstrong ML et al: Motivation for tattoo removal, *Arch Dermatol* 132(4):412, 1996.

Ashinoff R et al: Allergic reactions to tattoo pigment after laser treatment, *Dermatol Surg* 21(4):291, 1995.

Bondville J: Pain-free harvesting of skin grafts with EMLA, *Plast Surg Nurs* 14(4):231, 1994.

Brown CD, Zitelli JA: The prognosis and treatment of true local cutaneous recurrent malignant melanoma, *Dermatol Surg* 21(4):285, 1995.

Clamon J, Netscher DT: General principles of flap reconstruction: goals for aesthetic and functional outcome, *Plast Surg Nurs* 14(1):9, 1994.

Clark CP: Alpha hydroxy acids in skin care, *Clin Plast Surg* 23(1):49, 1996.

Dinman S, Giovannone MK: The care and feeding of microvascular flaps: how nurses can help prevent flap loss, *Plast Surg Nurs* 14(3):154, 1994.

Fleming ID et al: Principles of management of basal and squamous cell carcinomas of the skin, *Cancer* 75(2):699, 1995.

Forte R et al: Chemical peeling, *Plast Surg Nurs* 13(4):194, 1993.

Golden MA et al: Leech therapy in digital replantation, *AORN J* 62(3):364, 1995.

Guyuron B, Vaughan C: Medical-grade tattooing to camouflage depigmented scars, *Plast Reconstr Surg* 95(3):575, 1995.

Hodersdal M et al: Skin reflectance-guidance laser selections for treatment of decorative tattoos, *Arch Dermatol* 123(4):403, 1996.

James WA et al: Psychiatric reactions to leeches, *Acad Psych Med* 34(1):83, 1993.

Netscher D et al: Surgical repair of pressure ulcers, *Plast Surg Nurs* 16(4):225, 1996.

Netscher DT, Clamon J: Smoking: adverse effects on outcomes for plastic surgery, *Plast Surg Nurs* 205, 1994.

Nicol NH, Fenske NA: Photodamage: cause, clinical manifestations, and prevention, *Plast Surg Nurs* 16(1):9, 1996.

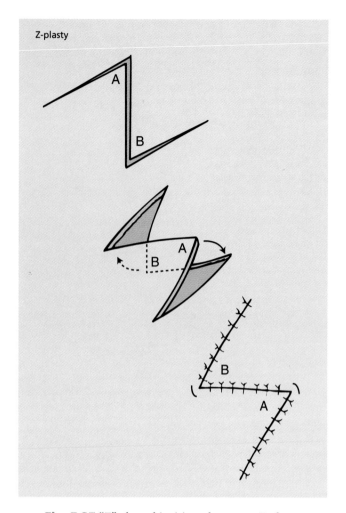

Z-plasty

Fig. 7-37 "Z"-shaped incisions, known as Z-plasty.

Ratner D, Grande DJ: Mohs' micrographic surgery: an overview, *Derm Nurs* 6(4):269, 1994.

Rosenbach A, Alster TS: Cutaneous lasers: a review, *Ann Plast Surg* 37(2):220, 1996.

Rosenberg GJ, Gregory RO: Lasers in aesthetic surgery, *Clin Plast Surg* 23(1):29, 1996.

Ryan F, LaFourcade C: Skin care, chemical face peeling, and skin rejuvenation, *Plast Surg Nurs* 15(3):167, 1995.

Spear SL, Arias J: Long-term experience with nipple-areola tattooing, *Ann Plast Surg* 35(3):232, 1995.

Vander Kam VM, Achauer BM: Laser resurfacing, *Plast Surg Nurs* 15(4):222, 1995.

Vander Kam VM, Achauer BM: Metastatic skin disease in an immunocompromised patient, *Plast Surg Nurs* 14(3):192, 1994.

Vander Kam VM, Achauer BM: Management of vascular premalignant nevi in the pediatric population, *Plast Surg Nurs* 14(2):79, 1994.

Walsh KC: Extinguishing burn injuries through public awareness, *Plast Surg Nurs* 12(4):164, 1992.

Westlake C: Commitment to function: microsurgical flaps, *Plast Surg Nurs* 11(3):95, 1991.

Williams L, Gregory R: Laser surgery, *Plast Surg Nurs* 13(2):106, 1993.

8 Subsurface Modification of the Trunk and Limbs

Reduction or augmentation of body parts with minimal scarring is the goal of using subsurface techniques. Some subsurface techniques such as fat removal or placement of an implant may require excision of excess overlying skin to give the body a sculpted, more aesthetic form.

Reconstructive procedures commonly involve subsurface techniques that utilize tissue expanders to increase skin volume and bulk. Additional skin is needed for reconstructive procedures to cover an adjacent defect without creating a separate donor wound for a skin graft. A tissue expander is also used for the creation of a subsurface space for the placement of a permanent implant. Some types of tissue expanders remain in place as the permanent implant after the expansion process is complete.

Some areas of the body are less receptive to diet and exercise and require surgical alteration to attain specific size and tone. Patients who have lipodystrophy or have lost large amounts of weight benefit from procedures such as suction-assisted lipectomy and excision of redundant skin. Retraction of skin and scars after these procedures gives the appearance of a more shapely, toned body. As a result, the patient feels a sense of self-improvement and increased confidence.

Areas of the body commonly reduced and reshaped by suction and/or excision include the upper arms, thighs, calves, flanks, abdomen, buttocks, neck, portions of the face, and chest. Etching and refinement of muscular features can be performed with minimal discomfort and scarring. Redundant skin can be excised from nearly every area of the body.

Augmentation of specific body parts by autografting, biomaterials, or synthetic implants vary according to sex. Males may request augmentation of specific muscle groups, such as the pectorals or gastrocnemius, by implants. Some request augmentation phalloplasty procedures, such as dermal-fat grafting for girth increase of 2 to 3 inches or suspensory ligament release of the corpora from the pubic bone for visual length of 1 to 2 inches.

Females request augmentation of the breasts (discussed in Chapter 10). Both sexes may request facial implants, such as cheeks, jaw line, or chin. Reconstructive surgeons use augmentation techniques and materials to rebuild physical features after significant tissue loss caused by a congenital defect, accident, or illness.

SUBSURFACE REDUCTION TECHNIQUES: SUCTION-ASSISTED LIPECTOMY

Excess fat can be removed by manual syringe, vacuum suction, and most recently, ultrasonic suction-aspiration. A minimal, well-placed scar less than 1 centimeter in size is all that remains after wound healing is complete. The risk of complications is minimal, and the results are very pleasing to the patient.

Anatomy and Physiology

The surface layers of the skin are the cutaneous epidermis and the dermis. Subcutaneous layers differ in thickness and composition by location on the body. Each level is separated by a layer of fascia (Fig. 8-1). Directly under the dermis and over the subcutaneous fascia is a layer of dense tissue referred to as Camper's fascia. Fibrous septa (retinacula cutis) form divisions in this layer between compact collections of adipose tissue containing nerves, blood vessels, and lymphatics that connect to the superficial dermal layers. Between the subcutaneous fascia and the muscle fascial layer is Scarpa's fascia. The adipose tissue in this region is looser with fewer septa. Distribution of adipose tissue over muscle is equal on both sides of the body bilaterally. These distribution patterns differ by race, sex, age, and physiologic structure.

Adipose tissue consists of adipocytes located in an areolar meshwork that store and release fatty acids in response to the body's need for energy. Every part of the body has variable deposits of adipose except the subcutaneous tissue of the eyelids, penis, scrotum, labia minora, cranial cavity, and lungs (except at the bases). Adipocytes are present in the fetus at 14 weeks' gestation and stabilize in number at adolescence. Under normal circumstances, adipocytes do not regenerate. An existing cell can increase by two to five times its normal size to store excess fat, but under normal circumstances new cells do not form. In morbid obesity in excess of 150% ideal body weight, adipocytes may increase in number.

Cellulite forms when the retinacula cutis expands and distorts laterally in response to enlarging adipocytes (Fig. 8-2). The superficial skin has the appearance of dimples and ripples because the underlayers are irregularly anchored to the skin by the septa. This phenomena is primarily characteristic of females. Some physicians have recently begun to treat areas of cellulite with minor suction, disruption of the fibrous attachments, and autologous injection of fat to smooth the defects (Fig. 8-3).

Indications

Fat removal from subsurface layers includes debulking flaps, reducing or removing lipomas, and lipectomy. Lipodystrophy can result from alteration of tissue at a specific site or predisposition

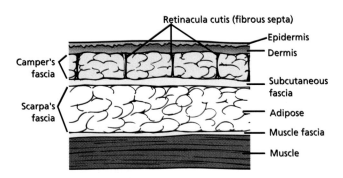

Fig. 8-1 Layers of adipose tissue in reference to fascial layers. Tissue thickness and structure vary according to anatomic location on body.

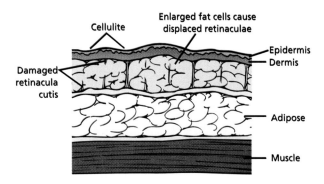

Fig. 8-2 Areas of damaged retinaculae and displacement by enlarged fat cells.

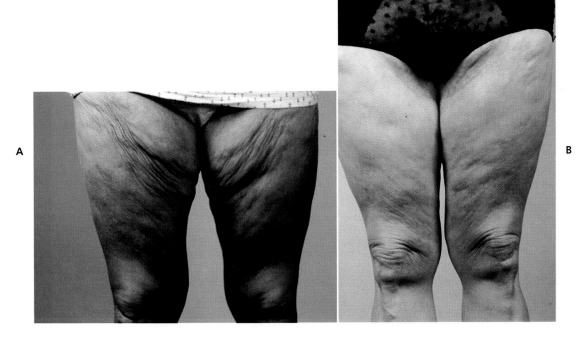

Fig. 8-3 Cellulite before (**A**) and after (**B**) liposuction. *(Courtesy Brian W. Davies, MD.)*

to localized areas of diet and exercise resistant fat. Weight gain tends to be centralized in these areas. Diet resistant fat is the target of suction-assisted lipectomy. Suction-assisted lipectomy is performed below the subcutaneous fascia to preserve the vessels, lymphatics, and nerves that run parallel to the fibrous septa.

This procedure is not intended to replace proper diet and exercise for weight reduction. Weight removed by suction-assisted lipectomy will range from 2 to 4 pounds. Self-image usually improves after the procedure, and the resultant positive attitude promotes a healthier approach to diet and exercise.

Patient Selection Considerations

Patients should be under 40 years of age (or over 40 with good skin elasticity) (Fig. 8-4), without serious health problems, and close to normal weight with good skin tone. Poor results

occur in patients with poor skin turgor, stretch marks, and/or cellulite. Suction-assisted lipectomy may result in the need for excision of loose skin, which leaves a scar. Criteria for suction lipectomy include the patient's realistic expectations of the results of the procedure.

Males commonly request suction-assisted lipectomy of submentum, anterior neck, bilateral flanks (love handles), epigastrium (spare tire), and hypogastrium (beer belly). Gynecomastia (Fig. 8-5) is often treated by suction-assisted lipectomy (see Chapter 10). Masculine body contouring emphasizes youth and health (Fig. 8-6).

Females frequently seek suction-assisted lipectomy of submentum, anterior neck, lower abdomen, thighs, buttocks, lateral trochanteric regions, and medial knees. Women tend to have thicker subcutaneous tissue, more stretch marks, cellulite, and denser areas of concentrated fat (Fig. 8-7).

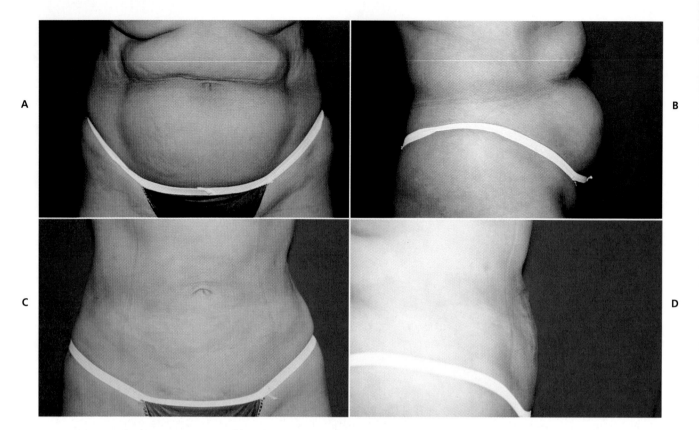

Fig. 8-4 Liposuction of female patient. Fat distribution over age 40 with good skin elasticity. **A and B,** Preoperative. **C and D,** Postoperative. *(Courtesy Brian W. Davies, MD.)*

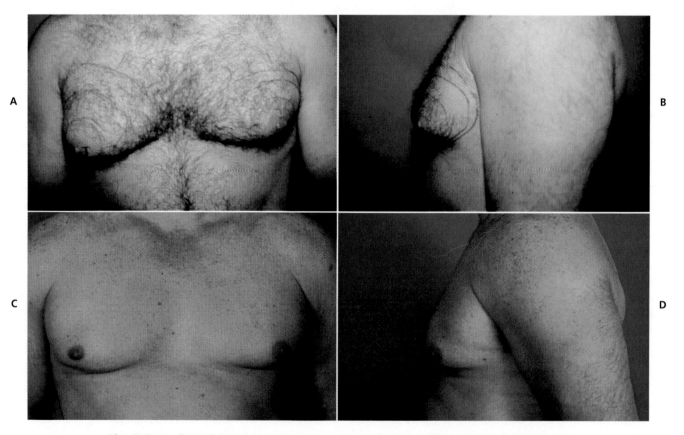

Fig. 8-5 A and B, Adult male gynecomastia patient with topographic markings for liposuction. **C and D,** Postoperative. *(Courtesy Brian W. Davies, MD.)*

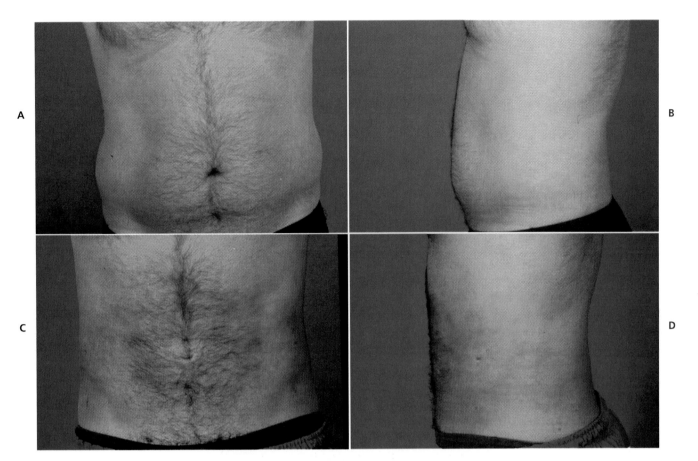

Fig. 8-6 Male pattern fat deposits for liposuction. **A and B,** Preoperative. **C and D,** Postoperative. *(Courtesy Brian W. Davies, MD.)*

Contraindications

A careful preoperative history and physical examination is performed to detect the potential for complications of the procedure. Psychologically, the patient should have a realistic view of the potential results. Physiologically, the patient should not be placed at risk for avoidable complications caused by preexisting infection, coagulopathy, diabetes, collagen disease, anemia, or nutritional deficit. Systemic diseases complicate the recovery from a suction lipectomy procedure. Healing time is prolonged, the potential for bleeding is increased, and infection is a serious threat.

Hernias can predispose the patient to penetration injury. Weakened areas of the abdomen such as a herniated umbilicus or inguinal canal can separate during cannula insertion causing damage to the bowel and underlying organs.

Extremely obese patients are not candidates for suction-assisted lipectomy. Suction lipectomy will not solve the problems associated with dietary intake in excess of nutritional requirements. Obesity may be a sign of a potential psychologic problem with self-image. Counseling and dietary modification should be considered. Use of lipectomy cannot safely or effectively remove large volumes of accumulated adipose tissue.

Preoperative Patient Care

Before the procedure, the patient is fitted with a compression garment if one is to be worn after the procedure. The patient is advised to stop smoking and refrain from alcohol consumption for at least 2 weeks before and after the procedure. Use of oral contraception may increase the risk of thromboembolism, and consideration is given to discontinue its use 1 month before the procedure. Some physicians plan to perform the procedure after the female patient has completed her menstrual cycle to minimize effects of hormonal influence on capillary fragility.

The area to be suctioned is contour marked in a standing position with curvilinear lines similar to a topographic map (Fig. 8-8). Incisions are planned to be hidden under a bathing suit (Fig. 8-9). Photographs are taken from anterior, lateral, and posterior views.

Intraoperative Patient Care

The patient is positioned for exposure of the site and secured with appropriate safety belts. The skin is prepped with an antimicrobial cleansing solution taking care not to scrub away the topographic markings. The surgical sites are draped to provide maximum surface exposure using sterile technique.

A bed or patient transport cart should be readily available if the patient is to be positioned in the prone position. In the event of an emergency such as cardiac arrest, repositioning the patient to a supine position may be a critical factor in patient stabilization. Appropriate numbers of personnel should be available for patient repositioning as necessary.

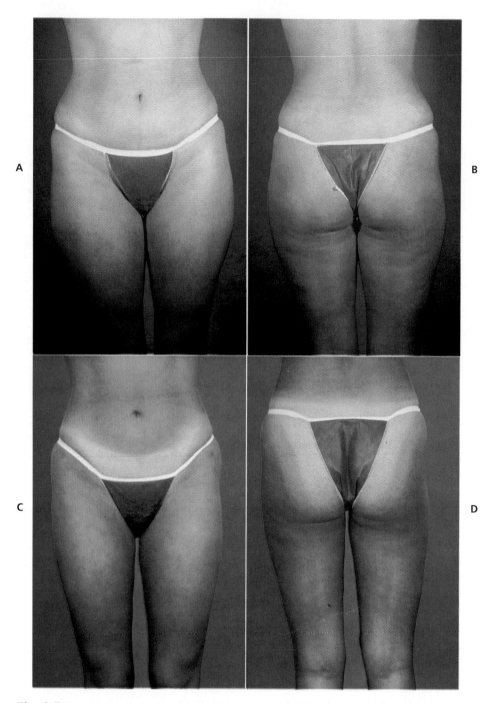

Fig. 8-7 Female pattern fat distribution. Suction-assisted lipectomy of hips, buttocks, and thighs. **A and B,** Preoperative. **C and D,** Postoperative. *(Courtesy Brian W. Davies, MD.)*

Anesthesia

Intravenous conscious sedation (IVCS) with local infiltration is commonly used with great patient satisfaction. In combination with tumescent technique, IVCS has proven to be highly effective for suction-assisted liposuction. Careful physiologic monitoring is performed one-on-one by an anesthesia provider or perioperative nurse. General anesthesia also is an acceptable method for the procedure.

Fluid volume replacement is given 2:1 or 2.5:1 (fluid to aspirate ratio). Crystalloid (Ringer's lactate) is the replacement fluid of choice, although 80% leaves the intravascular compartment and enters the interstitium. A Foley catheter is frequently used to monitor urine output and relieve a full bladder.

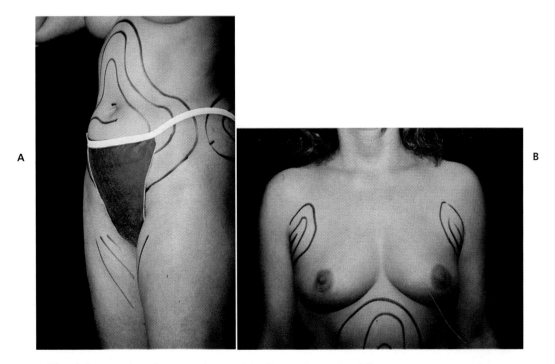

Fig. 8-8 Examples of topographic marking for suction-assisted lipectomy. *(Courtesy Brian W. Davies, MD.)*

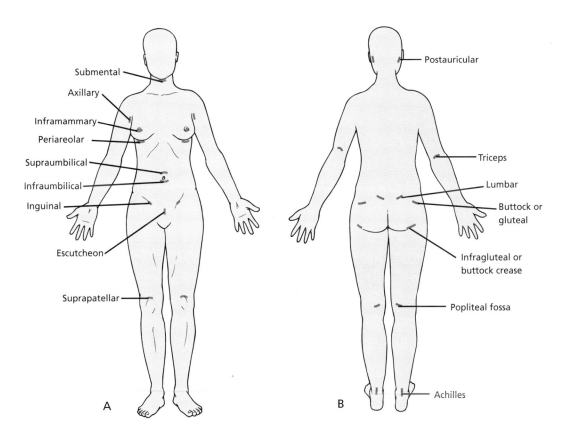

Fig. 8-9 Incision area for suction-assisted lipectomy. Incisions measure 1 cm or less.

Tumescent infusion

Large amounts of sterile saline irrigation containing lidocaine, epinephrine, bicarbonate, and/or triamolone are infiltrated into target adipose layers (Fig. 8-10). Fluid delivery devices include spring-loaded syringes, roller pump machines, and manual syringes for small areas (Fig. 8-11). The concentration of tumescent additives may vary, but the result is similar. Bicarbonate buffers and lidocaine provide an anesthetic effect. Epinephrine causes vasoconstriction, minimizing blood loss. Some physicians add a corticosteroid such as triamolone for an antiinflammatory effect. Desired vasoconstriction is evident when the overlying skin appears blanched. Ultimately, the fat becomes hydrated, allowing smoother passage of the suction cannula. Operator fatigue is decreased by less resistance in adipose layers during passage of the cannula.

Commonly used lidocaine solutions are composed of 100 ml 1% lidocaine with epinephrine 1:100,000 in 1 liter of sterile

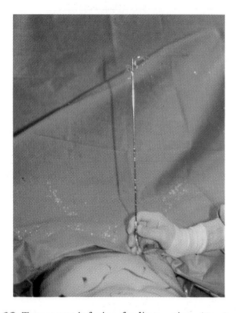

Fig. 8-10 Tumescent infusion for liposuction. *(Courtesy Brian W. Davies, MD.)*

normal saline (0.9%). This solution equals 0.1% solution with epinephrine 1:1,000,000. Some physicians prefer to use 0.5% lidocaine with epinephrine 1:200,000 in place of 1% lidocaine. Studies have shown that warming the tumescent solution to 40° C before administration increases patient comfort and may actually enhance the initial absorptive effects of lidocaine.

Using infiltration of large amounts of saline-based solution causes the tissue to become firm and easier to work with. High-pressure mechanical infusion systems can deliver 5 to 6 liters of fluid in 20 minutes. Infiltration with a small bore, blunt-tipped cannula is less traumatic and pretunnels the area for suction. Small sites can be infiltrated with an 18-gauge needle and a 20 to 60 cc syringe.

Blood loss in tumescent technique is minimal with an average mean hemoglobin loss of 9 mg/dl per 100 grams of adipose tissue removed as compared with up to a 20 mg/dl loss in a dry, noninfused liposuction procedure. Blood loss replacement therapy is uncommon. Patients who may be potential candidates for blood replacement can donate autologous blood up to 42 days before the procedure. The patient should be informed that most blood banking services charge a service fee for this storage service. No specific testing for human immunodeficiency virus (HIV) or hepatitis B virus (HBV) is performed because the donor is the same recipient. If the blood is not needed by the patient, it is discarded and not saved for use by another patient.

Tumescent technique enables the use of higher concentrations of lidocaine without toxicity. The average safe dose for tumescence is generally 35 mg/kg, but the literature reports use of 55 mg/kg without ill effect. Studies have shown that the lidocaine reaches its peak plasma level between 4 and 8 hours after infiltration. Some residual plasma lidocaine levels can be measured 24 hours after the procedure (see Chapter 4).

Procedures

Facial resculpting may be performed in combination with other procedures, such as rhytidectomy. As a primary procedure, removal of too much fat without excess skin excision can cause an aged appearance because of decreased skin elasticity. Tumescence can be used with favorable results at more controllable levels. The

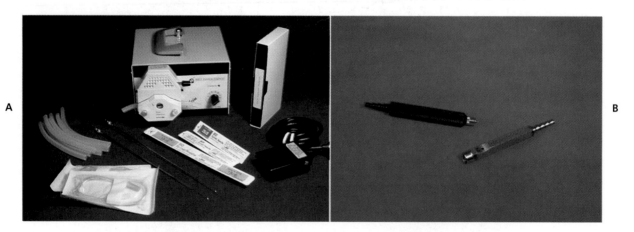

Fig. 8-11 Examples of fluid delivery devices for tumescent infusion. *(Courtesy Wells Johnson, Tucson, Arizona.)*

openings in the suction cannula should be directed away from the skin surface to preserve subdermal planes. Each pass of the cannula is performed in a criss-cross pattern to prevent linear deformities during healing. Care is taken to not reach the level of the facial nerve.

Neck liposuction works well with tumescence (between 200 and 500 ml) and small cannulae (1.5 to 3 mm). Small incisions are made behind the ears and in the central submentum. The cannula is passed with the openings away from the skin leaving at least a 2 mm margin of subcutaneous tissue to preserve elasticity. The average amount of neck fat removed is under 50 ml. The pinch test can help the surgeon determine equality of both sides of the neck. Undertreatment is recommended of the face and neck because it is easier to touch up the work later than to graft fat to fill in defects. Final touch-up can be performed with a syringe at a later date after the procedure if necessary (Fig. 8-12).

Upper arm contouring by suction, often referred to as suction brachioplasty, is performed using tumescent technique. Incisions are made into the axilla and antecubital fossa. Postoperative compressive dressings should be applied starting at the distal aspect of the arm wrapping upward to the proximal aspect.

Epigastric suctioning accentuates the chest and linea alba. The supraumbilical and inframammary incisions are easily concealed. The central groove created by the suction cannula in an upward-contouring motion through the umbilical incision gives definition to the upper abdominal lines. Hypogastric suctioning through infraumbilical and pubic line incisions is greatly facilitated by tumescence (Fig. 8-13). Care is taken to palpate the tip with each pass of the cannula. Untoward abdominal perforation can occur causing enteral injury.

Posterior thigh and buttock suctioning is performed through infragluteal crease and lateral gluteal incisions. The

fat is suctioned evenly and carefully using tumescent technique to protect fibrous attachments. The cannula is passed in a criss-cross pattern to create an even undersurface. Care is taken at the midline of the buttocks to avoid injury to anorectal tissue.

Anterior thigh suctioning is performed through lateral peripatellar and inguinal incisions. The cannula is passed along the axis of the thigh in a longitudinal fashion using tumescent technique. The medial knee and suprapatellar fat are approached through the same patellar incisions.

Ankle and lower leg fat is suctioned with extreme caution through incisions in the popliteal fossa and the lateral and medial borders of the Achilles tendon near the superior aspect of the heel. Anatomically, the subcutaneous tissue is extremely thin and subject to rapid edema. The lack of superficial fascia gives rise to bloodier aspirate. Tumescence is used, and the cannula is passed slowly with the opening directed away from the skin. Use of sequential compression stockings after the procedure can reduce the risk of complications. Tissue remodeling in this area can take 6 months or more.

Tissue aspirate appears yellow and pink-tinged as the suction lipectomy is performed. The aspirate appears bloodier as the end-point of adipose removal is reached. The skin is pinched to determine texture of the underlying areas (Fig. 8-14). The desired outcome is a thin, even surface. The surgeon can easily find contour irregularities by moistening his or her gloved hand with sterile saline before feeling the surface of the sculpted area. The suction cannula also can be rolled across the skin surface like a rolling pin to find any remaining lumps or bumps. Residual lumps can be resculpted to even out the area (Fig. 8-15). The average amount of aspirate ranges between 1500 and 2000 cc. Some patients can tolerate removal of 2500 to 3500 cc with the use of tumescence.

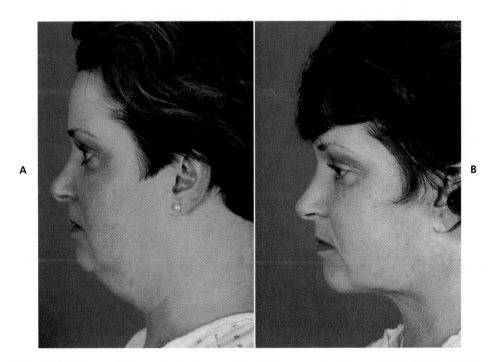

Fig. 8-12 Submental liposuction **A,** Preoperative. **B,** Postoperative. *(Courtesy Brian W. Davies, MD.)*

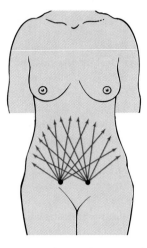

Fig. 8-13 Fan directional paths for lower abdominal suction-assisted lipectomy.

Equipment

Handles and hubs of the suction handpiece are made of stainless steel, aluminum, and other reusable materials (Fig. 8-16). Disposable and reusable stainless steel, blunt-tipped cannulae that fit into the handles and hubs are available in a variety of lengths (5 to 40 cm) and diameters (1.5 to 10 mm) with suction lumens aligned in specific patterns at varying distances from the tip. Blunt-tipped cannulae wedge into adipose tissue. They can enter just above the fascial plane without cutting nerves, vessels, lymphatics, and most importantly, the retinacula cutis. Three styles of blunt tips are commercially available (Fig. 8-17). Some are designed to remove more adipose tissue in bulk in the legs and trunk, and others are designed to sculpt finer features, such the neck and face. Smaller diameter cannulae produce the best results. Reusable models are cleaned with intralumenal brushes and terminally cleaned in an ultrasonic washer. Complex instrumentation

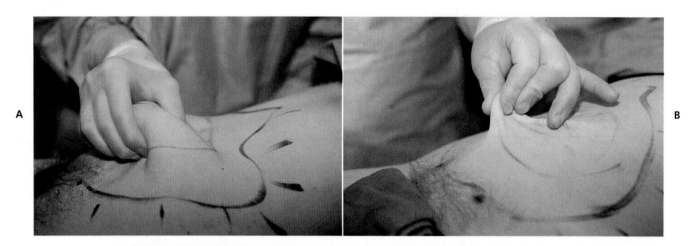

Fig. 8-14 **A,** Pinch test before procedure. **B,** Pinch test after procedure. *(Courtesy Brian W. Davies, MD.)*

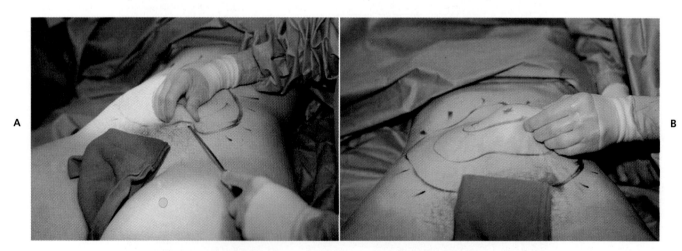

Fig. 8-15 Touch-up at conclusion of liposuction procedure. *(Courtesy Brian W. Davies, MD.)*

should be gas or steam sterilized. Stainless steel needles for use with Toomey syringes are available in 10- to 16-gauge. Custom designs with hooks, spatulae, and bifid (two prong) dissector tips also can be used for other applications, such as endoscopy (Fig. 8-18).

High-power, low-noise mechanical suction machines (Fig. 8-19) are commonly used for larger areas. Disposable suction liners and tubing are recommended for infection control. Disposable inline bacterial filters to 0.2 microns are used to minimize airborne biohazardous exhaust. Manual syringe aspiration is performed with tiny cannulas in smaller areas or as a finishing touch-up for facial lines (Fig. 8-20).

Ultrasonic, suction-assisted lipectomy is performed using ultrasonic probes that liquefy and aspirate fat, sparing nerves, vessels, and lymphatics. Ecchymoses and blood loss are minimal, and the result is a smooth surface contour. The ultrasonic probe, cannula, and handpiece are cooled by sterile normal saline to prevent heat build-up and tissue burns.

Postoperative Patient Care

Compression of the skin against the muscle helps secure hemostasis and control the final retraction of the skin envelope. Skin retraction secondary to scarring prevents drooping tissue

deformities. Wide bands of adhesive tape can be secured over the area for 7 to 10 days after the procedure to provide support to the healing tissue.

Compression garments are commercially available to help mold and shape the recontoured tissue (Fig. 8-21). They are only removed according to the surgeon's routine for showers and laundering. These are worn for several weeks after the procedure to control edema and support the healing tissue. The garment has openings for personal hygiene that are secured by hooks and Velcro.

Care is taken to ensure that the skin remains smooth under supportive tape or compression garment. Wrinkles and skin folds secured under pressure may cause a healing deformity and/or tissue damage. Sutures are removed 5 to 7 days after the procedure. Tissue remodeling takes approximately 3 months in most areas of the body, except the lower legs.

The patient is advised to avoid strenuous activity for several days after the procedure and may drive and return to work after 1 week. Light exercise such as walking may be resumed within 2 to 3 days. Sexual activity may resume after 2 weeks. Mild pain medication may be prescribed. Postoperative pain is usually caused by tissue edema. This gradually subsides over a period of 6 months.

Aspirin, vitamin E, nonsteroidal antiinflammatory drugs (NSAIDS), and other medications that affect coagulation are avoided because they may cause postoperative bleeding and hematoma formation, which is a potential source of infection. Smoking is prohibited because it interferes with oxygenation and tissue healing. Sun exposure is not advised because the iron content of hemoglobin under the skin can cause staining. Proper nutrition is emphasized because nutritional needs will increase by a minimum of 50% for wound healing.

Complications

Divots (dips in the skin surface) result when the tip of the suction is angled toward the surface creating a subdermal defect. This may happen when a suction cannula is passed through the subdermal layers with the openings toward the skin. Contour irregularity may not be apparent for several months because of swelling. Revision may be necessary at a future date. Some temporary numbness may exist for several months. Permanent nerve injury is uncommon.

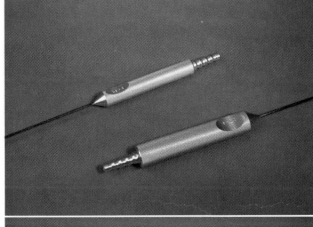
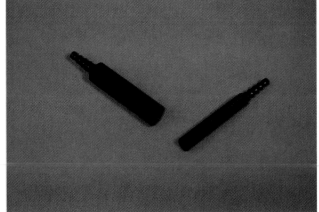

Fig. 8-16 Examples of handles and hubs of suction hand pieces. *(Courtesy Well Johnson, Tucson, Arizona.)*

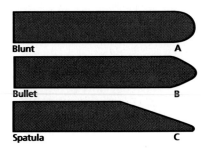

Fig. 8-17 Three styles of blunt cannulae tips. **A,** Blunt. **B,** Bullet. **C,** Spatula. *(Courtesy Wells Johnson, Tucson, Arizona.)*

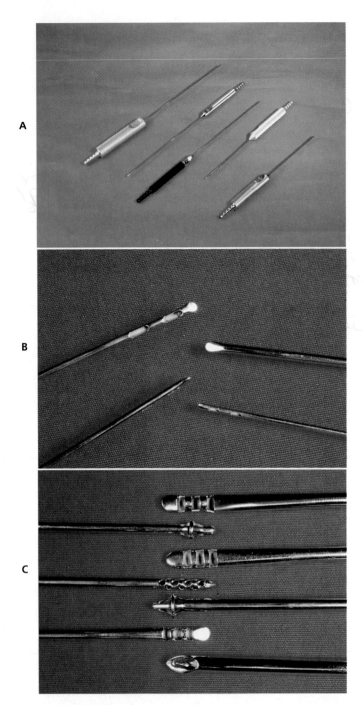

A

B

C

Fig. 8-18 **A,** Examples of custom-designed cannulae. **B and C,** Close-ups of cannulae tips. *(Courtesy Wells Johnson, Tucson, Arizona.)*

Prevention of thromboembolism begins with early mobilization and other antiembolic measures, such as support stockings and sequential compression devices. Sudden coughing, difficult respiratory effort, tachycardia, and hypoxemia may indicate pulmonary embolus and should be thoroughly assessed. Fat emboli is rare but can cause similar symptoms to pulmonary embolus. Thromboembolic symptoms can occur within hours to a few weeks after the procedure.

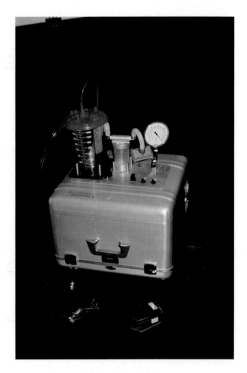

Fig. 8-19 Mechanical suction machine. *(Courtesy Wells Johnson, Tucson, Arizona.)*

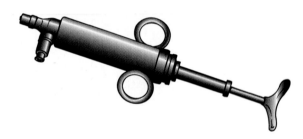

Fig. 8-20 Manual syringe.

Infection is a risk similar to any postsurgical wound. Redness, pain, and localized swelling 3 to 5 days after the procedure usually signal an infectious process. Purulent drainage should be cultured and antibiotic therapy started. Necrosis causes loss of devitalized tissue. The area should be debrided. Hematoma and seroma are minimized by the use of smaller cannulae and compression garments

ABDOMINOPLASTY

Cutaneous laxity of abdominal tissue in combination with diet and exercise-resistant fat interferes with aesthetic appearance and in extreme cases hinders personal hygiene. Physical and

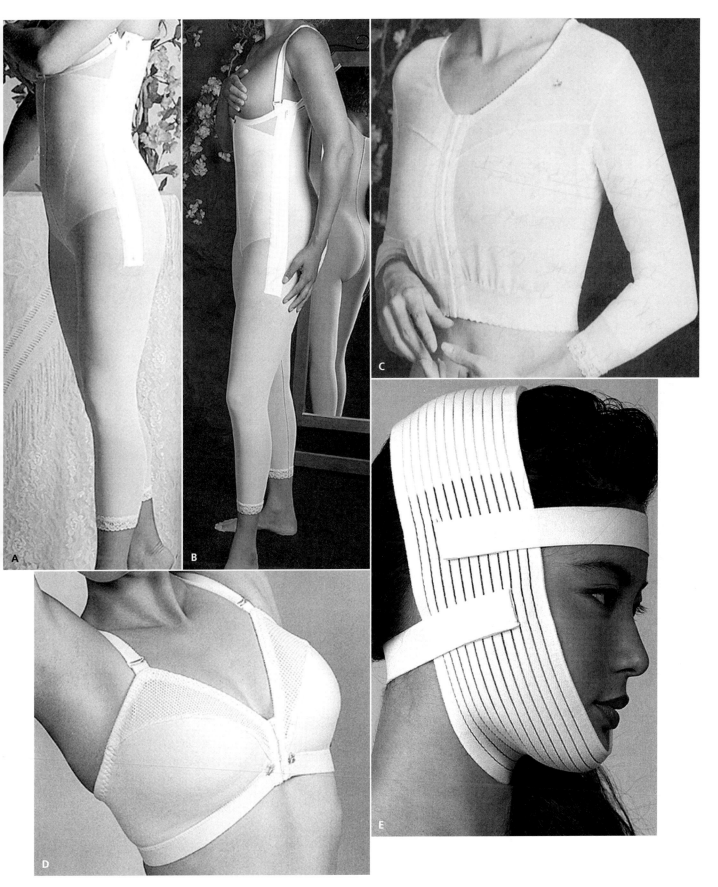

Fig. 8-21 Examples of compression garments. **A,** Full body. **B,** High back. **C,** Arm/vest. **D,** Bra. **E,** Neck and chin. *(Courtesy Design Veronique.)*

psychologic discomfort causes patients to seek surgical intervention for the problem (Fig. 8-22). Loss of tissue elasticity eliminates the use of suction-assisted lipectomy as a primary procedure, but it is still used in combination with sharp dissection. Abdominoplasty entails the same or a similar amount of dissection as a large myocutaneous flap but incorporates excision of a fatty skin segment and tightening of the underlying musculature. The procedure is performed to raise a large flap of abdominal tissue, pull it moderately taught, reposition it over the muscular recipient bed, and excise the excess. The rectus muscle is plicated as a subsurface modification before suturing the flap into place. The result is a smoother, tighter abdomen. Clothing fits comfortably with fewer bulges, and the silhouette is greatly improved.

Variations of this procedure include suction-assisted lipectomy in combination with sharp dissection of redundant skin. Suction lipectomy is not always advised if fat removal may jeopardize the flap. Mini-abdominoplasty is another option of lower abdominal tightening that extends sharp dissection between the pubis and the umbilicus for excision of redundant skin and fat. Classic abdominoplasty, described in more detail in this section, is commonly performed in combination with surgical procedures of other organ systems, such as hysterectomy or cholecystectomy, because visceral access is easier.

Anatomy and Physiology

The abdominal wall consists of muscles, fascia, blood vessels, and lymphatics outlined in a bony framework. This bony framework serves as a starting point for preoperative marking of surgical lines of dissection.

Surgical landmarks

Superficial landmarks of the exterior abdomen for preoperative marking include the following:

- Xyphoid
- Umbilicus
- Bilateral iliac crests
- Midline pubis
- Intermediate layers representing surgical landmarks
- Linea alba
- External oblique muscle
- Rectus abdominis muscle
- Aponeurosis rectus abdominis sheath

The outermost layer of abdominal skin and subcutaneous tissue overlies a strong, three-layered fibromembranous sheath, referred to as the *aponeurosis,* that covers and attaches the abdominal musculature. The linea alba is an essentially avascular tendinous band where the three layers of aponeurosis interlace in the midline from the xyphoid to the symphysis pubis. The umbilicus intersects the linea alba at the level of the iliac crests

The blood supply to the surgical layers associated with abdominoplasty arises laterally from the superficial epigastrics and the ascending and circumflex branches of the superficial iliac arteries and veins. The bilateral inferior and superior epigastric arteries and veins branch toward the midline. Innervation is from the anterior branches of the intercostal and subcostal nerves that arise from the level of T2 to T11 bilaterally. Lower portions are innervated by the bilateral anterior branches of the iliohypogastric and subcostal nerves that arise from the level of T12 to L1.

Indications and Contraindications

Abdominal skin and muscular tissue can become lax after weight loss and pregnancy. A panniculus, an apron of lax abdominal tissue, can bulge and hang over the pubic region causing disproportionate body dimensions. In other patients, the abdomen is the site of diet and exercise-resistant fat in combination with cutaneous laxity. Excision of loose skin and fat is

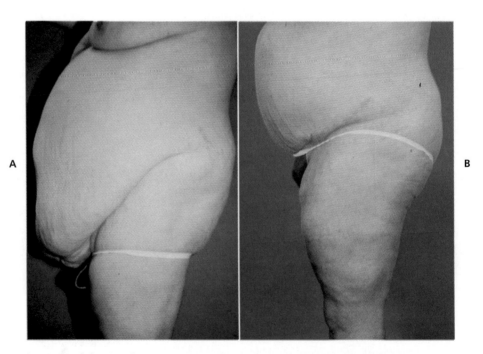

Fig. 8-22 Abdominoplasty. **A,** Preoperative. **B,** Postoperative. *(Courtesy Brian W. Davies, MD.)*

indicated if the patient is not planning further pregnancy, is within average weight parameters for height, accepts resultant abdominal scar, and is realistic about the results. Abdominoplasty is not the procedure of choice if the patient is planning future pregnancy, has had another abdominal incision that could interfere with circulation and wound healing, and/or has unrealistic expectations for the outcome.

A variation of this procedure is reverse abdominoplasty. This procedure requires an incision in the inframammary fold, and the loose skin of the upper abdomen is pulled cephalad to the inframammary line. This procedure may be done in combination with reduction mammoplasty.

Preoperative Patient Care

The patient is advised to avoid medications that would alter coagulation and to stop smoking for at least 2 weeks before the procedure. Risk factors that would adversely affect wound healing, such as diabetes, lupus, respiratory insufficiency, nutritional deficit, steroid use, and blood dyscrasias, are assessed. Uncontrolled systemic disease can cause tissue necrosis, slough, and the loss of the flap.

The patient is fitted for a postoperative compression garment. He or she is then marked with a surgical marker in a standing position because the full extent of abdominal laxity should be visualized. A midline vertical line is drawn from the xyphoid to the symphysis pubis, transecting the umbilicus in the center. Transverse lines may be drawn through the umbilicus at the level of the iliac crests and across the abdomen at the level of the anterior iliac spines. An oval-shaped line is drawn circumferentially around the umbilicus. Another line is drawn transversely along the pubic hair line before shaving to denote the proposed incision line. The surgical markings guide the lines of dissection and the subsequent reconstruction of the abdominal wall.

Intraoperative Patient Care

The bed should be padded with pressure-reducing material such as gel pads because the procedure may last between 2 and 4 hours. The patient is positioned supine and then into a modified beach chair position with the hips flexed and the arms secured on padded armboards as the procedure progresses (Fig. 8-23). A Foley catheter is placed to monitor urinary output and relieve bladder fullness. Antiembolism stockings or sequential compression devices should be used to prevent thromboembolism in the patient's legs. The leg strap is placed over the thighs.

The anesthesia provider usually administers regional or general anesthetic because of the extensive dissection associated with the procedure. Fluid replacement is closely monitored because the patient is at risk for volume deficit. Some surgeons request that the patient place one or more autologous units of blood in reserve. This blood is good for up to 42 days. The patient should be advised that most blood storage organizations charge an additional fee for maintaining autologous units.

Classic Procedure

The skin is carefully prepped from the nipple line to the anterior thighs, and the surgical site is draped using sterile technique. The primary incision is made to the fascial layer, extending from one iliac crest to the other (Fig. 8-24). Care is taken at the lateral margins because larger blood vessels intersect the intended incision line as they course superiorly. Smaller bleeders are coagulated with electrocautery, and larger vessels are ligated. Venous areas may seem to ooze persistently, but this is relieved by pressure. Excessive use of electrocautery can cause devitalization of tissue and promote flap loss.

Adequate exposure is critical to hemostasis. Retractors illuminated with fiberoptic cables are useful for deeper visualization. Blood loss from venous oozing can cause significant hypovolemia. Some surgeons and anesthesia providers request that blood loss be estimated throughout the procedure by weighing used sponges. Fluid replacement will be calculated according to patient condition, estimated blood loss, and urinary output. Irrigation and suctioned fluids should be calculated throughout the procedure.

The abdominal flap is progressively dissected free up to the umbilicus and raised, leaving as many vessels and nerves intact as possible (Fig. 8-25). A saline-moistened laparotomy sponge is placed over the exposed rectus muscle while the umbilical stalk is dissected free from the flap (Fig. 8-26). At this point, the operating bed is flexed to the modified beach chair position to decrease the tension on the patient's abdominal wall.

Dissection of the flap continues superiorly toward the xyphoid and bilateral costal margins. Exposure is particularly difficult because the dissection of the flap extends superiorly.

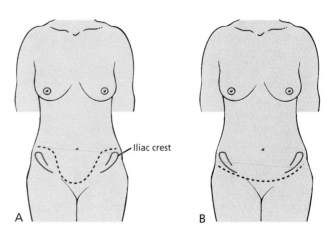

Fig. 8-24 Abdominoplasty incisions. **A,** Medial to iliac crest for patient who desires high "French cut" swimsuit. **B,** In natural abdominal skin creases below iliac crest.

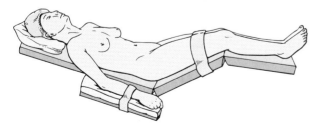

Fig. 8-23 Positioning of patient for abdominoplasty.

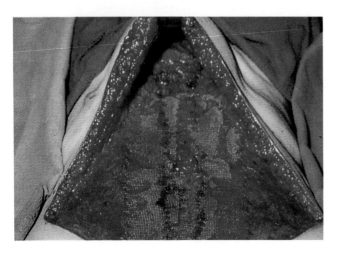

Fig. 8-25 Flap is raised. *(Courtesy Brian W. Davies, MD.)*

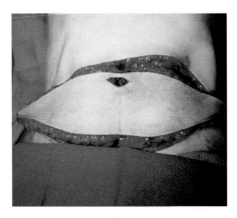

Fig. 8-27 Excess abdominal skin is excised. *(Courtesy Brian W. Davies, MD.)*

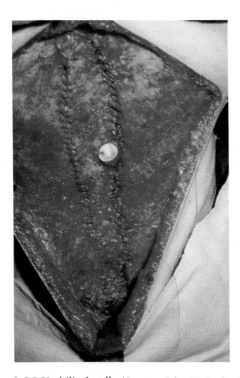

Fig. 8-26 Umbilical stalk. *(Courtesy Brian W. Davies, MD.)*

The flap is carefully lifted and pulled inferiorly toward the pubis. The distance between the superior and inferior edges will overlap demonstrating excess tissue. This excess is marked and trimmed off, leaving a freshly excised edge (Fig. 8-27). Musculoaponeurotic laxity is plicated between the xyphoid and pubis, and any existing diastasis is closed.

The umbilical stalk is measured to a new central position on an axis between the iliac crests and aligned on the line between the xyphoid to pubis. The umbilical placement lineup will resemble the cross hairs of a gunsite. The surface of the flap is marked with these topographic coordinates. A skin plug comparable in size to the circumference of the stalk is excised through the depth of the flap to create an umbilical insertion site. This opening resembles a keyhole. A stitch is placed on the

superior margin of the stalk, and the umbilical unit is drawn through the newly incised opening. The edges are approximated with interrupted sutures.

Closed suction wound drains are placed in the lower abdomen and sutured in place. The subcutaneous layer of the lower transverse incision is closed with a synthetic absorbable suture. The skin is closed with staples or a running subcuticular stitch. Care is taken to not invert hair follicles into the closure at the line of the pubis. Wound closure strips are placed over the skin edges as reinforcement, and saturated gauze, such as Xeroform, is placed in the umbilicus and over the closed wound edges.

An absorptive dressing, such as fluffed gauze, is placed over the wound and secured in position with an abdominal binder. A girdle or other compression garment may be used when the patient is ambulatory. Some surgeons prefer to use pressure taping over the area.

The patient is maintained in the hip-flexed position (beach chair) during transfer from the operating bed. Care is taken to not dislodge the Foley catheter or suction drains during the move. The flexure of the bed makes using a patient transfer roller difficult, and the move may necessitate extra help for a complete lift from one surface to the other to maintain a flexed position.

The patient is placed in a regular electric division or unit bed from the patient care unit. The bed is preflexed into the same beach chair position to receive the patient and serves as the recovery bed as well as the patient care division bed that the patient will occupy after the procedure. The flexure of the bed hinders patient movement; therefore the addition of an orthopaedic trapeze will be useful to the patient for self-repositioning during the first 24 to 48 hours of recovery. The side rails should be fully raised with the telephone, call light, and television controls easily within reach.

Postoperative Patient Care

The patient is maintained on bedrest in a hip-flexed supine position to relieve tension on the wound for the first 24 hours after the procedure. The wound is very snug because of the amount of excised tissue, and any undue tension would cause problems with wound healing. Antiembolic stockings or sequential compression devices are worn until the patient is fully ambulatory. Flexing exercises of the feet and legs will help prevent venous stasis. The patient is instructed to breathe deeply and use an incentive spirometry device. A pillow held firmly over the abdomen will help splint the incision for coughing.

The patient may remain in the hospital for 24 to 48 hours after the procedure. If the abdominoplasty is performed in combination with surgery of another organ system, the length of stay may be longer. Ambulation is permitted with the patient in a stooped position when the patient is stable. The drains are removed in 48 to 72 hours if the drainage has diminished. Sutures are removed in 1 week.

Complications

Serious complications are more common when abdominoplasty is performed in combination with surgery on another organ system, such as hysterectomy or cholecystectomy. The patient is at risk for thromboembolism and, to a lesser degree, fat embolism from the abdominoplasty procedure. Some surgeons prefer to administer a prophylactic IV alcohol solution during the procedure to decrease the risk of fat embolus syndrome.

Hematoma and seroma formation can compromise the abdominal flap. Adequate hemostasis and postoperative drains prevent pooling of blood under the flap. The abdominal binder will place even pressure on the flap and minimize serous pooling. Wound healing can be compromised by the same factors that affect any surgical wound, such as infection, tissue slough, and wound separation.

SUBSURFACE AUGMENTATION TECHNIQUES

Natural or synthetic materials placed in the subsurface layers of the body are used to enhance a contour, fill in or reconstruct a defect, or expand the superficial coverage of the skin. Many implants are permanent, but others are temporary, such as some tissue expanders. Subsurface implant material can be liquid, powder, gel, semisolid, liquid-filled or gel-filled elastomer shell, mesh, sheet, or solid. Desirable characteristics of subsurface augmentation materials are listed in Box 8-1.

The potential success or failure of the implant results depends on the technique of placement, the patient's generalized health condition, prevention of complications, and the composition of the implant. Studies have shown that implants placed for aesthetic enhancement had fewer complications than implants placed for reconstruction after chemotherapy or radiation treatments. This is due in part to the condition of the tissue in the area of implantation and the patient's health status.   Natural implant materials can be xenograft (different species), heterograft (homologous), or autograft (autologous). Examples include bone, skin, cartilage, membrane, fascia, collagen, fat, and whole organs. Synthetic implant materials can be of silicone, plastic, metal, Teflon, ceramic, acrylic, adhesives, and bioactive glass.

Documentation of any implant placed in a patient includes manufacturer, model number, type, size, lot number, and/or serial number as appropriate. Lot numbers should be listed in a retrievable departmental file that facilitates recall of the patient in the event of a manufacturer's alert per recommendations of the Joint Commission on Accreditation of Healthcare

---

Box 8-1 **Characteristics of Subsurface Augmentation Materials**

Nontoxic
Nonallergenic
Noncarcinogenic
Nonimmunologic
Nonreactive to tissue enzymes as appropriate
Biocompatible
Durable
Sterile for use
Size and shape accommodation
Removable as needed
Resorptive as appropriate
Position-stable
Texture-appropriate
Radiolucent
Noninterference with nuclear scans
Noninterference with health screening or surveillance
Nonconductive
Nonthermal
Nonplacement intensive

Organizations (JCAHO). Prehandling, such as rinsing with antibiotic solution, should be recorded according to institutional policy. If the patient is part of a controlled study, registration with the appropriate agency is done according to the program's protocol. Follow-up examinations are scheduled and explained to the patient. Some implant manufacturers include a wallet card for patient information. This can be important if the patient has magnetic, metallic, battery-controlled, or mechanical components in the implant. Characteristics of the implant could interfere with diagnostic testing with nuclear medicine scans or radiologic equipment.

Subsurface Augmentation by Injection

Subsurface injection augmentation is designed to plump up the subsurface layers and is usually done in an office but may be performed in combination with a surgical procedure. A smoother surface results in a more youthful appearance. Aging, exposure to weather, laugh lines, and facial creases over musculature respond well to soft tissue filler material such as commercially prepared collagen and autologous injectable fat cells. Other fibrous powders and gelatinous substances are available that are mixed with the patient's blood before injection. Subsurface dermal injection augmentation can be used in combination with facelifts or resurfacing procedures, such as peels, dermabrasion, and laser treatments.

Injectable subsurface augmentation with biologic material is not permanent. The body eventually degrades and resorbs the injected protein portion of the material through enzymatic action becoming nondetectable. Each patient will reabsorb collagen and/or fat cells at a different rate causing varying degrees of results; therefore the treated area is slightly overfilled to compensate for the absorption process. No injectable augmentation material is as effective as a facelift, blepharoplasty, or browlift. Reinjection with more of the same substance at a later date may be desired (Fig. 8-28).

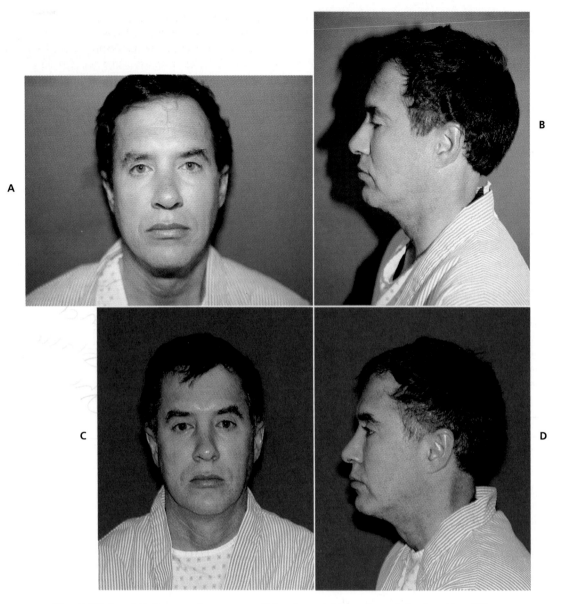

Fig. 8-28 **A and B,** Preoperative upper eyelid and nasolabial collagen injection. **C and D,** Postoperative views. Note that nasolabial fold is reappearing 6 months after the procedure. *(Courtesy Brian W. Davies, MD.)*

Complications include infection at the injection site, abscess, itching, sensitivity, uneven contour, and patient dissatisfaction. Sun exposure should be avoided during the healing phase, especially if bruising is evident, because free hemoglobin in the tissue can cause a permanent stained or discolored appearance referred to as *hemosiderosis*. This is the result of retained iron (hemosiderin) from reabsorbed hemoglobin. This phenomenon may occur in any tissue after any bruising event.

Collagen injection

Processed bovine collagen (Zyplast, Zyderm I, Zyderm II) was approved by the Food and Drug Administration (FDA) in 1981. Injectable collagen is available is several consistencies to meet the needs of each patient, but it is not recommended for injection into lips or near eye orbits. Local infiltration anesthetic would distort the terrain of the injection site and is not commonly used because lidocaine is incorporated into the collagen preparation. Topical anesthetic, such as eutectic mixture of local anesthetics (EMLA) may be applied to the skin to decrease the effects of the initial needle penetration if the patient desires.

Inflammatory reaction degrades bovine collagen and replaces it with human collagen. The augmentation results are not permanent. Zyplast works best in deeper dermal tissue in thicker-skinned persons and may last up to 6 months. It may cause encapsulation in the tissues. Zyderm works best in the superficial dermis, but it is absorbed within 4 months. It has less risk for the formation of contractures. Minimal traces are found in the body in 9 months. Some patients (1% to 5 %) may be allergic, and pretesting 48 hours before the procedure is advised.

Collagen can be prepared with other additives for varying degrees of texture and function. Studies are being done on collagen with fibrin and hydroxyapatite for hypotrophic mandibular and maxillary defects. Fibrel, in use since 1987, is a fibrin-based porcine collagen mixture that can be mixed with the patient's own plasma for coagulatory properties in wound healing. Other uses include injection for elevation of facial creases, wrinkles, and depressed scars.

Autologous fat injection

Fat can be procured from the patient and injected into subcutaneous layers of integument to fix facial contour defects but not fine wrinkles. Many of the adipose cells are destroyed in the procurement process. Fat resorbs within 6 to 12 months. Autologous fat donor sites include the following:

- Abdomen
- Buttocks
- Thighs
- Submentum

Local anesthesia is commonly used at both the donor and recipient sites. A syringe with a large bore needle or liposuction cannula with applied suction is used to procure the fat for injection. Recipient areas include augmentation of scars and lines in the face and lip-line enhancement. Most of the effects of injection are undetectable within 6 months. Fewer than 20% to 40% of injected cells survive 1 year in the recipient site. Allergy is not an issue because the fat is taken from the patient's own body. Initial inflammatory response supports phagocytosis and replacement with fibrous tissue.

Tissue Expanders

The use of tissue expansion has solved many problems caused by lack of available tissue cover needed to repair or reconstruct a body surface. Historically, physicians noted that the skin over an enlarging area, such as a pregnant abdomen or over a tumor, increased in quantity to accommodate the subsurface growth. After the baby was born or the tumor removed, the skin regained some of its original shape but not all. Some redundancy of skin remained. Various types of autologous flaps and grafts became available by using redundant skin created by tissue expansion.

A tissue expander is an expandable balloonlike device made of silicone elastomer (Fig. 8-29). It is placed under the subcutaneous tissue and progressively enlarged by injection of sterile normal saline through an integrated or remote injection port. The result of this process is a mechanically created redundancy of the overlying tissue and skin. This redundant skin can be raised as a flap or left in position to form a pocket for placement of a permanent implant.

Physiologic responses to tissue expansion

The epidermal layer of the skin does not undergo a significant change in thickness. However, the cells, although thinner, multiply quickly causing increased surface area. The dermal layer thins readily during the first month, then it slows for the

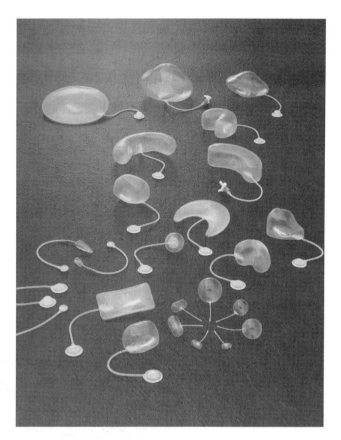

Fig. 8-29 Tissue expanders. *(Courtesy McGhan Medical Corporation, Santa Barbara, California.)*

duration of expansion. If the expander is placed under muscle, the muscular tissue thins and loses bulk without losing contractile function. Adipose tissue atrophies.

Skin appendages, such as glands, nerve endings, and hair follicles, are spread wider apart but do not increase in number. The surface over the expansion device feels cooler than the surrounding tissue. Circulation increases over the raised area as new blood vessels form. This formation may make the area over the expander appear bluish or darker pink. Extreme overexpansion can cause circulatory obstruction and death of the tissue.

Collagen proliferates, and fibrous tissues increase in volume forming a capsule around the expander. This capsule will gradually disappear over time when the expander is removed or can serve as a receptive pocket for a permanent implant. The surgeon may prescribe postoperative breast massage for fresh augmentation patients to prevent capsular contractures. Some capsules may contract and become tight around the permanent implant, causing pain. When examining a patient for early signs of possible contracture around a breast implant, ask the patient to raise her arms above her head. The breasts will appear globular with the arms raised and normal with the arms down. Some of these capsular contractures are surgically excised at a later date.

Types of tissue expanders

Tissue expanders are supplied sterile as single-use items from the manufacturer. The Lapin tissue expander has a surface-integrated injection port. The Radovan tissue expander has a remote injection port. Custom designs can be specially ordered. Examples of tissue expander shapes and fill-port locations include the following:

- Round with remote or surface integrated injection port
- Rectangle with remote or surface integrated injection port
- Crescent with remote or surface integrated injection port
- Elliptical (low profile) with remote injection port

Other types of tissue expanders can be left in place as permanent implants after insertion, such as for breast augmentation or reconstruction. Textured styles used for breast reconstruction are usually left in place after satisfactory tissue expansion.

Placement procedure

Placement of a tissue expander can be performed as an inpatient procedure or in an ambulatory setting. When performed in combination with another procedure such as mastectomy, the patient is usually admitted as an inpatient. Although IVCS with administration of local anesthesia can be used for uncomplicated procedures, general anesthesia is preferred for complex placement. The type and size of tissue expander used will be determined by the site of placement, the condition of the patient's tissue, and the amount of coverage needed. Mild tissue ingrowth will occur with textured implants to create stability. Some expanders are inflated and left in position to serve as permanent prosthetic implants.

Before the procedure, the area of expander placement is marked with a surgical marker, and an incision large enough to introduce the expander is made. The incision is generally hidden or incorporated for an aesthetic closure during the final phases of the procedure. The tissue is undermined enough to allow expander placement and positioning under the skin. Careful attention is given to hemostasis. Some surgeons may request antibiotic solution for irrigation.

A sterile insertion sleeve is supplied with textured tissue expanders for ease of placement. When in the final resting position, the inflation port should not be resting over a bony area because it may be the source of irritation or pressure necrosis. Care is taken to not place it near waistbands or bra straps for the same reason. Remote inflation ports are positioned approximately 5 to 6 cm away from the expander site. Lubrication is not used because it can interfere with the surface of the expander. The expander, as with all implants, should have minimal handling before placement. Only clean sterile gloves with all traces of powder and lint removed (or preferably, powderless gloves) should come in contact before placement. At all times, care is given to the prevention of lint and foreign bodies from contaminating the surface of the expander.

Fill technique. Before placement, all traces of air are removed from the expander with a syringe through the port. A fold or crease caused by an air pocket can allow a hematoma or seroma to form. When placed in the tissue pocket, measured amounts of sterile IV normal saline are injected into the port until the expander occludes all dead space. The scrub person is responsible for keeping track of the amount of saline injected. It is suggested that measured increments of 25 to 50 ccs are injected and tallied as they are used. A 60 cc syringe is useful for this purpose. Injection continues using capillary refill as a measure of skin and wound tolerance. Injection is halted before capillary refill or wound integrity is compromised. The final injection amount tallied is recorded in the patient's record for future reference.

Periodic injection intervals at 5 to 7 days using sterile saline into the injection port with a 23-gauge needle gradually cause the expander to enlarge. The injection port under the skin has a puncture-proof housing and a self-sealing silicone membrane that is located by palpation. Expander models are available that have an imbedded magnet (Fig. 8-30) for easier location using a magnetic detection device (Fig. 8-31) supplied with the expander. This magnet can detect the magnetic port through 60 mm of tissue. The additional amount of saline injected into the expander is documented in the patient's record.

Some surgeons prefer to add a surgical dye or tint to the saline before injecting. The manufacturer's recommendations state that combination of the saline with any substance before injection is not advised. This includes not adding antibiotics, anesthetic, or other chemical to the solution.

Contraindications

Expanders with a magnetic injection port should not be used for patients with an implantable drug infusion pump or a pacemaker. The magnetic field will interfere with the function of the

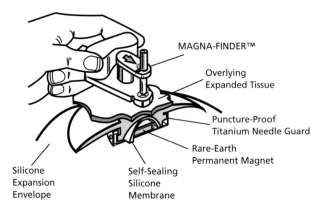

Fig. 8-30 MAGNA-SITE and MAGNA-FINDER integral port system. *(Courtesy McGhan Medical Corporation, Santa Barbara, California.)*

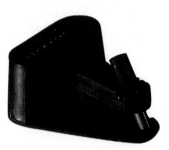

Fig. 8-31 MAGNA-FINDER tool. *(Courtesy McGhan Medical Corporation, Santa Barbara, California.)*

equipment. Patients with cancer and/or radiation at the potential insertion point are not candidates for tissue expansion.

Patient education about tissue expanders

The patient should be instructed that the tissue expansion process can take up to 6 months depending on the site and type of tissue to be expanded. The area of expansion will look abnormal and may cause social discomfort. In many cases, the temporary alteration in body image is minimal compared with the loss of self-esteem caused by the physical defect that is under reconstruction (Fig. 8-32).

The patient is instructed to avoid blunt impact or crushing of the expanding area. Signs that should be reported are changes in neurovascular status, such as sudden or gradual onset of numbness, tingling, coldness, or pins and needles sensation, especially distal to the insertion point, such as on a limb. Smoking adversely affects wound healing and should be avoided.

Tissue expanders with magnetic injection ports should not be used in patients who will undergo nuclear testing with a computerized tomography (CT) scan or magnetic resonance imaging (MRI). The test results would be affected and render a false reading.

Advantages and disadvantages

Advantages of using an expanded flap include color and texture match between donor and recipient sites. Disadvantages of tissue expansion are time mediated. The patient will need to return to the facility several times for instillation of sterile saline during the expansion process. Some pain and/or discomfort may be experienced by the patient as saline is added to the expander. When expansion is completed, a second procedure is performed to remove the expander and position a permanent implant or place the new skin. The skin over the expander will appear somewhat deformed during the expansion period, which can take from 3 to 6 months. The patient should be psychologically prepared for the temporary physical deformity associated with tissue expansion.

Complications

Complications include disruption of the insertion site wound caused either by overexpansion or infection. Extrusion of the expander is possible. Frank infection may necessitate explantation of the expander. Tissue reaction may occur if the expander comes in contact with lint, dust, talc, or other foreign body contaminant during the implantation process.

Hematoma and seroma are potential complications but are minimized by filling the expander to form a tamponade. Care is taken to not exert extreme pressure on the wound, because overinflation can cause tissue ischemia followed by necrosis. Meticulous hemostasis is important, but excessive use of cautery to control bleeders may generate devitalized tissue in the dissected pocket. If fluid accumulation is possible, closed wound suction drains may be necessary.

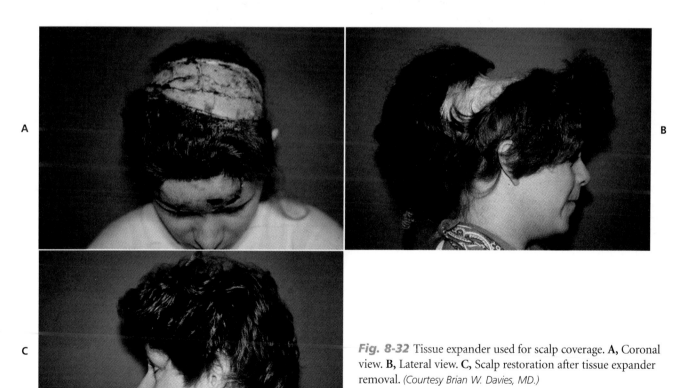

Fig. 8-32 Tissue expander used for scalp coverage. **A,** Coronal view. **B,** Lateral view. **C,** Scalp restoration after tissue expander removal. *(Courtesy Brian W. Davies, MD.)*

Reporting problems with medical devices

Tissue expanders are single-use items and cannot be resterilized or repaired. A leak in the expander will cause the expander to deflate. The damaged expander is removed and reported to the manufacturer if this happens. Some manufacturers request the return of the defective device for study. Reports are prepared for the FDA according to the Safe Medical Devices Act enacted in 1991. This act provided for voluntary reporting of problems with medical drugs and devices. The FDA has established a voluntary reporting mechanism referred to as MedWatch for problems with drugs and medical devices (Fig. 8-33). The FDA follows up with the manufacturer. MedWatch forms can be obtained from the FDA (Box 8-2). The report information should contain the following:
- Name and address of the facility
- Product name, model and serial numbers
- Manufacturer's name and address
- Brief description of the event as it was reported to the manufacturer

Subsurface Augmentation with Implants

Implanting a substance under the skin and/or subcutaneous tissues and muscle creates a new landscape over the surface (Fig. 8-34). Curvilinear surfaces such as the chin and cheeks can be reinforced with natural or synthetic implants giving more definition to facial lines (Fig. 8-35). Defects in bone can be filled and resculpted with a cement or semisolid plastic that hardens like ossified tissue. Bulk and ballottment can be created by placing a fluid or gel-filled sac below the subcutaneous tissue or muscle, such as with breast implants (Fig. 8-36).

Properties of natural and synthetic implants

Chemical and mechanical properties of an implant or implanted substance affect the biologic responses of the recipient site in several ways. Recipient tissue response is dependent on the origin of the implant.

Chemical properties. Absorbable materials reduce to a different chemical composition through dissolution, hydrolysis, and enzymatic action. All of these reduction methods involve intervention of white blood cells for phagocytosis. *Dissolution* of a compound involves breaking the implant down into simpler molecular components. Some elements literally liquefy and merge with surrounding tissue until chemically indistinct. *Hydrolysis* involves decomposition of synthetic implant material in the presence of body fluids. Water contained within the interstitial tissue causes molecules within the implanted substance to separate into component parts causing minimal tissue reaction. *Enzymatic action* takes place when naturally occurring chemicals (enzymes) act as catalysts to convert natural implant materials into individual molecular components at the cellular level.

Mechanical properties. The physical composition of the implant will also create some mechanical responses at the recipient site. Rough or irregular surface texture can cause an inflammatory reaction in surrounding tissue causing the formation of fibrous adhesions. Ingrowth of fibrous tissue anchors the implant in the recipient site. Smooth surfaces become encapsulated by a collagen envelope. Extreme density of the fibrous capsule can cause complications such as pain or displacement of the implant. Capsular contractures necessitate an additional surgical procedure to strip away tough adhesive tissue bands.

Natural implant materials

Natural implant materials are derived from autologous (self-generated), homologous (same species-generated, also referred to as allograft), or xenologous (different-species generated) sources. Implanted material of nonautologous origin can cause an inflammatory response or anaphylaxis. Autologous tissues are not rejected and cause minimal inflammatory response as a natural stage of wound healing.

Bone grafts. Bone grafts are used to repair acquired or congenital defects. The structure consists of a hard, cortical outer layer and an soft, spongy, cancellous inner layer (Fig. 8-37). The anatomic configuration is a system of tubular canals referred to as the Haversian system. Capillaries pass through these tunnels and nourish the bone. The bony tissue layers, referred to as *osteons,* are arranged in concentric layers around the Haversian canals. Osteocytes generate in the lacunae and thrive in this environment, continually laying down new bony tissue. The new bony tissue increases in radiographic density over a period of 6 months and is nearly normal in hardness by 1 year.

The serial process of bone healing requires bone to be in contact with bone. Small defects heal well using autologous or allograft bone. The process, known as *osteoconduction,* is the formation of granulation tissue that attracts osteoclasts for the degradation of dead bone. Osteoblasts infiltrate the bony (osteoinduction) area laying down new osseous material (osteogenesis).

Vascularization begins after osteoclastic activity and is functionally complete in 1 to 2 months. Capillary ingrowth from the recipient site starts at 4 days and is well established in 2 to 4 weeks. The sequence is faster in autografts than in allografts. Xenografts are not used for bone grafting because of rejection. Bone used in facial grafts usually vascularizes more quickly and resorbs to a lesser degree but usually requires a second surgical incision. Preferred sites for bone autograft and allograft procurement include the following (Fig. 8-38):
- Cranium (calvarial): usually procured for a wide variety of facial reconstruction procedures; commonly procured as a nonvascularized split graft for onlay or inlay; when large amounts are needed, the calvarium is procured as a full-thickness graft, then split into two layers; procurement carries the risk of injury to the brain and meninges
- Iliac crest (cortical, cancellous): most common site for large amounts of autologous bone graft
- Rib (cortical-cancellous, cartilage): used for cranial defects, facial onlay, and congenital ear deformities; the take is enhanced if the periosteum is left intact; easy to procure; resorption rate is fast when used as onlay
- Portions of radius or ulna: vascularized segments
- Portions of tibia or fibula

For **VOLUNTARY** reporting
by health professionals of adverse
events and product problems

Form Approved: OMB No. 0910-0291 Expires: 12/31/94
See OMB statement on reverse

FDA Use Only

Triage unit
sequence #

Page _____ of _____

A. Patient information

1. **Patient identifier**	2. **Age at time of event:** or_____ Date of birth:	3. **Sex** ☐ female ☐ male	4. **Weight** _____lbs or _____kgs
In confidence			

B. Adverse event or product problem

1. ☐ **Adverse event** and/or ☐ **Product problem** (e.g., defects/malfunctions)

2. **Outcomes attributed to adverse event**
(check all that apply)

☐ death _____ (mo/day/yr)
☐ life-threatening
☐ hospitalization — initial or prolonged

☐ disability
☐ congential anomaly
☐ required intervention to prevent permanent impairment/damage
☐ other: _____

3. **Date of event** (mo/day/yr)

4. **Date of this report** (mo/day/yr)

5. **Describe event or problem**

6. **Relevant tests/laboratory data,** including dates

7. **Other relevant history, including preexisting medical conditions** (e.g., allergies, race, pregnancy, smoking and alcohol use, hepatic/renal dysfunction, etc.)

C. Suspect medication(s)

1. **Name** (give labeled strength & mfr/labeler, if known)

#1 _____

#2 _____

2. **Dose, frequency & route used**

#1

#2

3. **Therapy dates** (if unknown, give duration) from/to (or best estimate)

#1

#2

4. **Diagnosis for use** (indication)

#1

#2

5. **Event abated after use stopped or dose reduced**

#1 ☐ yes ☐ no ☐ doesn't apply
#2 ☐ yes ☐ no ☐ doesn't apply

6. **Lot #** (if known)

#1
#2

7. **Exp. date** (if known)

#1
#2

8. **Event reappeared after reintroduction**

#1 ☐ yes ☐ no ☐ doesn't apply
#2 ☐ yes ☐ no ☐ doesn't apply

9. **NDC #** (for product problems only)

_ _ _

10. **Concomitant medical products** and therapy dates (exclude treatement of event)

D. Suspect medical device

1. **Brand name**

2. **Type of device**

3. **Manufacturer name & address**

4. **Operator of device**
☐ health professional
☐ lay user/patient
☐ other: _____

6.
model # _____
catalog # _____
serial # _____
lot # _____
other # _____

5. **Expiration date** (mo/day/yr)

7. **If implanted, give date** (mo/day/yr)

8. **If explanted, give date** (mo/day/yr)

9. **Device available for evaluation?** (Do not send to FDA)
☐ yes ☐ no ☐ returned to manufacturer on_____ (mo/day/yr)

10. **Concomitant medical products** and therapy dates (exclude treatment of event)

E. Reporter (see confidentiality section on back)

1. **Name, address & phone #**

2. **Health professional?**
☐ yes ☐ no

3. **Occupation**

4. **Also reported to**
☐ manufacturer
☐ user facility
☐ distributor

5. **If you do NOT want your identity disclosed to the manufacturer, place an "X" in this box.** ☐

Mail to: **MEDWATCH**
5600 Fishers Lane
Rockville, MD 20852-9787

or **FAX to:**
1-800-FDA-0178

Submission of a report does not constitute an admission that medical personnel or the product caused or contributed to the event.

FDA Form 3500 (6/93)

Fig. 8-33 FDA medical devices reporting form.

MedWatch forms can be obtained from the following address:
US Food and Drug Administration
5600 Fishers Lane
Rockville, MD 20852-9787
Phone: 1-800-332-1088
Fax: 1-800-332-0178
Website: www.fda.gov/medwatch

Vascularized bone autografts can be procured and grafted with a 90% success rate using microsurgical techniques (Fig. 8-39). Defects exceeding 6 cm heal best when a vascularized bone graft is used. Avascular autografts or allografts over large segments have a failure rate of 30%.

Allograft bone is taken from living or cadaver donors of the same species and may cause antigenicity reactions associated with foreign tissue. Microbial carriage of some diseases such as HIV or HBV is a risk. Avoidance of immunosupression is

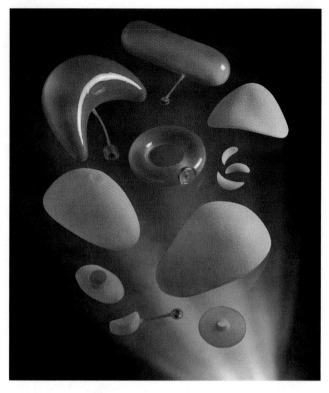

Fig. 8-34 Examples of custom implants. *(Courtesy McGhan Medical Corporation, Santa Barbara, California.)*

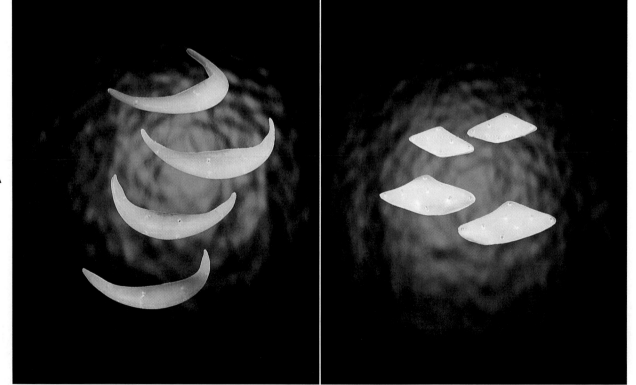

Fig. 8-35 **A,** Anatomical chin implants. **B,** Anatomical malar implants. *(Courtesy McGhan Medical Corporation, Santa Barbara, California.)*

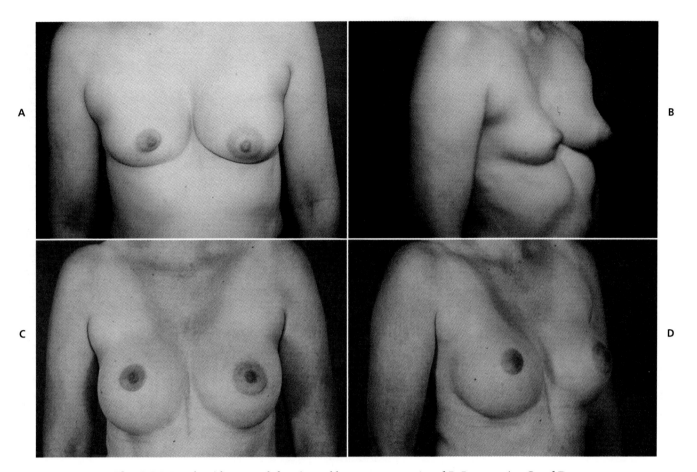

Fig. 8-36 Female with pectus deformity and breast asymetry. **A and B,** Preoperative. **C and D,** Postoperative. *(Courtesy Brian W. Davies, MD.)*

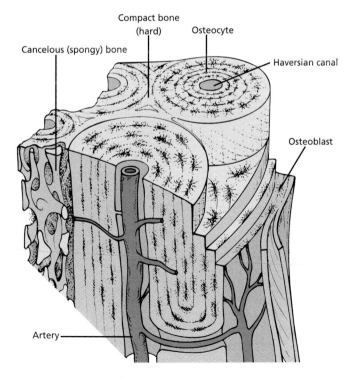

Fig. 8-37 Bone anatomy.

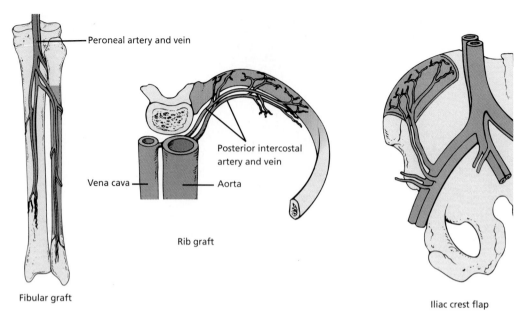

Fig. 8-38 Common donor sites for vascularized bone grafts. **A,** Fibular graft. **B,** Rib graft. **C,** Iliac crest flap.

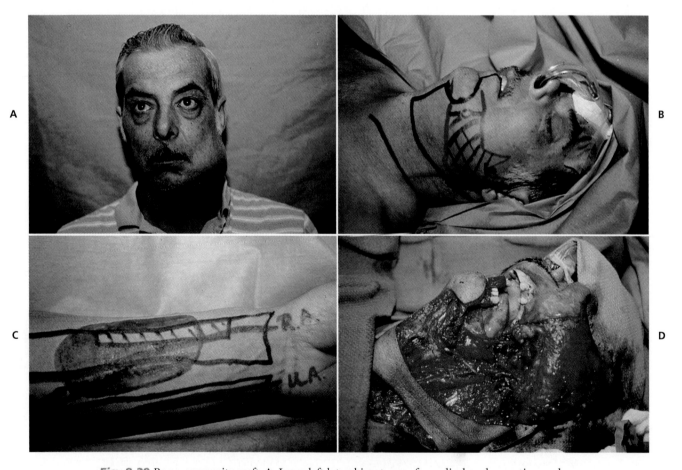

Fig. 8-39 Bone-composite graft. **A,** Large left lateral jaw tumor for radical neck resection and partial mandibulectomy. **B,** Skin marking on jaw for radical neck and mandibulectomy. **C,** Skin marking for left radial forearm muscle and bone flap. **D,** Resected neck and jaw.

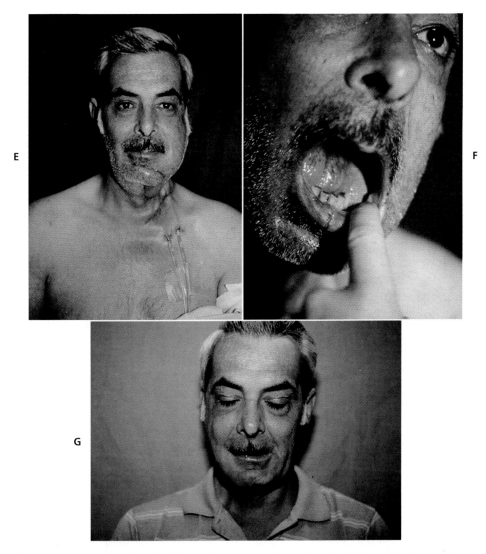

Fig. 8-39 cont'd **E,** Completed procedure external anterior view. **F,** Completed procedure internal floor of mouth view. **G,** Completed jaw line 6 months after the procedure. *(Courtesy Brian W. Davies, MD.)*

desired in the recipient to prevent complications associated with decreased immunity. Allograft bone works well as a replacement segment for long bones and serves a framework for osteoblastic ingrowth and neovascularization.

Cartilage grafts

Cartilage is a form of supportive connective tissue. The four types of cartilage found in the body are as follows:

- Hyaline
- Elastic
- White fibrocartilage
- Yellow fibrocartilage

Hyaline cartilage is translucent and is found in some articular surfaces, the nose, and the tracheal rings. Elastic cartilage is found on the nose, trachea, larynx, and the ends of the ribs. White fibrocartilage is the primary component of menisci and forms the articular surfaces between the vertebrae. Yellow

elastic cartilage is located in more flexible structures, such as the epiglottis, eustachean tubes, and the auricle of the ears.

Autologous cartilage is most commonly used for implantation. Additional sources of cartilage include treated allografts and xenografts. Cartilage is not available for autologous grafting in large quantities. Fortunately, the areas that require cartilage grafts are small, such as facial features. Cartilage is easily reshaped and transplanted and responds well to flexible forces, such as facial expression and ear flexibility. Unlike bone, it does not need to be placed against other portions of cartilage to remain viable.

Anatomically, cartilage is comprised of chondrocytes, proteoglycan matrix, and bound water covered with perichondrium. When used as an implant, the ability of the chondrocytes to produce collagen and maintain the matrix supports the viability of the graft. Cartilage has no intrinsic circulation and derives nutrition by interstitial diffusion. The chondrocytes continue to function within the graft. Autologous cartilage remains viable if the nutrients from the recipient site are able to diffuse into the graft. Poor integrity of the recipient tissue causes failure of the grafted cartilage. Allograft and xenograft cartilage cause immunologic responses that promote resorption. The foreign cartilage is destroyed by lymphocytes and antibody reaction. Some allografts have been treated to minimize antigenicity. This prolongs the resistance of the cartilage as a nonviable implant and encourages fibrous encapsulation with variable resorption over several years.

Resorption occurs when the chondrocytes no longer support viability of the matrix. Any destruction of chondrocytes, such as freezing, will cause the graft to resorb. Studies have shown that the condition of the perichondrium has a direct influence on nutrient diffusion between the cartilage graft and the recipient site. Disruption of the perichondrial surface by stripping or crushing causes variable rates of resorption. Fixed subperiosteal placement of elastic cartilage in a nonmobile position hastens resorption and supports ossification. Surfaces with intact perichondrium remain viable longer and reabsorb at a slower rate.

Costal elastic cartilage is frequently used in ear reconstruction for acquired deformities caused by illness or trauma and neoconstruction for congenital defects. Hyaline and elastic cartilage can warp after procurement. Thinner grafts distort more readily than thicker grafts. Perichondrium can influence the degree of warp encountered. Transverse scoring patterns created by sharp dissection against the concave surface of the costal elastic cartilage will cause natural curves to straighten.

Care of the patient with natural implant materials

Patient care associated with placement of an implant includes meticulous preoperative and postoperative assessment of the graft and recipient site, minimal handling of the implant, strict aseptic technique, and appropriate documentation according to policy and regulatory agency guidelines. During the procedure, the graft procurement and recipient sites are prepped and draped separately. Preferably, separate sterile fields and instrument setups are established for each surgical site to prevent the potential for cross contamination. Implants that require reshaping or sculpting, such as cartilaginous grafts, should be procured and prepared away from the recipient field. Autologous grafts should be moistened frequently with sterile saline to prevent drying.

The patient is instructed to not manipulate the implant after the procedure unless specifically instructed to do so by the plastic surgeon. Postoperative assessment of the implant placement and/or graft procurement wounds includes observing for redness, swelling, drainage, and integrity of the sites. Erythema, rash, and localized swelling in the presence of an allograft or xenograft may indicate an allergic or sensitivity reaction to a foreign substance and should be investigated.

Alloplastic implant materials

Alloplastic implants are synthetic materials considered permanent and without reabsorptive properties. They can reduce operating and anesthesia time by not requiring the patient to have a surgical donor source, such as for bone or other autologous tissue. The risks associated with homologous or allograft procedures are eliminated. Most subsurface implantation of alloplastic material is performed to replace or build up the foundation for autologous biologic tissue. Examples of alloplastic materials for implantation are listed in Box 8-3.

Most alloplastic materials can be inexpensively produced in many shapes and consistencies. Many are inert in vivo (in position in living tissue). Any area of the body can be enhanced, augmented, or reconstructed by subsurface implantation. Examples of implant characteristics and body implant sites include the following:

- Tissue expansion: any body surface (hair bearing, any skin adjacent to a defect)
- Solid implant: facial contours and structural reconstruction
- Flexible solid: penis
- Flexible with conversion to solid: acrylic, cement for neoconstruction of hard surface
- Flexible sheeting: structural reinforcement, prevent adhesions
- Mesh: structural reinforcement, bridge defects, scaffold for ingrowth of tissue
- Powder: osseous integration material
- Gel-filled/fluid-filled sacs: breasts, testicles, submuscular augmentation (pectoral and gastrocnemius in males)
- Liquid or semiliquid injectable: subsurface augmentation of creases

Silicone

Silicone is derived from the organic chemical element silicon and is available as a medical grade liquid, gel, or solid. Variations in consistency can be manipulated to accommodate differing subsurface structural needs. The generalized smooth surface of silicone deters adherence. Tissue ingrowth does not occur unless a secondary specialized surface has been applied by the manufacturer.

Liquid silicone is no longer injected into soft tissue for augmentation because it may migrate to other areas of the body, including major organ systems, causing various systemic complications. Expandable reservoirs made of silicone sheeting are commonly filled with saline for subcutaneous or submuscular augmentation. Reservoirs prefilled with medical grade silicone gel are used for mammary reconstruction or augmentation as part of controlled adjunctive studies. Smaller versions of prefilled silicone gel implants are used as testicular implants.

The FDA banned silicone breast implants in 1992 with the exception of those in use for clinical studies. Studies have not conclusively shown silicone implants responsible for the wide range of atypical symptoms attributed to their use. In 1997, the

---

Box 8-3 **Alloplastic Materials Used for Implants**

Silicone-based
Polytetrafluoroethylene
Acrylic
Metal
Biologic glass

Mayo Clinic study showed that 24% of women with silicone breast implants require additional surgery for medical reasons within 5 years of implantation. Problems found in the study group were breast deformity, necrosed breast tissue, capsular contractures, and implant rupture.

Solid silicone implants are used to augment soft tissues and bony surfaces. When solid silicone is placed below the periosteum (subperiosteal), such as in the chin and cheeks, bone resorption occurs because of inflammatory response and direct pressure. Placement of solid silicone implants above the periosteum (preperiosteal) demonstrates less bony resorption. Fibrous encapsulation caused by mild inflammation response gives the solid implant stability.

Advantages. Silicone can be fashioned into nearly any shape or size. The available variations in consistency make it a suitable choice for many augmentation procedures. It can be sterilized by steam or dry heat per the manufacturer's recommendations.

Disadvantages. Although considered inert, an inflammatory response does occur after implantation. Silicone oil used to lubricate hypodermic needles and plungers in disposable syringes has been found encapsulated in the skin, subcutaneous, and lymphatic tissues of diabetics who use daily insulin injections. Actual antibodies have not been isolated, but silicone synovitis and siliconoma have resulted from silicone foreign body reactions. Extrusion may occur if the implant is placed in thinner tissue layers close to the skin surface such as the nose or chin.

The gel from a ruptured silicone implant is difficult to remove. The silicone particles measure 20 to 60 μm in size and can be phagocytosed by macrophages during an inflammatory response. The macrophages can transport the particle to the lymphatic system.

Polytetrafluoroethylene carbon

Polytetrafluoroethylene (PTFE) is a carbon fluorine bond that is stable, biocompatible, and resistant to enzymatic breakdown in the body. PTFE has low tensile and compressive strength making it unsuitable for bony tissue replacement but excellent for subsurface soft tissue augmentation.

The first PTFE implant for plastic surgery was Teflon, but currently it is used primarily for vocal cord reconstruction. Gore-Tex is a form of Teflon used for aesthetic soft tissue augmentation that has been shown to be nonallergenic and reasonably inert. It is soft and flexible with small pores that allow for tissue ingrowth. Other uses for Gore-Tex include chest and abdominal wall reconstruction, vascular prosthetics, and suspension of ligaments in facial asymmetries. Gore-Tex can be sterilized by ethylene oxide or steam according to manufacturer's recommendations.

Proplast I was a PTFE composed of Teflon and carbon, formerly used for maxillofacial and temporomandibular joint reconstruction. Proplast II was a combination of PTFE and aluminum oxide particles. These were removed from the market because of the complications associated with biodegradation and particle migration. Patients commonly present for explantation of this material and request alternate forms of reconstruction of the formerly implanted area.

Acrylic

Methyl methacrylate is a powdered polymer that when mixed with a liquid monomer becomes a good material for reconstruction of bony skull defects. In orthopedics, it is also used as a bone cement for prostheses. It solidifies in 6 to 8 minutes allowing for contouring during its soft state. During the solidification process, an exothermic reaction is created. When solidified, a high-speed drill with a burr is used to sculpt the desired surface shape. This acrylic polymer is also available as a preformed, heat-treated implant.

Hydroxyapatite

Composed of calcium phosphate, hydroxyapatite is used for inlay and onlay grafting of orthognathic defects. This substance is a mineral component of both bone and coral. When placed against bone, it bonds and promotes osteogenesis by stimulating the growth of new bone. The need for autologous graft procurement is decreased, eliminating the need for a second surgical site.

Hydroxyapatite is sometimes referred to as a bioceramic, or bioglass. Although not a perfect replacement for bone, it does allow for bony ingrowth for bone formation. Brittleness and low pressure strength are disadvantages of this material. Varieties of orthopedic implants are coated with hydroxyapatite to promote fixation and bony ingrowth. Studies have shown that this coating promotes a firmer fixation and rapid healing.

Metals

Metallic implants are primarily used for procedures performed on bony surfaces. Commonly used metal alloys include titanium, cobalt, stainless steel, chromium, nickel, and tantalum. Most metal implants, such as bone screws, cause only a limited inflammatory response. Chromium-cobalt alloys (vitallium) when blended with nickel can cause a delayed hypersensitivity response (metal allergy). Studies have shown a possible tendency for carcinogenicity of some combinations of metals, especially hematologic and lymphatic, caused by the release of metallic ions into the system. Some of the corrosion and metallic release can be minimized by special oxide coatings. Macrophages adjacent to titanium implants show ingestion of titanium particles but to date have not shown oncogenicity.

Alloplastic implant handling

Implant materials should be supplied sterile from the manufacturer. The package should remain sealed until the recipient site is prepared. After double-checking the integrity of the package and the type and size of the implant, the package is opened by the circulator and the item is retrieved by the scrub person. If the product becomes contaminated, it should be prepared and resterilized only according to manufacturer's recommendations. Appropriate biologic indicators should be processed with the load.

The implant itself should not be flipped onto the sterile field because it may become damaged or contaminated during transfer. The scrub person should once again carefully check the implant for integrity, type, and size before passing it to the surgeon. The implant should have only minimal handling before placement because lint and debris on surgical gloves can cause granulomas and other foreign body complications. Placing the implant in sterile saline or antibiotic solution before implantation can help prevent adherence of potentially harmful material to its surface.

Nursing care of the patient with an alloplastic implant

The patient should be advised to not place excessive pressure on the surgical incision or over the implant because ischemia of the tissues may cause failure in wound healing or extrusion of the implant. The skin over a fluid-filled implant may feel cooler than surrounding skin but should not feel progressively cold. Mild to moderate pain and swelling is expected, but severe pain or frank edema is abnormal and should be investigated. Hot and red skin with exquisite pain may indicate infection and should be treated with antibiotics and probably explantation.

Patients with breast implants are advised to continue routine self-breast examinations and examination by a clinical practitioner. Breast implants are not a contraindication for mammography. (See Chapter 10 for more information on breast examination and surgery.)

PLASTIC SURGERY OF THE HAND

A hand injury or deformity is devastating both physically and psychologically. Physically, the hand is a highly visible part of the body. It is a primary means of reacting to and manipulating the environment. Social and cultural aspects include touching others and sensing by tactile communication. Some injuries or deformities can prevent even the act of shaking hands, which is a sign of acknowledgement in the community. Some hand injuries and deformities cause the patient to be dependent upon other people for personal needs, such as eating or toileting.

Psychologically, a hand disfigured by trauma is highly visible and is a constant reminder of inconvenient restrictions in motion and productivity. Usually the patient has witnessed the actual trauma to his or her hand. As a result, the damage of crushed or missing digits is immediately seen and the sight can produce posttraumatic stress syndrome, nightmares, and flashbacks. The patient tends to remember images of the injured hand immediately after the trauma and what it looked like in the emergency department before going into surgery.

Anatomy and Physiology

The posterior aspect of the hand is referred to as the *dorsum* and is covered with hair-bearing epidermis over dermis. Underneath, thin subcutaneous fascial layers loosely traverse to the distal portions of the hand attaching to the extensor tendons over the posterior aspect of the digits. The anterior aspect of the hand is covered with non–hair-bearing epidermis and dermis with thick palmer fascia arranged in vertical, oblique, and longitudinal fibers. Transverse layers of fascia cover the flexor tendons on the anterior aspect of the digits. The muscles of the hand are separated into three groups. The first is the muscle group of the thumb on the radial aspect of the hand. This muscle group forms the thenar mound at the base of the first digit (thumb). The second group is along the ulnar aspect of the hand forming the hypothenar mound at the base of the fifth digit. The third muscle group forms the midportion of the palm, filling the

interosseous spaces. The tendons of the dorsal and palmar surfaces are arranged in sheaths that cover the bones.

In anatomic position, the ulnar bone is medial to the radial bone in the forearm. Eight small carpal bones of the wrist are arranged in two rows and are held together by ligaments. The distal portion of the forearm bones articulate with the first row of three carpal bones referred to as the *scaphoid* (navicular), the *lunate,* and the *pisiform.* This complex is known as the *radiocarpal joint.* Five carpal bones forming the second row distal to this complex are referred to as the *capitate,* the *hamate,* the *triquetral* (triangular), and the *multiangular* (trapezoid [greater] and trapezium [lesser]). The five bones of the hand known as the *metacarpals* (one through five) align along the carpals to form the carpometacarpal joint (Fig. 8-40).

Digits one through five, referred to as *phalanges* (singular: phalanx), are distal to the metacarpals. The first digit (thumb) has two bones distal to the first metacarpal. Digits two through five are each composed of three bones distal to the corresponding metacarpal of the hand. Flexion of the carpometacarpal joint is the ability to grasp between the thumb and finger, referred to as *opposition,* which is a form of circumduction. This thumb motion distinguishes humans from the rest of the animal kingdom.

Each phalanx has a proximal base, a shaft, and distally, a head. The articulations of the proximal phalanges are at the level of the metacarpals in the metacarpophalangeal (MP) joints. The middle row of phalangeal bones articulates at the proximal interphalangeal joints (PIP). The distal phalangeal bones articulate at the distal interphalangeal joints (DIP).

The arterial blood supply is from the radial and ulnar arteries branching into the deep and superficial palmar arterial arches. The deep palmar arch supplies the first digit (thumb) and the radial aspect of the second digit. The superficial palmar arch supplies the ulnar aspect of the second digit (index finger) and all of digits three, four, and five. Venous drainage is through the dorsum into the cephalic and basilic venous systems (Fig. 8-41).

Motor and sensory innervation are derived from branches of the radial, ulnar, and median nerves. The superficial branch of the radial nerve arises from the level of nerve roots C6 to C7 and provides sensation to the dorsum of the hand. It divides into four dorsal digital nerves that supply the radial side of the dorsum of the hand at the level of the wrist. The median nerve arises from nerve roots C6 to C7 to T1 and innervates the lateral aspect of the palm and the first, second, and third digits. This nerve enters the hand through the carpal tunnel. Distally to the wrist, the recurrent branch of the median nerve divides into four or five volar (palmar) digital nerves. The ulnar nerve arises from nerve roots C7 to T1 and innervates the intrinsic muscles, the palm, and the fifth digit (Fig. 8-42).

Lymphatic vessels drain superficially from the digits to the thenar and hypothenar compartments along the path of the basilic and cephalic veins. These lymphatic vessels drain through the clavipectoral and supraclavicular nodes. Deep lymphatic drainage is along the radial and ulnar vessels.

Carpal Tunnel Syndrome

Carpal tunnel syndrome (CTS) is a hand neuropathy caused by the entrapment or compression of the median nerve by the transverse carpal ligament (Fig. 8-43). Other causes include

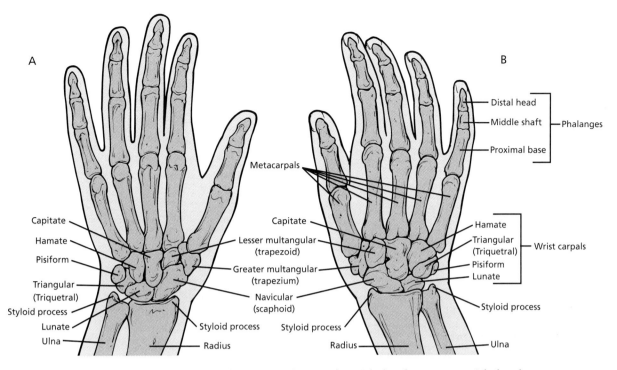

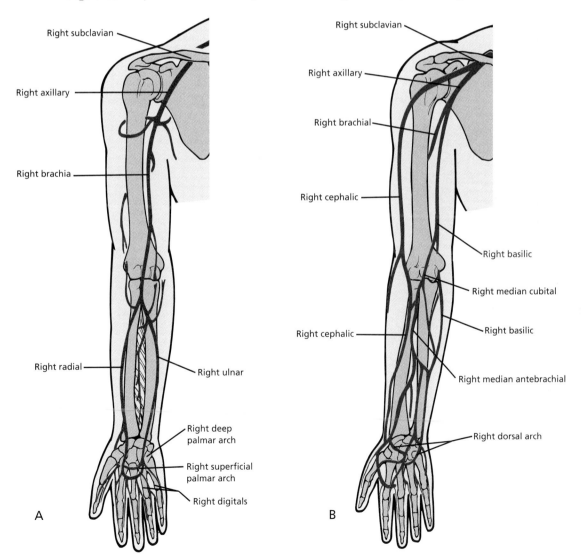

Metacarpals

Distal head
Middle shaft } Phalanges
Proximal base

Capitate
Hamate
Pisiform
Triangular (Triquetral)
Styloid process
Lunate
Ulna
Radius

Lesser multangular (trapezoid)
Greater multangular (trapezium)
Navicular (scaphoid)
Styloid process

Capitate
Hamate
Triangular (Triquetral) } Wrist carpals
Pisiform
Lunate
Styloid process
Styloid process
Radius
Ulna

Fig. 8-40 Bony structure of hand. **A,** Palmar surface right hand. **B,** Dorsum right hand.

Right subclavian
Right axillary
Right brachia
Right radial
Right ulnar
Right deep palmar arch
Right superficial palmar arch
Right digitals

Right subclavian
Right axillary
Right brachial
Right cephalic
Right basilic
Right median cubital
Right basilic
Right cephalic
Right median antebrachial
Right dorsal arch

Fig. 8-41 Anterior view of vascular structures of right arm. **A,** Arteries of right arm. **B,** Venous drainage of right arm.

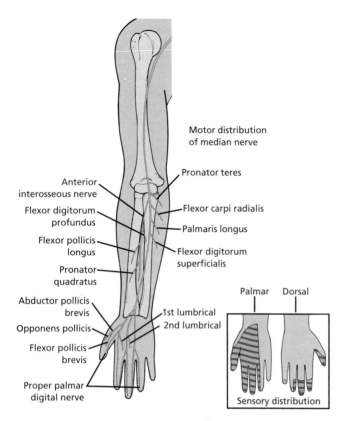

Fig. 8-42 Innervations of the median nerve of right arm.

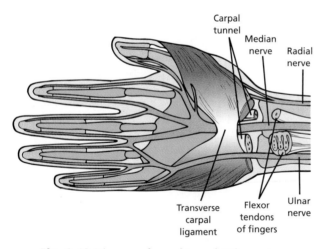

Fig. 8-43 Diagram of carpal tunnel. Palmar view.

displacement of the lunate bone or an enlarged volar (palm side) carpal ganglion. The result of pressure at the transverse carpal ligament is numbness of the hand and fingers, tingling, and a burning sensation. Some patients complain of nocturnal symptoms that rouse them from sleep. These sensations are usually accompanied by radiating pain and an inability to function properly, primarily in the dominant hand.

The advent of computer keyboards and video games started a trend of bilateral repetitive stress injury that is treated with surgical carpal tunnel release procedures. Repetitive stress can

generate inflammation that causes adhesions and scar tissue. Other theories state that CTS may be caused by trauma, fluid retention associated with the hormones of pregnancy or oral contraceptives, or rheumatoid arthritis. Some patients are relieved by antiinflammatories and splinting; others require surgical decompression.

Preoperative patient care

Diagnosis is made by a complete patient history and a physical examination. The patient's occupation and hand use patterns are evaluated. Noninvasive and invasive neurologic testing provides the diagnosis. The Phalen's test is performed by asking the patient to raise his or her arms in a vertical direction and flex the wrists for 30 to 60 seconds. The test is considered positive if the patient complains of parasthesia in the area of median nerve distribution. Tinel's test is performed by gently tapping on the median nerve to elicit a tingle over the distal hand and finger distribution. Electronic nerve conduction study is an invasive diagnostic test that provides an electrophysiologic confirmation of neuropathy by testing each nerve branch.

Anesthesia considerations

The procedure can be performed using local, regional, or general anesthesia. The choice of anesthesia is dependent on surgeon or patient preference and the involvement of the surgical procedure. Regional block anesthesia is commonly preferred because the procedure can be performed without excess fluid from infiltration anesthesia interfering with visualization of tissue at the surgical site. When the procedure is completed, the carpal canal can be infiltrated with local anesthetic, such as bupivacaine, to help with postoperative discomfort.

Intraoperative patient care

Carpal tunnel release is neurolysis performed by an open procedure or endoscopically. The median nerve is freed from the band of transverse carpal ligament to relieve pain and restore sensation and function.

The patient is positioned supine with his or her arm extended on a hand/arm table. A double bladder pneumatic tourniquet cuff is placed over padding on the upper affected arm. Anesthesia personnel will perform an anesthetic block, such as a Bier block, if general anesthesia is not used. An IV catheter is inserted into a vein close to the surgical site. The arm is elevated and an elastic compression bandage (Eshmarch) is applied starting distally at the hand and wrapped proximally up the arm to exsanguinate the extremity. The upper bladder of the tourniquet cuff is inflated to between 200 to 300 mm Hg depending on the patient's diastolic blood pressure and the elastic bandage is removed. Anesthetic is injected into the IV catheter to produce regional anesthesia. The anesthetic effect is effective as long as the tourniquet is inflated. A Bier block is commonly used for procedures that are performed in less than an hour and a half.

The hand and arm are prepped with antimicrobial solution, and the surgical site is draped leaving the hand and forearm exposed. All members of the team should sit for the procedure to preserve the integrity of the sterile field. The surgeon will perform either an open or endoscopic carpal tunnel ligament release. The tourniquet is often released before the portals are closed to double-check for the potential of a bleed. There is potential for a release of an inadvertent bolus of local anesthetic when the tourniquet is released. Physiologic and neurologic monitoring and observation should continue until the procedure is complete and the patient is ready to leave the room. The incisions are closed, and a palmar splint is applied.

Open carpal tunnel release

CTS syndrome is a common clinical entity, and the procedure to release the carpal tunnel is one of the most frequently performed surgical procedures of the hand. Current trends in the treatment of CTS have progressed from the open technique to an advanced endoscopic approach.

The open procedure is performed by two surgical methods. One method is to decompress the carpal tunnel by dividing the carpal ligament through a longitudinal skin incision that extends from the middle of the palm to the wrist. After the procedure, a bulky dressing and an immobilizing splint are used to promote healing. Most surgeons perform an open carpal tunnel release using some variation of this method.

Another open method less commonly used is the transverse wrist incision placed in a natural skin fold. An advantage is that the incision heals quickly with minimal postoperative pain and a shorter recovery period. There is less scar contracture and adhesion formation. A disadvantage is that this method offers limited exposure with the possibility of only partial ligament release and potential for injury to surrounding structures.

Endoscopic carpal tunnel release

The endoscopic approach for carpal tunnel release was first introduced in 1989 by J.C. Chow. This variation utilized a two-portal technique. This technique has proven to be a safe, simple, and effective method. Benefits of this method include a significant reduction in postoperative pain, less palmar swelling and tenderness, and a rapid return of the patient's grip and pinch strength. The result is a quicker return to work and the activities of daily living.

A transverse incision is made along the volar crease in the wrist and in the center of the palm (Fig. 8-44). The incision proceeds through the skin and the subcutaneous tissue creating a tunnel to the forearm fascia. The exploration extends from the palmaris longus to the flexor carpi ulnaris. The fascia is incised in two locations about 1 cm apart. This flap is carefully transected proximally to create a distal flap that will allow an adequate view of the carpal tunnel. A Freer elevator is used to separate adherent tissue from the transverse carpal ligament. The endoscope is inserted, and the median nerve is visualized. An endoscopic blade is used for dissection of the transverse carpal ligament under direct visualization. The Carposcope, one form of an endoscope, functions as a lighted retractor, dissector, guide, and V-Blade knife. Endoscopic procedures for the release of the carpal tunnel have been refined as an easy and safe approach to repairing CTS.

The perioperative nurse's role in endoscopic carpal tunnel surgery is to ensure proper handling, maintenance, and care of the equipment, and adequate knowledge of the procedure to ensure patient safety and facilitation of a successful surgical outcome.

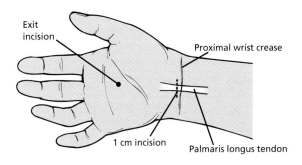

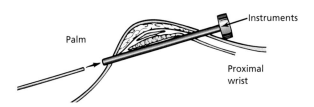

Fig. 8-44 Endoscopic carpal tunnel release. **A,** Incisions for endoscopic carpal tunnel release. **B,** Instrument placement for endoscopic carpal tunnel release.

Postoperative Patient Care

Postendoscopic patients do well after the procedure with little or no complaint. A simple dressing is applied with a supportive palmar splint at 30 degrees to 45 degrees extension to minimize pressure on the median nerve during finger motion exercises. Mild narcotic agents or nonaspirin over-the-counter (OTC) analgesics are usually sufficient.

Patients are encouraged to keep the hand elevated for 36 to 48 hours. Postoperative finger exercises are started on the first day while the hand is in an elevated position. The patient is instructed to spread and flex fingers several times every hour while awake. The palmar splint can be removed on the second to third postoperative day, but the patient is instructed to use the splint when sleeping for about 2 weeks. Exercises continue and include squeezing a soft foam rubber ball.

Potential complications

A complication of endoscopic carpal tunnel release is an incomplete release of the transverse carpal ligament. Other potential problems with both open and endoscopic methods include injuries to the median, ulnar, and digital nerves and/or damage to the flexor tendon. Reflex sympathetic dystrophy (RSD) can result from nerve damage. Vascular complications include injury to the superficial palmar arch causing hematoma.

Hand Trauma

The patient's body image is threatened by appearing and performing outside of the norm, which has a tremendous psychological impact. The patient may not want anyone to see the injured or deformed hand. The patient is concerned how others will see the injury and may feel that it will cause the loss of livelihood. Some patients will feel depression and self-blame for failing to avoid the injury. After the procedure, the patient will be concerned about the outcome of surgical repair and/or reconstruction and how the hand will look to others. Patients who require multiple procedures may fear a failure of the procedures to restore form and function.

Microsurgical repair is critical for successful digital replantation. Replantation of digits should occur within 4 to 6 hours after the injury (Fig. 8-45). The literature reports successful replantation of multiple digits 24 hours after injury when the amputated parts are still vital and have been carefully cooled. Larger segments of amputated hands and arms have a lower success rate because they are comprised of higher amounts of muscular tissue and require increased amounts of perfused oxygen for survival. Amputated parts maintained at room temperature reach critical ischemia at 6 hours.

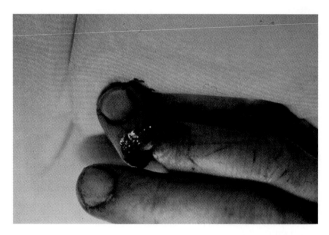

Fig. 8-45 Trauma to digit. *(Courtesy Brian W. Davies, MD.)*

Preoperative patient care

Preoperative assessment of the patient includes history and physical examination, x-ray examination of the injured part, complete blood count, and urinalysis. The patient is assessed for generalized health status and health-related considerations that would adversely affect wound healing, such as diabetes or smoking. The details of the injury are assessed for complexity (level of amputation), mechanism of injury (slice, burn, crush, explosion), wound edges (jagged, clean, avulsion), contamination, remaining skin/soft tissue cover, blood supply, or muscle/tendon/ligament damage. If the injury is a partial or complete amputation, the severed part is assessed for completeness and major structures, such as blood vessels, bone edges, skin, and muscle damage.

Antibiotics and tetanus toxoid are administered as appropriate. If completely severed, the part is placed in a dry, sterile container, which is then placed in regular ice. Fluid should not be added to the part because the tissue may macerate.

Contraindications to replantation include prolonged warm ischemia (over 6 to 8 hours), severe bruising or crushing injury, degloving injury, multiple fractures, and associated systemic injuries or illness that preclude further effort. Some surgeons exclude geriatric patients from replantation because of vascular changes associated with aging. However, the literature reports a patient aged 85 years who had a digital replantation with success.

Anesthesia considerations

Replant procedures may be performed under IVCS; Bier, axillary, or supraclavicular block; or general anesthesia. Long procedures for both children and adults are usually performed under general anesthetia.

Intraoperative Patient Care

Patient comfort and positioning with adequate padding are essential because the procedure may be prolonged. A gel-filled or air mattress can be used to relieve pressure areas, and a small pillow can be placed under the knees to decrease lower back strain. The injured arm is extended on a padded hand/arm table attached to the operating bed. Care is taken to not abduct the arm more than 90 degrees or brachial plexus nerve injury may result. A pneumatic tourniquet is applied over padding on the upper aspect of the arm. An elastic compression bandage is used to exsanguinate the arm before the tourniquet is inflated. The

elastic bandage is removed after the cuff is inflated to between 200 to 300 mm Hg. The hand and arm are prepped with antimicrobial solution, taking care not to abrade the wound edges. Additional sites of the body such as the iliac crest may be prepped if an autologous bone graft may be procured. The affected arm is draped with the hand and lower arm exposed.

Anastomosis of amputated digits is a lengthy procedure that can last 8 to 10 hours. The surgical team should be seated to preserve the integrity of the level of the sterile field. Two surgical teams may be used. One team prepares the amputated distal digit and the other team prepares the proximal recipient site (stump) under pneumatic tourniquet hemostasis. Operating loupes and/or a microscope are used to identify and work with small structures during the procedure. Small drills and saws are used to prepare the bone for fixation. Microsurgical instrumentation is used. Small cellulose eye-type spear sponges (Weck cells) are helpful for use on the microsurgical field. Heparinized irrigation is used to prevent coagulation, and lidocaine may be used to prevent vasospasm.

The amputated distal part of the digit is kept cool and moist as the transected end is carefully debrided. Vertical, 2 cm, longitudinal incisions are made on the midlateral aspects of the dissected portion for ease of identification of major structures (Fig. 8-46). Vessels, nerves, and tendons are isolated and tagged with small vessel clips. The proximal segment of the patient's stump is prepped, debrided, and functionally incised 2 cm on the bilateral longitudinal aspects. Major structures are identified and tagged. The bony end of the distal segment is smoothed, and the proximal bony tip is shortened several centimeters to enable the dissected blood vessels to span the defect. The bones are approximated with steel sutures or K-wire. Short vein grafts can be procured from other areas of the body to bridge vascular anastomoses.

The procedural steps in preparing a digit for replantation may be performed by a two-team approach; team one prepares the amputated digit, team two prepares the proximal reattachment site:

- Severed part prepared (cleaned)
- Blood vessels, nerves, and tendons identifed and tagged
- Tissue edges trimmed and debrided, bony edges trimmed, and the shaft slightly shortened

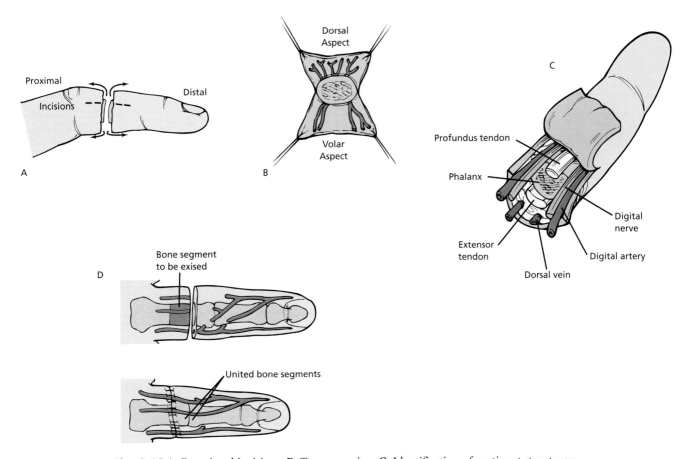

Fig. 8-46 A, Functional incisions. **B,** Transvese view. **C,** Identification of pertinent structures. **D,** Bone repair and arterial anastomosis.

- Proximal edge of the finger prepared (hand and arm are prepped)
- Bleeding controlled
- Blood vessels, nerves, and tendons identified and tagged
- Tissue edges trimmed and debrided
- Bony edges trimmed and mated to amputated part
- K-wire or steel suture fixation of the two bone edges
- Anastomosis of tendons (extensor and flexor)
- Arterial anastomosis followed by vein anastomosis and/or graft
- Nerve repair
- Muscle and skin closure

Toe-to-hand transfer

Another method of digit reconstruction for a traumatic amputation is the toe-to-hand transfer. This procedure is a free neurovascular flap and is most commonly performed when an amputated thumb cannot be salvaged. This procedure is referred to as pollicization.

The great toe with its accompanying tendons, vascular attachments, bone, and second web space is grafted to the hand. The transfer procedure is performed in the same order as replantation. After the fixation of bone and tendon anastomosis, the arterial and venous circulation is microscopically reestablished. Anastomosis of the digital nerves is established as possible to provide a potential for return of sensation and function (Fig. 8-47).

Postoperative patient care

Postoperative wound monitoring is very important. Frequent circulatory checks are important for careful observation of capillary refill, color, temperature, and wound drainage. Venous congestion can cause the loss of the replanted part. Some surgeons use leech therapy to relieve collections of deoxygenated blood for 4 to 7 days until venous circulation is reestablished. The wound dressing and splints may be modified to prevent pressure or constriction of circulation. The replanted part will be immobilized for up to 3 weeks. After this time, simple passive exercises will be started. The patient is cautioned about inadvertent injury because the part will be insensate for an indefinite period of time, perhaps permanently.

At 8 weeks, active range-of-motion exercises are added to the rehabilitation schedule. When bony healing is confirmed by x-ray examination, strengthening exercises are begun (Fig. 8-48). Some patients may experience abnormal neurologic sensation, such as tingling and burning in the replanted digit. Desensitization programs for sensation retraining are added to physical and occupational rehabilitation programs.

Congenital Hand Deformities

Some congenital deformities of the hand may be more easily adapted to daily living because the child has not experienced the use of whole, intact hands. However, the appearance of

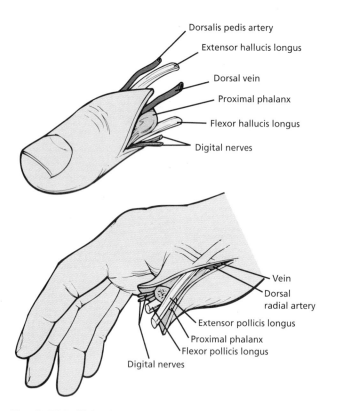

Fig. 8-47 Pollicization: great toe transplant for thumb reconstruction

deformed (macrodactyly), fused (syndactyly), missing, or extra digits (polydactyly) can be the source of dismay and embarrassment. As the child grows older, the differences of his or her hands will become more acutely evident. Other children will ask questions and many, unfortunately, will offer ridicule. Further concerns include how the deformity will impact daily life and ability to perform in school. Parents of a child with a congenital hand deformity may blame themselves. The extent of congenital deformity will determine the effectiveness of the repair, reconstruction, or neoconstruction.

Syndactyly

Syndactyly is the most common congenital anomaly that is characterized by the fusion of two or more fingers or toes. Fusion of digits can be simple or complex. Separation is not performed until the child is 1 year old. Simple fused digits are primarily soft tissue webbing without tendon, nerve, or bony involvement. Separation of a simple syndactyly is performed by soft tissue dissection and Z-W plasty. Some simple separations require a full-thickness skin graft.

Complex fusion incorporates various levels of bone deformity that is separated by a powered saw. Tendons are sometimes absent, and the conjoined digit may share a nailbed or critical vascular structures. Skin closure for complex deformities are similar to simple closure (Fig. 8-49).

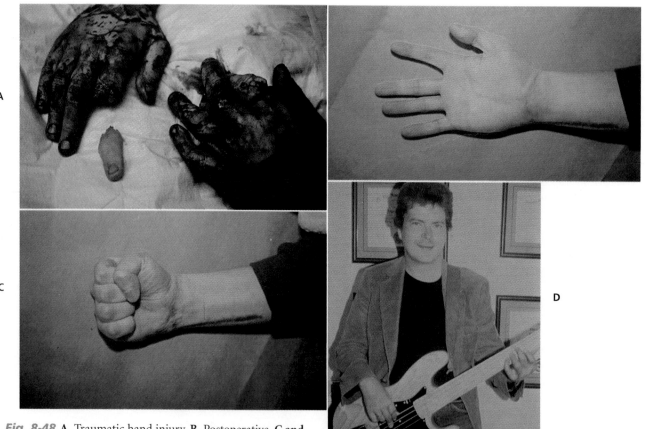

Fig. 8-48 A, Traumatic hand injury. B, Postoperative. C and D, Almost complete recovery. (Courtesy Brian W. Davies, MD.)

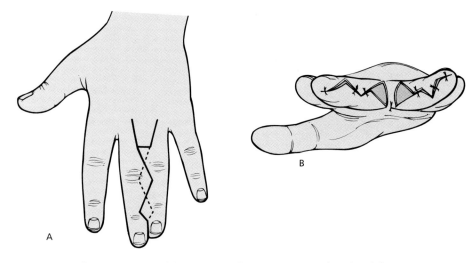

Fig. 8-49 View of the incisions for separating syndactylized digits.

Bibliography

Atroshi I et al: Endoscopic carpal tunnel release: prospective assessment of 250 consecutive cases, *J Hand Surg* 22(1):42, 1997.

Babovic S et al: Effects of tissue expansion on secondary ischemic tolerance in experimental free flaps, *Ann Plast Surg* 34(6):593, 1995.

Burk RW et al: Lidocaine and epinephrine levels in tumescent technique liposuction, *Plast Reconstr Surg* 97(7):1379, 1996.

Gabriel SE et al: Complications leading to surgery after breast implantation, *N Engl J Med* 336(10):677, 1997.

Gibbs KE et al: Open vs. endoscopic carpal tunnel release, *Orthopaedics* 19(12):1025, 1996.

Goel A et al: Replantation and amputation of digits, *Am J Phys Med Rehabil* 74(2):134, 1995.

Golden MA et al: Leech therapy in digital replantation, *AORN J* 62(3):364, 1995.

Hallock GG: Preexpansion of free flap donor sites used in reconstruction after burn injury, *J Burn Care Rehabil* 16(6):646, 1995.

Hollinger JO et al: Role of bone substitutes, *Clinical Ortho,* (324):55, 1996.

Hunstad JP: Addressing difficult areas in body contouring with emphasis on combined tumescent and syringe techniques, *Clin Plast Surg* 23(1):57, 1996.

Ishikura N et al: Repair of complete syndactyly by tissue expansion and composite grafts, *Brit J Plast Surg* 48(6):396, 1995.

Kale AA, DiCesare PE: Osteoinductive agents: basic science and clinical applications, *Am J Ortho* 24(10):752, 1995.

Kaplan B, Moy RL: Comparison of room temperature and warmed local anesthetic solution for tumescent liposuction: a randomized double-blind study, *Dermatol Surg* 22(8):707, 1996.

Malata CM et al: Tissue expansion: clinical applications, *J Wound Care* 4(2):88, 1995.

Malata CM et al: Tissue expansion: an overview, *J Wound Care* 4(1):37, 1995.

Modena S et al: Mastectomy and immediate reconstruction: oncological considerations and evaluation of two different methods relating to 88 cases, *Eur J Surg Oncol* 21(1):36, 1995.

Papay FA et al: Comparison of ossification of demineralized bone, hydroxyapatite, Gelfoam, and bone wax in cranial defect, *J Craniofac Surg* 7(5):347, 1991.

Peters W et al: Analysis of silicon levels in capsules of gel and saline breast implants and of penile prostheses, *Ann Plast Surg* 34(6):578, 1995.

Pomerance J et al: Replantation and revascularization of the digits in a community microsurgical practice *J Reconstr Microsurg* 13(3):163, 1997.

Queen TA, Palmer FR III: Gore-Tex for nasal augmentation, *Ann Otol Rhinol Laryngol* 104(11):850, 1995.

Silverman PM, Gordon L: Early motion after replantation, *Hand Clin* 12(1):97, 1996.

Soloman RP et al: The new implant tracking regulations: Defining, implementing, documenting, *AORN J* 58(6):1142, 1993.

Springer RC: Liposuction: an overview, *Plast Surg Nurs* 16(4):215, 1996.

Suh H, Lee C: Biodegradable ceramic-collagen composite implanted in rabbit tibia, *ASAIO J* 41(3):M652, 1995.

Thomas WO III et al: Explantation of silicone breast implants, *Am Surg* 63(5):421, 1997.

Thursen B et al: Capsular contracture after breast reconstruction with the tissue expansion technique, *Scan J Plast Reconstr Surg Hand Surg* 29(1):9, 1995.

Van Heest AE: Congenital disorders of the hand and upper extremity *Pediatr Clin North Am* 43(5):1113, 1996.

Von Schroeder HP, Botte MJ: Carpal tunnel syndrome *Hand Clin* 12(4):643, 1996.

Vuyk HD: Augmentation mentoplasty with solid silicone, *Clin Otolarngol* 21(2):106, 1996.

Yassi A: Repetitive strain injury *Lancet* 349(9056):943, 1997.

Head and Neck Surgical Procedures

Facial expression is nonverbal communication with the outside world. Patients who have sagging jowls and baggy eyelids appear older than their actual age. Loose facial structure creates a look of a scowl and unfriendliness, which can give the mistaken impression of anger. The media-based culture is youth-oriented and can present a barrier to psychologic self-esteem. Laxity of the skin and underlying structures can give the impression of anger, tiredness, or boredom. A more youthful appearance evokes a sense of energy and spirit. Males and females commonly seek surgical intervention to tighten facial skin and underlying tissues. Facelift, brow, and eyelid procedures are more commonly performed for females between 51 to 64 years of age than for males. Most of these are performed as outpatient procedures.

Over the past few years, more middle-age men have requested facial rejuvenation procedures. Males are finding that a younger, more rested facial appearance gives a more energetic and attractive appearance, which may provide an advantage in the corporate environment and for career change options.

ANATOMY AND PHYSIOLOGY OF THE HEAD AND NECK

Musculature of the head and neck includes the following (Fig. 9-1):

- Temporalis
- Occipitalis
- Frontalis
- Masseter
- Mentalis
- Orbicularis oris
- Orbicularis oculi
- Zygomatic major
- Zygomatic minor
- Sternocleidomastoid
- Platysma

The lateral aspects of the parotid glands and cheeks are covered by the fascial layers referred to as the *superficial musculoaponeurotic system* (SMAS). This tissue layer is the key structural element in a facelift procedure. It is continuous with the zygomatic muscle laterally, frontalis muscle superiorly, and the platysma muscle inferiorly (Fig. 9-2). The SMAS overlies the facial motor nerves and vasculature and begins to sag and change in response to dermatochalasis (relaxation of the skin) with age. The galea fascia overlies the frontal bone and supports the brow. This tissue loosens with advancing age causing the brow to sag and wrinkle.

Innervation of the face is derived from three cranial nerves. Eye muscles are innervated by the occulomotor nerve (cranial nerve III), with the exception of the lateral rectus and the superior oblique. Cutaneous sensory innervation is supplied by the trigeminal (cranial nerve V) and cervical nerve plexus. Branches of the trigeminal nerve supply sensory innervation of the lateral face, ears, and cheeks. The muscles of facial expression are innervated by the facial nerve (cranial nerve VII). Motor activity of the forehead, eyebrows, cheeks, lips, ears, and scalp are supplied from this source.

Primary facial vasculature arises from branches of the common, external, and internal carotid arteries. Major secondary arteries include the facial and the temporal arteries (Fig. 9-3). Venous drainage flows into the internal and external jugular veins. Lymphatic drainage flows from the nodes of the head and neck into the cervical plexus.

PREOPERATIVE FACIAL MARKING

Improvement possibilities of sagging facial lines are determined during initial photo sessions. Life-size photos are used to plan and map out the surgical approach. Each facial perspective is measured, and the surgical plan is developed using transparent overlays. Preoperative facial marking is performed to create a skin surface template similar to the overlay for the surgical lines of dissection and undermining.

The patient should be marked in a sitting position before the anesthetic is administered. Natural expression and gravitational effects on the cheeks, jowls, forehead, and eyelid tissue are well demonstrated while the patient sits upright looking straight forward. Local infiltration anesthesia can distort the facial lines and markings leading to irregular lines of incision. The sitting position allows the lateral aspects of the face to sag in response to laxity. Upper lid redundancy is more prominent, and fat disposition can be more accurately determined. The proposed incisions are placed in areas of concealment if possible. The natural fold of the eyelid is an example. Some surgeons will photograph the procedure in process per personal preference. Photographs are taken after the procedure for the permanent record. Photography permission should be obtained and documented per facility policy.

RHYTIDECTOMY (FACELIFT)

Rhytidectomy (facelift) is the surgical smoothing of deep wrinkles (rhytids) of the lower portion of the face. It is performed to

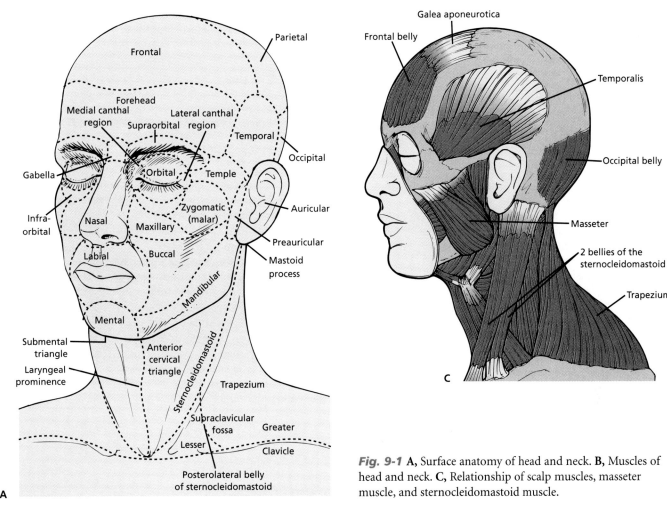

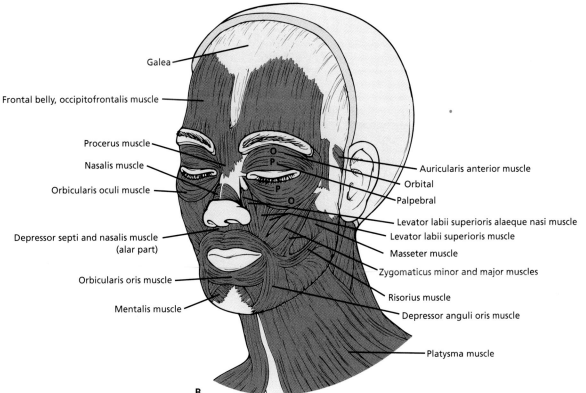

Fig. 9-1 A, Surface anatomy of head and neck. **B,** Muscles of head and neck. **C,** Relationship of scalp muscles, masseter muscle, and sternocleidomastoid muscle.

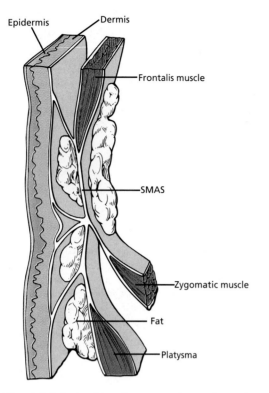

Fig. 9-2 Relationship of SMAS to skin and muscle.

remove redundant skin caused by the loss of elasticity and lax underlying support structures.

Historically, the facelift has been performed since the turn of the century and only involved tightening of the skin of the face. The results lasted 3 to 5 years. In 1901, Hollander made a vertical incision in front of the ear that extended into a curvilinear incision to the neck. In 1920, Bettman published preoperative and postoperative photos of temporal and periaurical incisions currently used in modern facelift procedures. In 1927, Bames recommended subcutaneous undermining and suturing to the relatively immobile underlying fascia. This remained the technique used for rhytidectomy until the 1970s. Lexer used two S-shaped incisions, one along the temple and the other over the mastoid area. He was the first to undermine the skin in the subcutaneous plane. In 1974, Skoog advocated a deep-layer suspensary technique.

Numerous variations in technique have appeared in the literature that incorporate the subcutaneous or the SMAS technique. Methods currently used for facelift involve tightening all layers of the skin, fascia, muscle, and subcutaneous tissue of the face and neck. The results last 5 to 10 years but will vary according to the health, lifestyle, and activity of each individual patient. Modern methods, including endoscopy and laser application, have augmented the facial rejuvenation process.

If the procedure is performed when the patient is too young, the results will be less obvious and the need for revision every 5

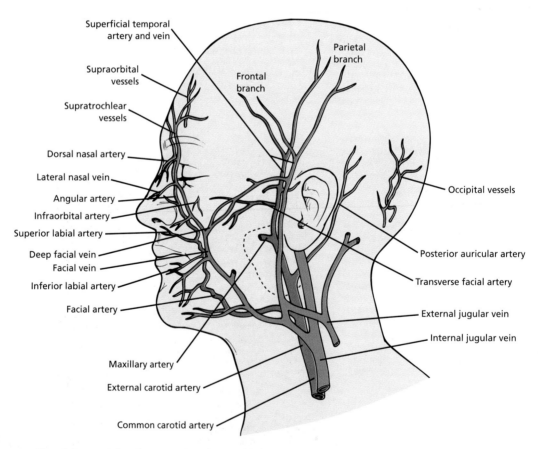

Fig. 9-3 Arterial and venous distribution of head and neck. Branching of internal carotid artery from common carotid artery is not shown but occurs just inferior to the point at which the external carotid artery is indicated.

to 10 years will decrease the effectiveness of the procedure. Results are best if the skin of the face is not too wrinkled and lax, as commonly seen after 70 years of age (Fig. 9-4).

Preoperative Patient Care

The surgeon should explain the procedure and discuss any associated complications. The patient's health condition is evaluated for the selection of anesthesia. The patient is given written preoperative and postoperative instructions, such as facial cleansing and skin care, postoperative medications, diet, and events for the day of surgery. The patient is instructed to not smoke for at least 2 weeks before and after surgery because the associated vasoconstriction interferes with wound healing. An elastic head garment is fitted for postoperative use.

The physician should take a careful health history to determine if the patient has any bleeding condition that can create postoperative complications. Current medications and nutritional habits may alter coagulation, such as some Chinese foods, fish oils, anti-inflammatory drugs, and vitamin E. Aspirin and alcohol can cause bleeding and are avoided for at least 2 weeks before and after the procedure. Hair dye and bleach may be applied up to 1 day before the procedure but not again until 4 weeks after.

The patient should have realistic expectations about the surgical outcome. Postoperative appearance may shed 5 to 10 years from the patient's visual age. Dissatisfaction stems from approaching the procedure with the belief that the fountain of youth is in the operating room (OR).

The patient should arrive at the surgery department with clean hair (no hairspray or oils) and no facial makeup. He or she is also reminded to not eat or drink after midnight the night before surgery. Vomiting can cause a disruption of the wounds. Smoking is prohibited as it is in all plastic surgery patients (Fig. 9-5).

Anesthesia Considerations

General anesthesia is commonly used, but intravenous conscious sedation (IVCS) or monitored anesthesia care (MAC) are other options in combination with local infiltration containing epinephrine. If general anesthesia is used, the endotracheal tube is not taped to the face because it interferes with the planes of surgical dissection. Some surgeons secure the tube to the patient's front teeth with suture. Other surgeons prefer nasotracheal intubation. The anesthesia provider monitors the patient under general anesthesia or MAC using electrocardiogram (ECG), pulse oximetry, temperature probe, and carbon dioxide (CO_2) monitoring. IV antibiotics and steroids are given during the procedure at the request of the surgeon.

Intraoperative Patient Care

The patient is positioned on the operating bed in the supine position. A pressure-relieving foam mattress or gel pad is used to minimize pressure areas on the patient's back. A gel-filled or foam donut is used to position the head. Application of sequential pneumatic compression stockings or antiembolism stockings can help to prevent deep vein thrombosis. The patient's arms are secured on armboards or tucked in at his or her sides with the drawsheet. The safety belt is placed across the patient's thighs.

If general anesthesia is used, the eyes are protected with corneal protectors, moist gauze pads, and/or ophthalmic ointments. Cotton balls are placed in the ears during the prep to prevent pooling of prep solution. The hair is partitioned from the face and shaved from the incision line. The face and hairline are prepped with antimicrobial solution. Chlorhexidine (4%) is not recommended for the facial prep because it can cause irreversible eye damage, but it can be used in the hair because it is less damaging to dyed or chemically treated hair. The patient's head is draped with care to not dislodge the endotracheal tube if general anesthesia is used.

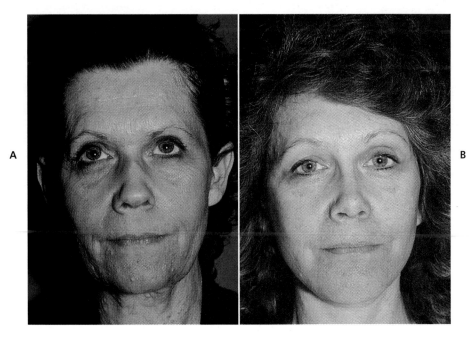

Fig. 9-4 Browlift, rhinoplasty, blepharplasty, facelift. **A,** Preoperative. **B,** Postoperative. *(Courtesy Brian W. Davies, MD.)*

Procedure

Current rhytidectomy combines skin undermining and the creation of several flaps composed of muscle, fascia, fat, dermis, and epidermis. This procedure tightens and repositions deeper structures to vertically advance the facial skin in a horizontal plane. This prevents shifts in the hairline both temporally and postaurically. The molar cheek fat is repositioned providing dramatic improvements in the midface plane, jowls, and nasolabial folds. Facial nerves and the parotid ducts are protected beneath the SMAS.

The procedure is performed through standard incisions made in the hairline anterior to the tragus of the ear (preauricular) and around the posterior aspect of the ear lobe (postauricular) (Fig. 9-6). The bilateral incisions are made parallel to the hair follicles to prevent hair loss. The skin of the cheeks and bilateral neck is undermined and lifted from the fascia and muscle. The raised flap is measured to the ear incision, and the excess skin is trimmed away. The underlying muscles are tightened, and the skin flap is sutured in place. Excess fat is removed from the chin and anterior neck through a small, separate submental incision. Liposuction is commonly used (Fig. 9-7).

The subperiosteal approach follows a deeper plane adjacent to bone along the orbit, brow, and midface. This method provides support for the deeper tissue to reduce the gravitational

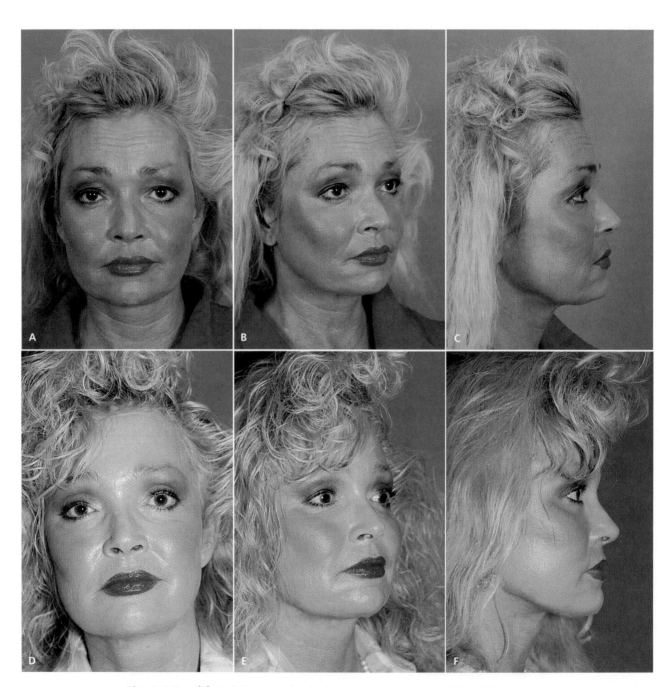

Fig. 9-5 Browlift. **A-C,** Preoperative. **D-F,** Postoperative. *(Courtesy Brian W. Davies, MD.)*

load on the skin. The tightening of exterior as well interior muscles adds years to the efficacy of the procedure.

Most current approaches of facial rejuvenation include techniques to improve the appearance of the neck. One surgical approach includes advancement of the SMAS and the platysma muscle while either reshaping or excising the neck fat. The aesthetic goal is to produce a smooth and youthful contour to the neck. Over-resection can cause a hollowed-out appearance. Good technique includes sharp dissection accompanied by lipectomy. The remaining fat provides a smooth contour to the neck and submandibular area.

Superficial small skin wrinkles are not removed by a facelift procedure. Some patients require an additional superficial chemical peel or CO_2 laser treatment around the lip line in combination with or after rhytidectomy. The peel can be performed at a later date if needed over an area of elevated flap.

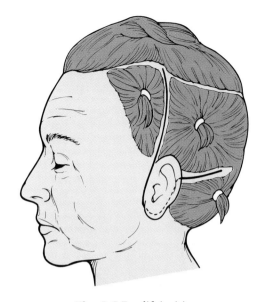

Fig. 9-6 Facelift incision.

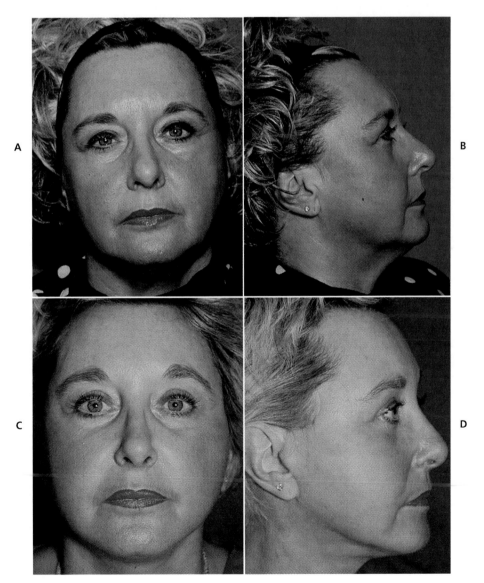

Fig. 9-7 Browlift, blepharoplasty, neck liposuction. **A and B,** Preoperative. **C and D,** Postoperative. *(Courtesy Brian W. Davies, MD.)*

Postoperative Patient Care

The patient will remain in the postprocedural recovery area for approximately 1 1/2 to 2 hours depending on his or her physical condition. The head should remain in a neutral position, elevated 30 degrees for 24 to 48 hours after the procedure. Excess strain on the incision lines is avoided. Cool compresses are applied to decrease postoperative bleeding and swelling. The head dressings and closed wound suction drains, if used, remain in place for 24 hours. The elastic head garment is worn continuously for 1 week and at bedtime for 3 weeks. The patient is instructed to sleep on his or her back to avoid putting pressure on the flaps. Excessive compression on the incision line may impair circulation and interfere with wound healing.

The patient may experience moderate pain for several days after surgery. Oral analgesia, narcotic or nonnarcotic, will be prescribed by the physician. Aspirin is avoided because it interferes with clotting mechanisms and may cause hematoma formation. Bruising and discoloration can last for up to 1 month or longer.

The face, cheek, and neck areas may be insensate because of the facial flap resection. Sensation should improve over time. The patient is warned about the potential for facial, neck and scalp burns by hairdryers or curling irons. Extreme heat can also cause vasodilation and promote bleeding. Mild activities are resumed 2 days after the procedure. Sexual activity can resume after 1 week. Any strenuous activity such as sports is avoided for at least 1 month.

Male patients may find that scars are best concealed by wearing the hair slightly longer. They may have more superficial bleeding because of the vascularity of the beard line. The hair-bearing facial surface may be shifted causing the need to shave lower onto the neck and closer to the ears. Hair loss along the incision line is common but usually returns after 3 months if the follicle has not been damaged.

Complications

Hematoma is the most common complication of rhytidectomy. Hypertension increases the risk of bleeding. Men have a slightly higher incidence than women. The patient should be advised that normal swelling feels softer to the touch, but hematoma feels firm and progressively becomes harder. Small localized areas can be drained with a syringe and needle. Pressing on the flap or "milking" the hematoma is not advised and may cause the loss of the flap. Sutures are released to evacuate the hematoma to prevent compromise of the blood supply. Skin slough at the wound site caused by tension on the incision line may leave a healed scar that later needs surgical revision. This may result in incision line alopecia.

Wound separation and necrosis can be caused by inadequate blood supply. The patient should be cautioned that postoperative smoking and exposure to passive smoke interferes with wound healing causing a wider, discolored scar. Injury to temporal and marginal mandibular nerves can be caused by infiltration of local anesthetic, cautery, suture, edema, and hematoma. Most of these injuries recover spontaneously.

Parasthesia or numbness of the lower two thirds of the ear is caused by damage to the great auricular nerve. Sensation is usually altered 2 cm anterior to the preauricular incision caused by undermining of the flap.

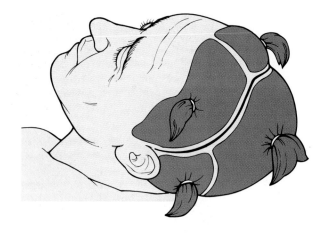

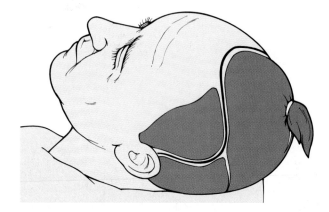

Fig. 9-8 Incisions for forehead/browlift.

Postoperative depression and dissatisfaction with the surgical outcome can be psychologic complications. If the patient has been adequately informed and prepared before the procedure, postoperative depression is a rare event. Patient education should focus on the time elements of the postoperative recovery period and the return to usual activities. Realistic expectations of the surgical procedure and its intended results are important to stress and reinforce.

BROWLIFT

The upper third of the face between the eyebrows and the natural hairline (the border of the scalp and superior portion of the face) becomes lax, wrinkles, and develops creases along the glabellar surface and across the bridge of the nose. The corrections can be made by creating a beveled coronal incision at or behind the hair line (Fig. 9-8), undermining the forehead tissue and trimming the redundant skin (Fig. 9-9). A sterile comb is useful for combing through the hairline to remove stray hair along the incision line. The incision is closed with subcuticular stitches or skin staples (Fig. 9-10). Some surgeons use an endoscopic approach, which is described as follows.

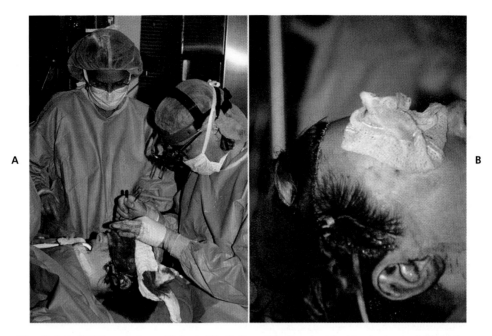

Fig. 9-9 A, RNFA assisting with browlift. **B,** Browlift closed with skin staples and 1/4 inch penrose drain in place. *(Courtesy Brian W. Davies, MD.)*

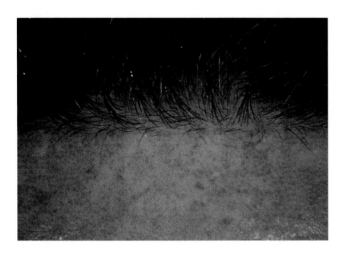

Fig. 9-10 Healed browlift incision. *(Courtesy Brian W. Davies, MD.)*

Patient Care Considerations

Preoperative evaluation includes height of the forehead, hair loss pattern, and thickness of the scalp. The height of the forehead is measured. The average desired forehead measures 5 cm from eyebrows to hair line. Preoperative instructions are the same as those for facelift patients. Browlift is commonly performed in combination with facelift and blepharoplasty (Fig. 9-11). Some patients have an autologous fat injection to fill furrows or solid silicone implants placed to augment cheeks or chin.

ENDOSCOPIC FACELIFT AND BROWLIFT

Endoscopic technique in plastic surgery is an evolving method of facial rejuvenation. The endoscopic technique provides a precise surgical field, allowing a view of the subsurface structural anatomy

of the face in a highly specific perspective. The corrugator and procerus muscles are resected through endoscopic instruments. Minimal skin incisions for the introduction of instrumentation are challenging because all surgical alterations are subplanar (Fig. 9-12). No excess superficial skin can be excised.

Instrumentation

The equipment for endoscopic facelift consists of the following basic components:

- Endoscopic unit composed of a camera and light source (xenon)
- Television monitor
- Video recorder and printer
- Endoscope 4 or 5mm; 30-degree down-angle rigid
- Instrumentation, periosteal elevators, and manipulators

The subperiosteal technique is the most popular endoscopic method because this surgical plane allows a better field of vision for dissection (Fig. 9-13). It also permits better illumination because of the reflection between facial bone and the periosteum. The field becomes bright and almost bloodless, permitting enhanced visualization. The bony landmarks and fascial attachments to specific areas of the bone help the surgeon maintain orientation during the dissection. Superficial liposuction or chemical peeling is sometimes performed in the same surgical session.

BLEPHAROPLASTY (AESTHETIC EYE SURGERY)

The eyes are the most expressive region of the face. They express human emotions very effectively and play an important role in interpersonal communication. The skin of aging eyelids

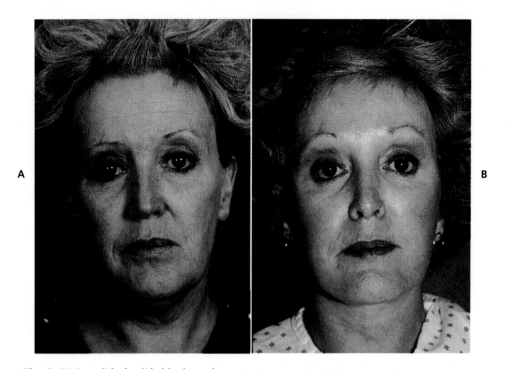

Fig. 9-11 Browlift, facelift, blepharoplasty. **A,** Preoperative. **B,** Postoperative. *(Courtesy Brian W. Davies, MD.)*

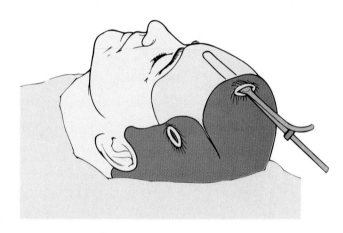

Fig. 9-13 Endoscopic browlift.

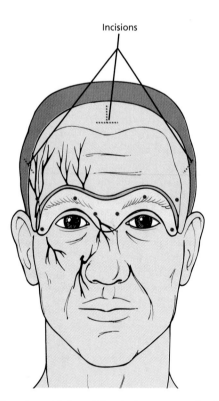

Fig. 9-12 Endoscopic browlift. The lines across the face show the procerus/corrugator resection.

becomes redundant, losing elasticity. Orbital fat accumulates between the muscle fibers. Baggy, drooping eyelids cause disfigurement, producing a weary and dull appearance (Fig. 9-14).

Blepharoplasty is the surgical removal of redundant skin of the upper and/or lower eyelids. It is the third most commonly performed cosmetic procedure (Box 9-1). It is often performed on women between the ages of 35 and 64 years of age. Eyelid surgery is considered reconstructive when the skin of the upper eyelid interferes with vision and may be covered by some health insurance plans (Fig. 9-15). Blepharoplasty is commonly performed in conjunction with rhytidectomy. This procedure can be performed under local anesthesia with IVCS or general anesthesia. General anesthesia is usually preferred if combined with rhytidectomy.

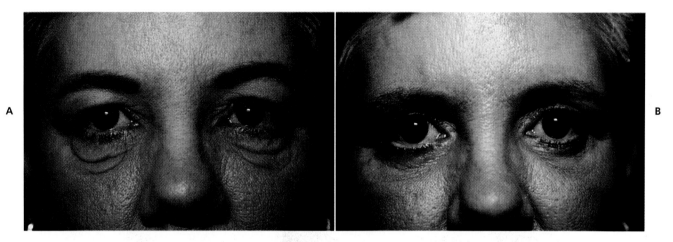

Fig. 9-14 Blepharoplasty. **A,** Preoperative. **B,** Postoperative. *(Courtesy Brian W. Davies, MD.)*

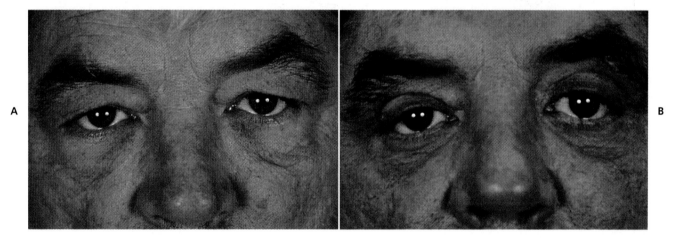

Fig. 9-15 Upper lid blepharoplasty. **A,** Preoperative. **B,** Postoperative. *(Courtesy Brian W. Davies, MD.)*

Anatomy and Physiology

The upper eyelids consist of three layers: skin, circular orbicularis palpebral muscle, and the tarsoconjunctival connective tissue layer. The tarsus of the upper lid is a 10 mm band of tissue extending from the lid margin (palpebral fissure) to the cephalad margin, where it is joined by the Muller's muscle and the levator aponeurosis muscle (Fig. 9-16). The tarsus of the lower lid measures 4 mm. The superior and inferior tarsal tissue is somewhat rigid, but flexible enough to conform to the shape of the globe and cornea. The eyelids are innervated by the facial nerve and fibers of cranial nerve III.

Innervation of the eye is derived from cranial nerves II through VI. Cranial nerve II (optic nerve) is for vision. Cranial nerve III (oculomotor nerve) is a motor nerve serving the pupils and all ocular muscles except the lateral rectus and superior oblique. Cranial nerve IV (trochlear nerve) innervates

---

Box 9-1 **Indications for Blepharoplasty**

PTOSIS
Laxity of the levator muscle from the tarsal plate; difficulty raising eyelid; congenital or senile

AGED EYE
Excess skin and protrusion of periorbital fat; may occur simultaneously with senile ptosis

ELECTIVE WESTERNIZATION
Asian upper eyelids have no supratarsal fold; the horizontal level of the lateral canthus is 3 mm superior to the medial canthus; the lateral canthus of Western eyes is only 1 to 2 mm superior to the medial canthus

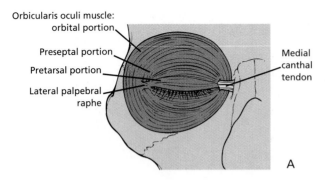

Orbicularis oculi muscle:
   orbital portion
   Preseptal portion
   Pretarsal portion
   Lateral palpebral raphe

Medial canthal tendon

A

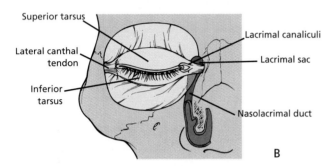

Superior tarsus

Lateral canthal tendon

Inferior tarsus

Lacrimal canaliculi

Lacrimal sac

Nasolacrimal duct

B

Fig. 9-16 The orbital, preseptal, and pretarsal portions of the orbicularis muscle.

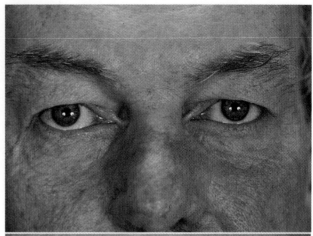

A

B

Fig. 9-17 Blepharoplasty. A, Preoperative. B, Postoperative. *(Courtesy Brian W. Davies, MD.)*

down and inward motions. Cranial nerve V (trigeminal nerve) is a sensory nerve providing sensation to the upper and lower lids and cornea. Cranial nerve VI (abducens nerve) provides motor impulses for lateral elevation. Blood is supplied by the internal and external carotid arteries.

Preoperative Patient Care

Preoperative photographs are used for preoperative procedural planning (Fig. 9-17). Recommended photographs include a full-face view, a close-up of the eyelids in response to smiling, and a close-up of the eyelids with the periorbital structures in an upward and downward gaze.

Detailed information should be provided regarding the location and extension of any postoperative scars, how visible they may be, and how long will it take for them to fade. Skin assessment of previous surgical sites or injuries can be indicators of potential scarring. Eyelid scars are usually well hidden and are not as conspicuous as long as they do not surpass the eyelid skin. Discussion of the techniques available before the procedure will help allay any concerns that the patient may have. Physical examination of the skin and subcutaneous tissue of the eyelids and periorbital areas is essential to rule out any tumors or lesions.

The tone of the upper lids should be assessed during the preoperative evaluation. The "squint test" is done by asking the patient to squint as if looking at the sun. This test is done to check for major relaxation of the orbicularis, which produces festoons (bulges) that appear at the orbital and preseptal areas. The skin is pinched between the thumb and index finger. The amount of skin that remains folded or tented upward after the pinch is released will display laxity of both muscle and skin tension.

Skin marking is performed before injection of local anesthetic using a skin marker with the patient in a sitting position. Incisions are placed in natural skin folds if possible.

Anesthesia Considerations

Some surgeons select general anesthesia to have total control during the blepharoplasty procedure if the patient is intolerant of IVCS with local infiltration. Lidocaine with epinephrine is usually injected to decrease intraoperative bleeding.

Intraoperative Patient Care

The patient is positioned supine on the operating bed with his or her head positioned on a foam or gel-filled donut. After the administration of anesthesia, the eyes are prepped with a mild antimicrobial solution that is not harmful to the ocular tissue. Corneal shields are placed to prevent accidental injury. The head is draped in sterile fashion, and the sterile field is established.

Procedure

The elliptical upper lid incision is created along the surgical markings by sharp dissection (Fig. 9-18, *A*). Low-temperature, battery-operated cautery can be used to control pinpoint

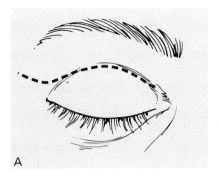

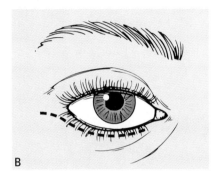

Fig. 9-18 **A,** Incision for upper eyelid blepharoplasty.
B, Incision for lower eyelid blepharoplasty.

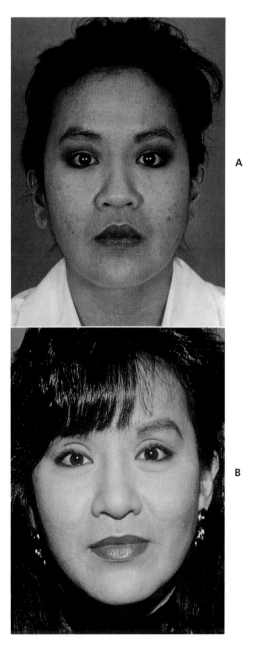

Fig. 9-19 Upper blepharoplasty on the Asian eyelid.
A, Preoperative. **B,** Postoperative. *(Courtesy Brian W. Davies, MD.)*

bleeders. The orbicularis oculi muscle is isolated, and a strip of preseptal muscle and protruding periorbital fat is removed. The upper lid suture line is at the level of the suprastarsal fold. This creates the "Westernization" effect of the upper eyelids sought by some Asian patients (Figs. 9-19 and 9-20).

For the lower eyelid, the incision is made close to the inferior ciliary margin, usually within 2 millimeters of the lower palpebral rim (see Fig. 9-18, *B*). This method is referred to as *transpalpebral blepharoplasty*. These incisions are sutured closed in one single layer. The transconjunctival approach (incision into the inner aspect of the lower lid) is used for fat removal, leaving the skin, orbicularis muscle, and orbital septum intact.

A margin of 2 millimeters may separate the palpebral fissure (the opening of the eye) immediately after the procedure, but this will diminish as swelling and infiltrative anesthetic effects fade, usually within 1 week. The finished upper lid should measure 26 to 30 mm to have optimal form and function. Females or patients with smaller eyes may require less upper lid tissue for an aesthetic result. A slight asymmetry may be apparent after the procedure. A revision may be indicated if a noticeable asymmetry persists after 9 months to 1 year after the procedure. It may be necessary to excise a small portion of skin and or muscle on the side that has a smaller-appearing fold. This is more common in cases of ptosis.

Postoperative Patient Care

For the first 24 hours after surgery, the head should be elevated 30 degrees, and cool compresses are applied to alleviate swelling. Antibiotic ointments may be prescribed. The eyes may feel dry and blurry for a few days, but a commercial tear solution can be used to moisten the conjunctiva. Contact lenses may irritate the eyes and should be avoided for a few weeks after the procedure.

There is usually minimal postoperative discomfort. Severe pain may indicate a serious complication, such as retroorbital bleeding, and should be evaluated by the physician immediately. Bruising and discoloration are prominent but will fade within approximately 2 weeks. The sutures are removed in 3 to 5 days after surgery (Fig. 9-21).

Complications

Some patients may experience persistent numbness of the eyelids. Other complications include the need to repeat the

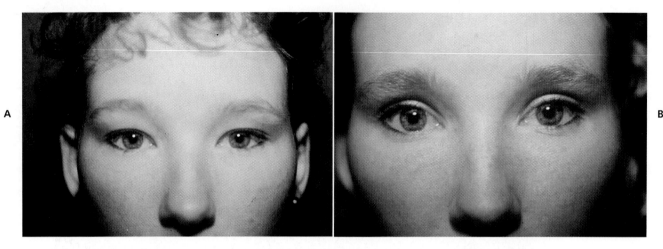

Fig. 9-20 Caucasian female with epicathal folds (oriental eye). Upper lid blepharoplasty. **A,** Preoperative. **B,** Postoperative. *(Courtesy Brian W. Davies, MD.)*

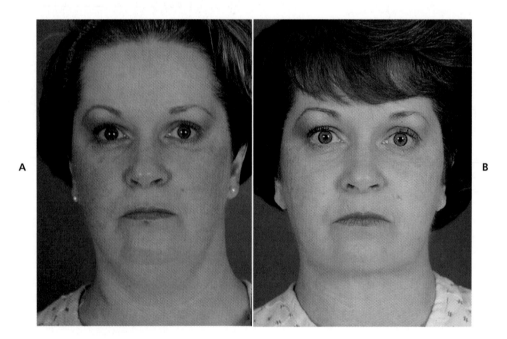

Fig. 9-21 Browlift, blepharoplasty, neck liposuction. **A,** Preoperative. **B,** Postoperative. *(Courtesy Brian W. Davies, MD.)*

procedure to remove more tissue. Iatrogenic problems, such as removal of too much skin or orbicularis muscle, can result in an incomplete eyelid closure after the procedure and subsequently, "dry eye." If excess fat is removed, the eye may appear sunken and aged. Ectropion, or everted eyelid, can result if eye tissue remains lax causing the eye to lay open. The cornea can be damaged by environmental factors if there is no protection by the eyelid. Some patients can benefit from lid massage to stretch the skin. Severe cases may need skin grafting.

Milia may appear at the suture line. These usually disappear within several weeks without intervention but can be removed with a fine sterile needle or electrosurgery. Early suture removal within 2 to 3 days can help prevent this.

Injury to the lacrimal system can include interruption of the tear duct causing "dry eye." Patients who have intrinsic dry eye not caused by iatrogenic intervention are not good surgical candidates. If surgery is absolutely necessary, a conservative resection is done. Some patients may have a pooling of tears in the space between the globe and the lid referred to as *epiphoria.*

AESTHETIC RHINOPLASTY

The nose balances the facial aesthetic appeal (Fig. 9-22). Variations in nasal contour are found in different races, ethnic groups, and sexes. Aesthetic procedures of the face commonly involve multiple procedures that include recontouring of the nose.

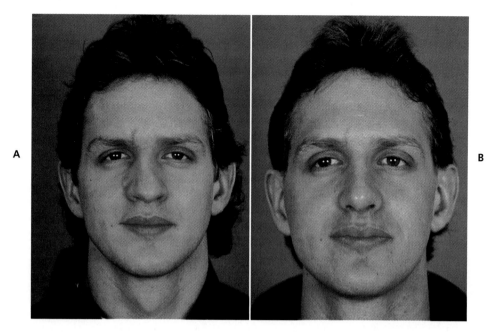

Fig. 9-22 Rhinoplasty. **A,** Preoperative. **B,** Postoperative. *(Courtesy Brian W. Davies, MD.)*

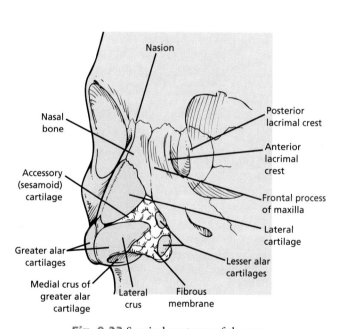

Fig. 9-23 Surgical anatomy of the nose.

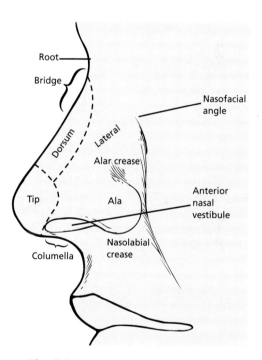

Fig. 9-24 Surgical landmarks of the nose.

Anatomy and Physiology

The aesthetic anatomy of the nose is divided into subsurface and superficial structural components. The subsurface consists of segmental cartilage and bone (Fig. 9-23). The superficial components include creases and projections (Fig. 9-24).

Preoperative Patient Care

Realistic expectations are reinforced for the patient seeking aesthetic rhinoplasty. The patient is evaluated in a seated position. Facial measurements are taken from anterior and lateral views comparing the alae, eye canthus, nasal pyramid, and the buccal commissures. From the anterior perspective, comparison is made between the medial canthus of the eyes and the alar borders. The alae of broader-based noses extend beyond the intercanthal distance of the eyes. Extension beyond 2 mm usually requires resection of the nasal sill. The dorsum should appear as two straight or slightly concave rows that extend from the eyebrows to the tip of the nose. The round protuberances of the alae should rise slightly above the dorsum. The tip of the nose appears as an inverted triangle with the point resting over the superior angle of the collumella and the base extending between the medial aspects of the alae.

Lateral, or profile, evaluation of proportion and balance is made. The face is divided into four imaginary horizontal planes: hairline, browline, collumella, and chin. The length of the nose is measured from the nasion to the tip. Projection of the tip is measured by comparison to the alar-cheek junction. The angle of the collumella and the upper lip should be 95 to 105 degrees for a feminine appearance and 90 to 95 degrees for a masculine look. The nasal bone is palpated by the surgeon, and the cartilaginous elasticity is tested. Multiple full-face and 3/4-sized photographs are taken from anterior, lateral, and basal views (Fig. 9-25).

Anesthesia Considerations

Aesthetic rhinoplasty can be performed using local anesthesia with IVCS or general anesthesia. Lidocaine with epinephrine is usually injected along incision lines to minimize bleeding. Cocaine 4% or lidocaine 2% may be added if intranasal incisions are planned.

Intraoperative Patient Care

The patient is placed on the operating bed in a modified beach-chair position (low Fowler's with flexed knee-gatch). The safety belt is placed over the thighs and secured. While the local anesthetic is taking effect, the face is washed with an antimicrobial solution, taking care to not allow the solution to enter the eyes or ears. Males may need to have excess nasal hair trimmed.

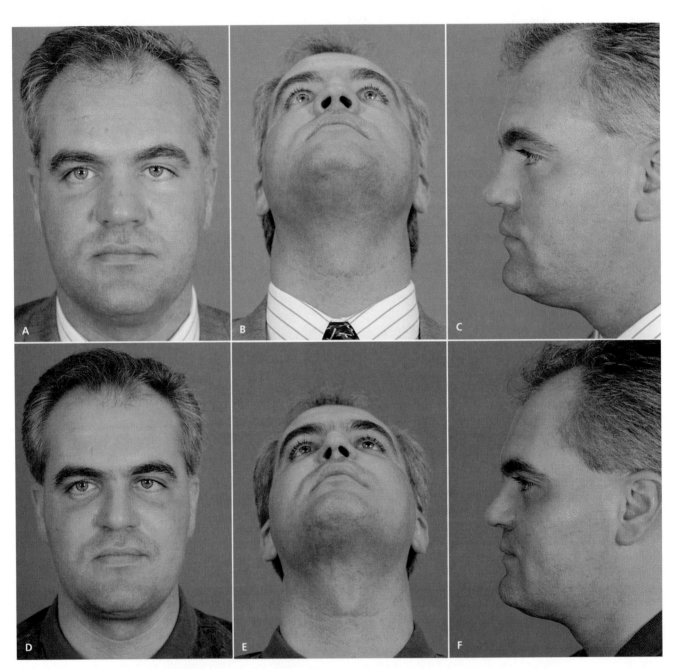

Fig. 9-25 Rhinoplasty. **A-C,** Preoperative. **C-F,** Postoperative. *(Courtesy Brian W. Davies, MD.)*

Procedure

An incision is made on the intranasal surface along the rim of the infracartilaginous ridge. The mucous membrane is reflected downward for the introduction of additional surgical instruments, such as a periosteal elevator or a rasp. Through this incision the nasal tip can be reduced or corrected. The incision can be continued along the inner aspect of the columella if a functional procedure such as septoplasty is planned (Fig. 9-26). Cartilage grafts can be inserted through a small, transverse, supranasal incision to reshape the dorsum (bridge) of the nose. Small-gauge wire suture may be used to attach the cartilage graft to the nasal bone.

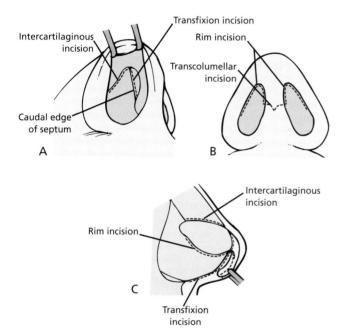

Fig. 9-26 A, Intracartilaginous and transfixion incisions. **B,** Incision for open rhinoplasty. **C,** Intercartilaginous and rim incisions to create a bipedicle flap.

Other reinforcement can be accomplished by inserting a cartilage graft into a central intracolumellar pocket (Fig. 9-27).

Resection of a dorsal hump is performed through incisions that are only large enough to introduce a rasp. The bony hump can be dissected through a subperiosteal incision (Fig. 9-28). Using a limited incisional approach spares neurovascular structures. A splint may be used to stabilize the nose for 5 to 7 days. Overcorrection can result in secondary deformities, such as concave dorsum, collapse of the nasal projection, or nasal tip misdirection.

The alar base can be reduced by taking a wedge from the nostril alar-lip junction (Fig. 9-29). The incision is closed with a monofilament nylon suture. The sutures are removed in 3 days for minimal scarring (Fig. 9-30).

Postoperative Patient Care

The patient may complain of nasal puffiness, congestion, headache, and pain after the procedure. This may be relieved by the application of ice. Nasal packing may be used for 24 to 48 hours, and the patient should remain in bed with the head of the bed elevated at least 30 degrees for the first day after the procedure. The patient may experience black eyes. Postoperative instruction should include not blowing the nose for at least 1 week to 10 days.

Some residual swelling will be evident for several months after the procedure. Some patients will require a secondary revision at a later date.

AESTHETIC OTOPLASTY

Aesthetic otoplasty procedures to decrease the angle of prominent or large ears are commonly performed on an outpatient basis for both children and adults. In some individuals, the ears protrude straight out on right-angles to the head causing self-consciousness and low self-esteem. Moderate to short hair styles do not hide the ear projection for either sex. Prominent ears stick out through the hair of long-haired individuals. For some

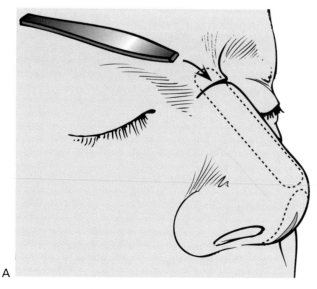
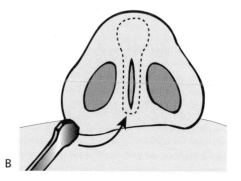

Fig. 9-27 A, Graft inserted into dorsal pocket. **B,** Graft inserted into columella pocket.

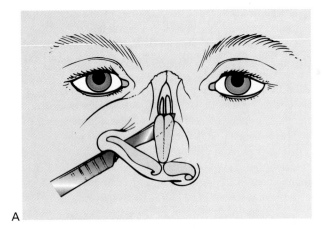

A

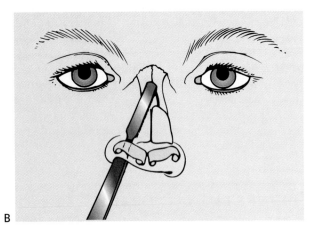

B

Fig. 9-28 Methods of reducing the dorsal hump of the nose.
A, Reduction of cartilagenous hump with #19 blade.
B, Reduction of bony hump with a rasp.

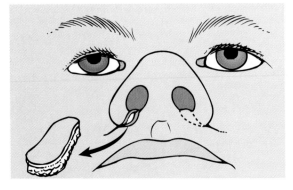

Fig. 9-29 Reduction of the alar base.

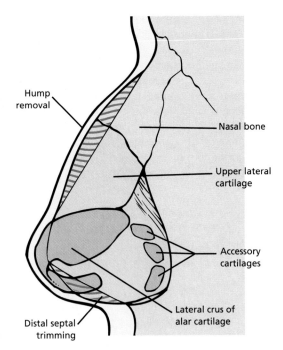

Fig. 9-30 The lateral anatomy of the nose showing a level of hump removal and distal septal trimming.

The external framework of the ears can be reconstructed using autologous rib or cartilage grafts or porous polyethylene implants. This type of procedure can be performed for congenital absence or deformity of the external ear or for ears lost by trauma, such as burns or violence. The goal in this type of reconstruction is to create a natural-looking ear that appears as normal as possible, can withstand average environmental contact, and can support the use of corrective eyewear. Psychologically, the appearance of the ear elevates the patient's self-esteem and sense of well-being. Children with ear deformities benefit from reconstruction starting around 4 years of age (before school starts). Additional finalizing and refining procedures can be performed as the child matures.

Anatomy and Physiology

The external ear is composed of a sheet of yellow fibrocartilage arranged in folds covered with muscular tissue, dermis, and epidermis. The surface of the ears is covered by fine hair and sebacceous glands. Thicker, coarser hair is more plentiful on the tragus and antitragus. Specific structures of the external ear are identified in Figure 9-32.

The arterial blood supply is derived from external carotid, temporal, and occipital arteries. Venous drainage follows the specific arteries. Sensory innervation is from cranial nerve V, cervical plexus, branches of the pneumogastric, and maxillary nerves. Motor innervation of the auricular musculature is supplied by the facial nerve (Fig. 9-33).

The ears should be positioned symmetrically bilaterally. The attachment of the auricle (also referred to as the pinna) should not deviate by more than 10 degrees from the vertical axis. The top of each auricle should align with the canthi of the

adults, this is a source of embarrassment. For children, this is the focus of ridicule and teasing. Approximately 85% of ear growth is established by 3 years of age, and adult-sized reconstruction can be performed by 6 years of age. Although some growth and change take place in the external ear into adulthood, growth is usually completed by 9 years of age (Fig. 9-31).

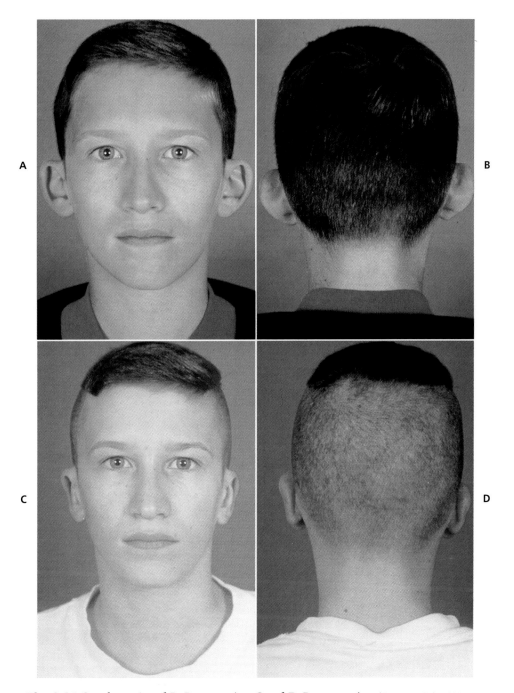

Fig. 9-31 Otoplasty. **A and B,** Preoperative. **C and D,** Postoperative. *(Courtesy Brian W. Davies, MD.)*

eyes horizontally. Typical prominence is commonly caused by failure of the antihelical fold to form properly by 20 weeks' gestation. Other forms of prominence are caused by conchal hypertrophy.

Preoperative Patient Care

Age-specific psychologic considerations and rationale for aesthetic otoplasty should be discussed before the procedure. Realistic outcomes include the potential for scarring, changes in

sensation, sensitivity to changes in the weather, and the potential for overcorrection or undercorrection. Life-size photographs are taken in direct anterior and posterior views for use in planning the procedure.

Anesthesia Considerations

Pediatric procedures are usually performed under general anesthesia. Older children and adults may prefer local anesthesia with IVCS.

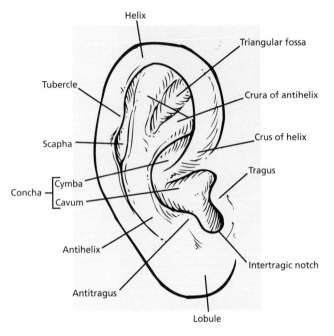

Fig. 9-32 Anatomy of the ear.

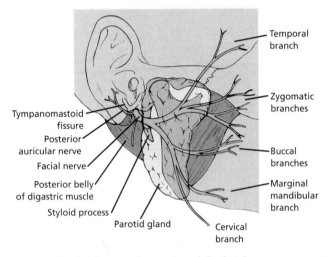

Fig. 9-33 Normal anatomy of the facial nerve.

Intraoperative Patient Care

The patient is placed on the operating bed in a supine position with the head resting in a donut. Some surgeons may prefer to use a Mayfield headrest. The head of the operating bed is elevated 30 degrees to decrease arterial pressure and improve intraoperative positioning. The ear canals are occluded with cotton balls. The hair is combed away from the field and secured with rubber bands. Coarse hair growing on the tragus/antitragus should be trimmed with iris scissors dipped in water-soluble lubricant. The lubricant catches most of the clippings preventing stray hairs from entering the surgical wound or ear canal. Cotton-tipped applicators dipped in antimicrobial solution are used to clean exposed aspects of the ear canals and auricular folds. The ear and surrounding hair-bearing surfaces are prepped with antimicrobial solution taking care to not allow solution to pool under the patient or to enter the eyes.

Procedure

Correction of antihelical deformity can be performed by scoring or removing cartilage behind the ears through a small posterior incision. A small oto/dermabrader tip can be used to score and thin the posterior cartilage to create a smooth fold. Care is taken to avoid thinning the cartilage too much. Permanent nylon fixation sutures are attached to strategic anatomic cartilaginous landmarks to secure the ear frame towards the head to reduce the prominence. The skin is closed with absorbable suture.

Conchal reduction is performed by excision of a wedge of cartilage through an anterior or posterior approach. The anterior incision is placed 1 cm below the antihelical fold. Some plastic surgeons use a combination of both methods. A tiny suction drain may be placed for 24 hours after the procedure.

Postoperative Patient Care

Protective ear dressings of gauze fluffs are applied and secured to mold the ears snugly against the head. Care is taken to not place extreme pressure over the surgical area. Ischemia would hinder wound healing and cause failure of the procedure. To protect the ears some surgeons use firm plastic ear shields that attach to the head with elastic straps. Two days after the procedure, the bulky dressing is removed and replaced with a headband that fits securely over the ears. The headband is worn at bedtime for 3 to 6 weeks. The patient is instructed to sleep with the head elevated and to use a soft foam pillow when reclining. Nonabsorbable nylon skin sutures, if used, are removed in 7 days.

The patient is instructed to avoid heavy lifting (more than 10 to 15 lb), extremes of temperature, contact sports, wearing a hat or helmet that touches or covers the ears, and any activity that pulls or presses on the incisions. Increases in arterial pressure can cause hematoma formation.

Complications

Potential complications include hematoma, infection, and dissatisfaction with the result. Hematomas that do not resorb can be surgically aspirated. Infection can cause loss of tissue or scarring. Pockets of pus can be drained with a syringe and needle. Antibiotics are commonly used.

Pulling on the incisions can cause reprotrusion of the auricles. Increased pressure from increased arterial pressure or a hematoma can put strain on the subsurface stabilizing sutures and cause failure of the procedure. Reoperation may be necessary.

CLEFT LIP AND PALATE PROCEDURES

Cleft lip is the result of the lack of fusion of the soft tissue of the upper lip during embryonic life. These clefts can be unilateral or bilateral in nature. They may vary in degree of deformity and severity from a notching of the upper lip to a more extensive cleft that continues into the floor of the nose. Extreme clefts can extend to the inferior aspect of the eyes. The upper lip consists of skin, orbicularis oris muscle, and mucosa. Two skin ridges near the midline of the upper lip outline the central philtrum. The red portion of the lip, or the vermilion, peaks at the philtral ridge and curves downward to form what is known as *Cupid's bow*. An absence of one or both of the philtral ridges will result in a distortion of the lower nose. Cleft lip is often associated with bony deformity and/or soft tissue deformity referred to as cleft palate. These two deformities are usually closed in separate procedures (Fig. 9-34).

The palate is composed of tissues that constitute the hard bony palate anteriorly and the soft palate posteriorly, which if not fused appropriately will result in a cleft. A cleft palate is a separation in the midline roof of the mouth that originates in the soft palate. It can involve the hard palate and maxilla, extending superiorly into the nose. Extreme occurrences may involve facial clefts that extend to the inferior aspect of the eye. Cleft palate may occur with or without the presence of cleft lip.

Etiology of Cleft Lip and Palate

The alveolus, which borders the hard palate, may fail to fuse during the first trimester and cleft on one or both sides involving soft and bony tissues resulting in unilateral or bilateral splits. Multifactoral components contribute to the incidence of cleft lip and palate. Common associations include environmental exposure, genetic factors (Fig. 9-35), increased parental age, and low socioeconomic status with the main focus on poor nutrition. Family history can be an indicator as well as associated anomalies, such as club foot, cardiac deformity, central nervous system (CNS) neural tube malformations, exposure to rubella, or folic acid deficiency. Combined cleft lip and palate occurs more often in males with a higher incidence in Asians. Isolated cleft lip is more common in Caucasian females.

Maternal contributing factors during gestation include the use of anticonvulsants, steroids, or sedatives, such as Valium. Exposure to rubella or toxoplasmosis from handling soiled cat litter is also implicated.

Preoperative Patient Care

Early neonatal assessment is crucial to determining the extent of the defect. Severe clefts will interfere with feeding and ability to survive. The extent of neoconstructive surgery or reconstruction will be dependent on the type of defect, the health condition of the neonate, and the method of feeding planned. The parents commonly blame themselves for the neonate's defect and should be reassured that restoration is possible. Special long nipples are available to help with bottle feeding, and methods have been outlined for modification in breast feeding. Sucking provides exercise for strengthening oral-facial musculature used for speech. Adequate nutrition will promote wound healing of the surgical incisions.

Anesthesia Considerations

The anesthetic of choice is general endotracheal anesthesia. Local anesthetic with epinephrine is injected to control bleeding.

Intraoperative Patient Care

The room should be warmed as for any pediatric procedure. Radiant lights and limb wrapping are useful for maintaining

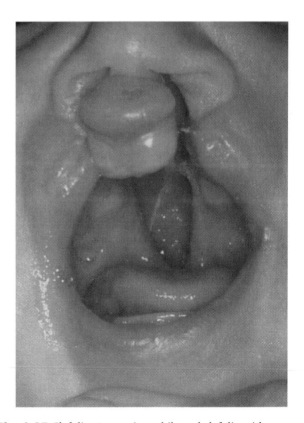

Fig. 9-35 Cleft lip. A prominent bilateral cleft lip with a complete cleft palate is seen in an infant with trisomy 13. The cleft extends from the soft to the hard palate, exposing the nasal cavity. *(From Zitelli: Atlas of pediatric physical diagnosis, ed 3, St Louis, 1996, Mosby.)*

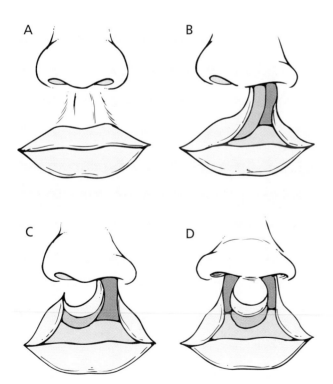

Fig. 9-34 **A,** Normal lip **B,** Complete unilateral cleft of the lip and palate. **C,** Bilateral cleft lip (incomplete on the right, complete on the left). **D,** Bilateral complete cleft lip and alveolus.

core temperature. The child is placed supine on the operating bed with his or her head secure in a donut. The parents are often allowed into the OR for induction and escorted to the family surgical waiting lounge after the child is asleep. Some anesthesia providers allow the parent to hold the child during the induction process. The child is intubated orally in a supine position, and the tube is secured centrally to the chin with tape. The position for the procedure is supine with a roll under the shoulders and the head positioned lower on the headrest (Fig. 9-36).

During the procedure, a gauze sponge pack is placed in the back of the throat to prevent aspiration of blood and irrigating solutions. The airway is thoroughly suctioned, and the gauze pack is removed from the throat before extubation at the conclusion of the surgical procedure. Elbow restraints are placed after closure to prevent grabbing at the repaired lip and mouth during emergence from anesthesia.

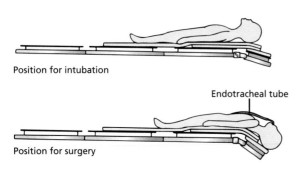

Fig. 9-36 Positioning for cleft palate repair.

Cleft Lip Repair

Primary closure of an isolated cleft lip, referred to as *cheiloplasty*, can be performed a few days after birth. This procedure can be done to facilitate feeding in the absence of cleft palate and to help the parents cope with the deformity. Formal cleft lip repair is performed after the infant is 3 months of age. Many surgeons prefer to wait and follow the "Rule of 10s": 10 weeks, 10 grams of hemoglobin, and 10 pounds of body weight.

Cleft lip repair is the rearrangement of existing tissues and musculature to recreate the normal lip line form and function as closely as possible. Muscular control is important for sucking, swallowing, learning speech, kissing, and creating facial expression. The goal is to achieve symmetry and create a functional lip repair that will appear normal from a conversational distance and provide adequate unhindered function and animation when the patient is speaking. The surgical procedure utilizes a rotation-advancement flap that is used to correct a complete unilateral cleft lip. The degree of tissue lengthening determines the direction of the flap (Fig. 9-37). Additional surgical procedures may be necessary to correct asymmetry of the nose by elevating the tip to correct a deviation caused by the cleft. This procedure is performed before the child is 4 years of age.

Palatoplasty

A palatoplasty is the closure of the soft palate. This is commonly done at 6 months of age before speech is learned. The soft palate closes the nasopharynx during swallowing and allows the production of normal speech sounds. An intact hard palate is essential for sucking and to prevent the escape of air via the nose during normal speech.

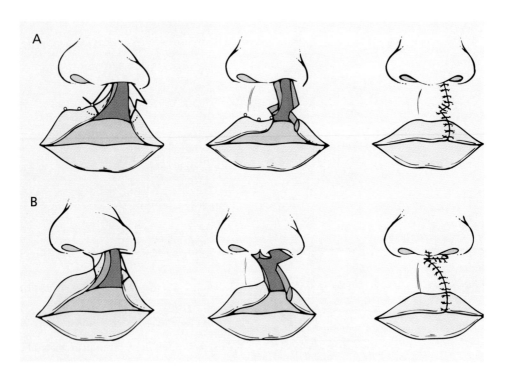

Fig. 9-37 Cleft lip repair. **A,** Randall-Tennison triangular flap method. **B,** Millard rotation-advancement method.

The repair of the cleft palate is usually performed when the child is between 1 year and 18 months of age. Tissue adjacent to the cleft is used in the form of flaps. The surgeon's goal is to reestablish an anatomic and physiologic environment that will be conducive to the development of a normal speech patterns and swallowing for the patient.

A common method of cleft palate repair consists of the closure of the soft palate by the V-Y or the Wardill-Kilner palatoplasty (Fig. 9-38, *A*). This is achieved by making a V-shaped incision on the oral side of the palate and elevating the mucoperiosteal flaps on both the oral and nasal sides. The blood vessels are carefully preserved during this phase. The Y-shaped closure in three layers closes the cleft while lengthening the palate.

Another approach is the Furlow technique, which is better known as the double opposing Z-palatoplasty (Fig. 9-38, *B*). This method has successfully normalized the velopharyngeal mechanism while minimizing the adverse effects on maxillary growth. This technique lengthens the velum while retrodisplacing and constructing the levator sling. The mucoperiosteal flaps are not elevated; therefore scarring is minimized in the hard palate.

Pharyngoplasty (pharyngeal flap) may be necessary to correct hypernasal tones in speech caused by air escaping through the nasal cavity when speaking. This procedure decreases the size of the pharynx and nasopharynx. This is usually done when the child is in his or her early teens but can be done as part of the primary repair.

Postoperative Care

Postoperative care in the postanesthesia care unit (PACU) is focused on prevention of airway obstruction, aspiration, and wound protection. Elbow restraints should be in place on arrival from the OR. Care is taken in suctioning oral secretions. A child with a palate repair will have nasal packing and may have ineffective airway clearance. The child should be maintained on his or her side, preferably the right side, to facilitate airway maintenance. Placing the child on his or her back may cause choking.

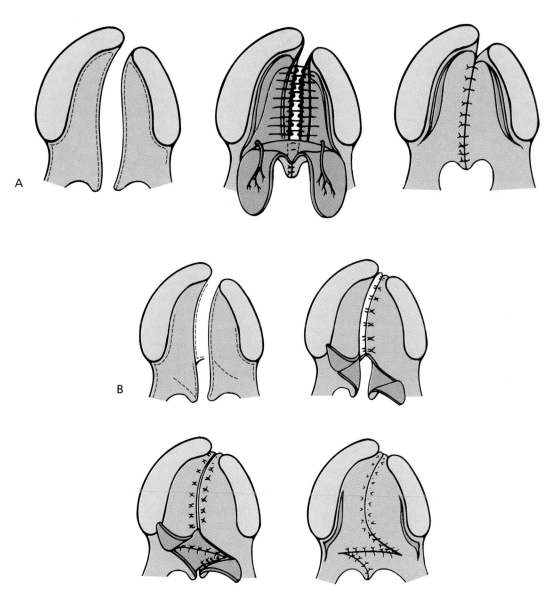

Fig. 9-38 Methods of cleft palate repair. **A,** Wardill-Kilner. **B,** Furlow double Z-plasty.

To stabilize and relieve tension on the incision, a small curved frame known as a Logan's bow is often applied over the repaired lip area to provide protection during the healing process. The parents are the key element of the child's postoperative care. They are taught how to care for the wound and how to assess for complications, such as hematoma, wound disruption, or infection. The parents are taught how to clean the wound and apply topical antiseptic or antibiotic ointment. Skin sutures are removed in 5 to 7 days.

The parents are taught to not allow objects into the child's mouth that could injure the healing palate. Avoidance of drinking straws, spoons, forks, tooth brushes, and sharp toys is important. The child should be fed in a seated position and in small amounts. Infants should be burped frequently because they tend to swallow air as they feed.

Children with cleft palate frequently have ear involvement causing middle ear infections. Parents should be advised that the child may need a myringotomy with ventilation tubes in the future. Some surgeons prefer to place the tubes at the time of the palate repair to avoid additional anesthesia or hospitalization.

Complications

The most common complication is wound disruption. Disturbance of the surgical site may necessitate additional procedures or a revision of previous work. Fistula formation between the nasal floor and the palate is a potential complication. Prolonged crying caused by pain is often a source of wound disruption. Preemptive pain control on a routine schedule is often needed. Acetaminophen is adequate for lip repairs, but the addition of codeine or other opioid may be needed for pain associated with palate repair. Infection is possible and is treated with antibiotics as needed. The parents are instructed to rinse the child's mouth after each feeding to prevent the accumulation of material in the oral cavity.

HAIR REPLACEMENT

Hair loss is caused by hormone changes, aging, and genetic predisposition. Becoming bald at a younger age usually indicates more extreme losses of hair. Other forms of hair loss may be caused by trauma, accidents, or burns. Natural hair replacement is considered cosmetic surgery. Replacement of hair lost because of accident or injury is considered reconstructive surgery and may be covered by health insurance in some situations.

Autologous hair transplantation was first performed by the Japanese in the late 1930s. The original hair replacement procedures were developed for eyebrow restoration in women. In the 1950s, American surgeons and dermatologists developed techniques for autologous transplantation of scalp hair to eliminate or diminish balding. The process of hair transplantation does not increase the number of hairs but redistributes the existing hair.

Surgical Hair Replacement Procedures

Patients having hair restoration surgery should be instructed that the process may take several years to complete. Additional procedures may be needed to compensate for continuing natural hair loss. Patience on the part of the patient and the surgeon helps avoid irregular hair lines, patchy growth, excessive scars, and misdirected hair growth. Careful planning can be beneficial for successful redistribution of existing hair.

Hair grafts

Hair grafting involves moving hair-bearing scalp from one area of the head to another. The size and shape of the graft may vary according to the donor site and the site of graft placement. The most common hair-bearing grafts consist of the following:

- Micrograft (1 to 2 hair follicles)
- Minigraft (2 to 4 hair follicles)
- Slitgraft (4 to 10 hair follicles)
- Punch graft (10 to 15 hair follicles)
- Stripgraft (30 to 40 hair follicles)

Hair is surgically removed or repositioned from an area of the scalp where hair is more abundant and is transplanted to an area where hair is thinned or absent. The temporal and occipital areas of the scalp are most frequently used because those areas do not experience the same degree of genetically mediated thinning or balding. The newly transplanted hair graft is not affected by the continually thinning hair in the transplant site (Fig. 9-39).

Early hair grafts were performed in punch graft fashion in sessions of 30 to 50 full-thickness plugs per procedure. These grafts looked like tufts of rooted doll hair. Today, the most current techniques involve micrografts and minigrafts, which may utilize up to 700 grafts per session. The hairline is blended into the crown of the head by starting with the smallest micrografts of single and double hairs. Tiny grafts look more natural and appear aesthetically pleasing. The number of grafts needed is partially dependent on the color and texture of existing hair and the availability of donor hair. Lighter, coarse, or gray hair gives better coverage than darker hair.

Scalp reduction

Surgical removal of an area of bald scalp may be performed in conjunction with grafts.

Advantages. Immediate results can seen as far as diminishing the area of baldness. Fewer grafts are required, and the patient's scalp hair will have greater density.

Disadvantages. The procedure may need to be repeated in order to remove the desired amount of scalp. Spreading of the scar can be caused by tension needed for wound closure. Scarring can be both visible and permanent.

Scalp flaps

Scalp flaps are larger, hair-bearing, vascularized pedicles of scalp that are moved from one part of the head to another. A vascular attachment is maintained. Before procuring the flap, a tissue expander may need to be placed under the skin to enlarge the surface area (Fig. 9-40).

Advantages. The density of hair in the flap is consistent and remains the same as it was at the original site. The newly grafted hair does not change in texture and will not fall out after the procedure. Scarring is not usually a problem. The scars that result from surgery are more readily covered by hair. One flap can take the place of over 350 or more punch grafts.

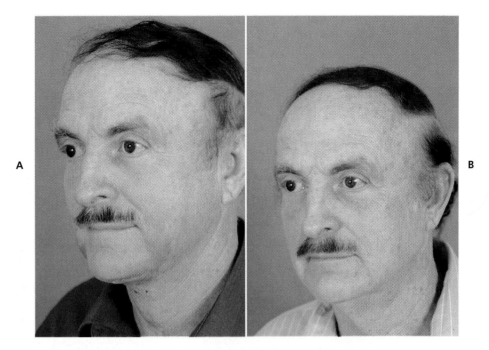

Fig. 9-39 Scalp advancement. **A,** Preoperative. **B,** Postoperative. *(Courtesy Brian W. Davies, MD.)*

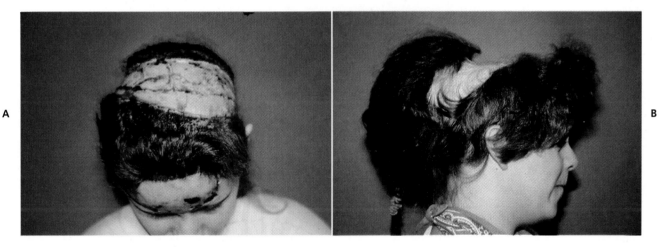

Fig. 9-40 Tissue expander used for scalp coverage. **A,** Coronal view. **B,** Lateral view. *(Courtesy Brian W. Davies, MD.)*

Disadvantages. This surgical procedure requires more than one staged procedure. This expensive and complex procedure may need to be performed in a hospital. Complications, such as tissue necrosis or graft failure, are more common. The direction of hair growth can be distorted by malpositioning the flap.

Patient Selection Considerations

Patient selection is important to the success of the procedure. The patient should have realistic expectations and understand and accept the limitations of the result. Most individuals with areas of baldness or very thin hair can expect some improvement with hair transplantation. A careful history and physical examination will determine the patient's suitability for the procedure and help to establish the potential outcome. Some surgeons use computer imaging as a tool to demonstrate to the patient the proposed new hairline. For some patents, this may be misleading and should be used judiciously.

After the initial examination, an individualized plan of care is developed including measurements of the proposed hairline, the type and number of grafts to be used in a session, and the number of sessions that will be needed (Fig. 9-41).

Available donor hair

The patient is assessed for available donor sites. Donor hair can only be taken from specific areas. The volume of hair in these sites will directly influence the amount of hair that can be procured.

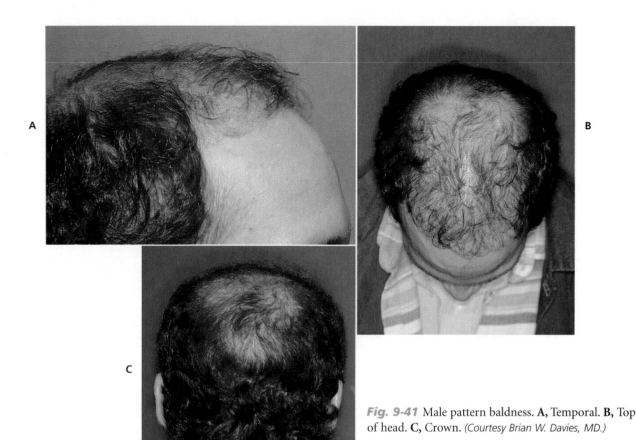

Fig. 9-41 Male pattern baldness. **A,** Temporal. **B,** Top of head. **C,** Crown. *(Courtesy Brian W. Davies, MD.)*

Degree of hair loss

The surface area of baldness may be too large for adequate coverage. A scalp reduction procedure may be needed. Some patients may be satisfied by only grafting hair in the front to fashion a hairline and frame the face.

Age

Young male patients are not necessarily suitable candidates for hair transplantation. Although the hair that is transplanted may not be affected by continual balding patterns, the hair indigenous to the area will continue to fall out. The available donor hair may not be enough to cover future balding areas. As the patient ages, he may have full hair patterns on top at the graft sites but patchy bald areas around the circumference of his head.

Preoperative Patient Care

The patient should be instructed to not take aspirin several weeks before the scheduled procedure because of the risk for increased bleeding. Smoking should be discouraged for at least 2 to 3 weeks before and after the procedure because it causes vasoconstriction that impairs circulation and inhibits wound healing.

Hair transplantation is usually performed in an office-based surgery setting. Before the procedure, the patient is given an oral sedative, such as Valium, which provides light sedation. Baseline vital signs are taken, and the patient is encouraged to relax. The hair at the donor site is trimmed very short to make the hair graft easier to obtain. The donor and recipient scalp is marked for the procedure (Fig. 9-42). The scalp is prepared with an antimicrobial solution.

Intraoperative Patient Care

Local anesthetic with epinephrine is injected into the donor site. Ice may be applied to the donor area before injection to decrease the discomfort associated with multiple needle punctures. The ice causes vasoconstriction, thereby minimizing blood loss at the site; however, the resultant vasoconstriction may incidentally slow the anesthetic absorption. A thin strip of hair-bearing scalp is excised (Fig. 9-43, *A*). The donor scalp wound is closed with an absorbable subcuticular suture. After this area heals, the scar is usually thin and well concealed by the surrounding hair.

Next, the strip of hair that was taken is cut into many small micrografts and minigrafts under magnification (Fig. 9-43, *B*). When preparation of the grafts is complete, the recipient sites are prepared (Fig. 9-43, *C*).

The grafts are carefully placed in the recipient sites using specially designed instruments (Fig. 9-43, *D*). Care is taken to place each graft in the correct position for directional hair growth. The hairline is usually grafted with single hair micrografts for a more natural appearing hairline. Minigrafts are used in successive rows behind the hairline towards the crown of the head. Each graft fits

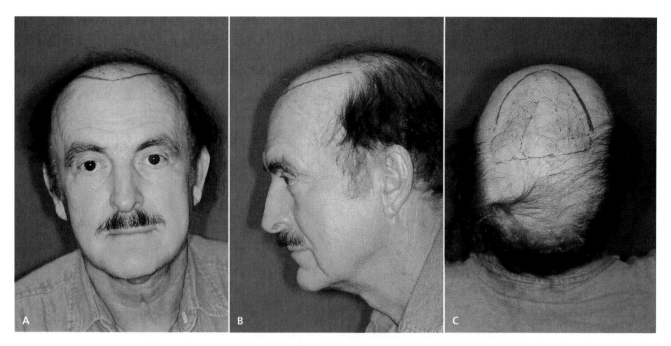

Fig. 9-42 Head markings for hair transplant. *(Courtesy Brian W. Davies, MD.)*

precisely without suturing or other fixation (Fig. 9-43, *E*). Some surgeons prefer a light dressing after the procedure.

Postoperative Patient Care

The patient should not drive or perform strenuous activity for 48 hours. An appointment is made for follow-up examination 2 to 3 days after the procedure. The sutures are removed in 1 week to 10 days. Subsequent sessions for additional grafting are planned 3 to 4 months apart. In some patients, the whole process may take several years and can be quite costly. The patient is informed that the transplanted hair will fall out and new growth will reappear from the follicle within 6 weeks to 3 months. The rate of growth is $1/4$ to $1/2$ inch per month (Fig. 9-44).

Complications

The risks of complications from hair transplantation surgery is minimal. Complications may include bleeding, infection, graft failure, and granulomatous cyst formation. Some patients experience numbness or parasthesia of the scalp or scarring, and some patients may have erratic hair regrowth at the graft site.

Nonsurgical Treatment for Hair Loss

Rogaine (minoxidil 2%)

A topical solution of minoxidil 2% (Rogaine), a drug usually used to treat hypertension, has been proven to cause moderate amounts of hair growth caused by a condition known as *androgenic alopecia,* or male pattern baldness. Each milliliter contains 20 mg of minoxidil. The results varies between individuals. It is used indefinitely for continued effect and costs between $35 and $45 per bottle, which contains several applications. This is an ongoing treatment for hair loss, not a cure. It is recommended for use on healthy, intact scalp and not for use on irri-

tated or sunburned surfaces. This solution should not be used on other areas of the body or with other topical preparations because absorption could be altered. Patients using guanethidine for high blood pressure, pregnant patients, and nursing mothers should not use this product. The safety and efficacy have not been studied in patients under 18 years of age. Patients can be referred to the manufacturer (Upjohn Company, 1-800-952-1616) for further information and are often offered rebate coupons. Rogaine is available over-the-counter.

Advantages. Rogaine (1 ml) is applied to a clean, dry scalp twice a day for a 4-month trial. The solution must remain in contact with the scalp for at least 4 hours before allowing the head to be washed. Instruct the patient to wash his or her hands thoroughly. If new hair growth is apparent after the trial period, then the drug is continued. It is not cost prohibitive as a short-term precursor to hair transplants and can be tried when other options such as surgery are not feasible. This may be beneficial for younger patients who have not realized the full extent of hair loss patterns.

Disadvantages. Rogaine does not provide dramatic results and is not effective in all cases of frontal hair loss. In many individuals, this may be the area of hair loss that disturbs them the most. Slight to moderate degrees of improvement may be expected in approximately 10% of users. If the drug is discontinued, the new hair growth will fall out within a few months. Prolonged use can become expensive. Side effects from the drug are minimal and seem to be dose related. They include itching and minor irritation because the solution has an alcohol base.

Women and Hair Replacement

One in five women will experience thinning hair. The pattern of hair loss in women is different than that of men who typically

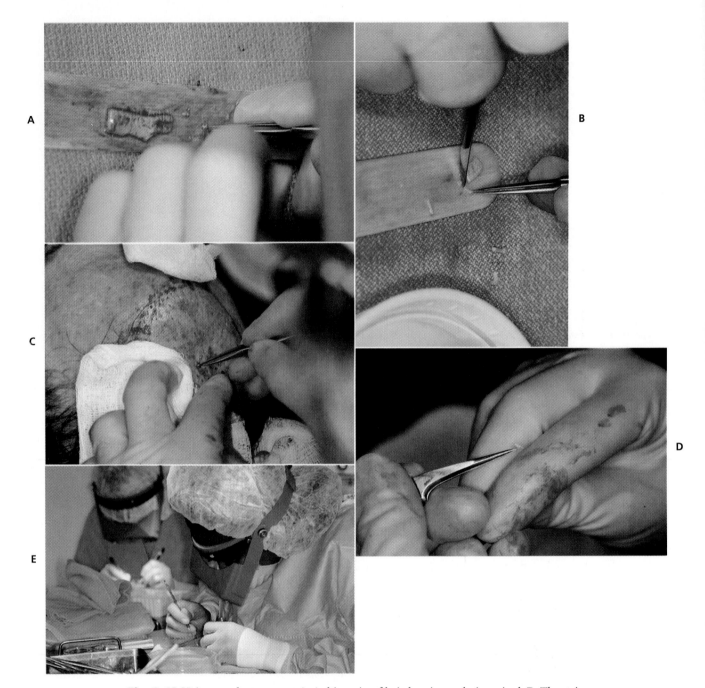

Fig. 9-43 Hair transplant process. **A,** A thin strip of hair-bearing scalp is excised. **B,** The strip is cut into many micrografts and minigrafts. **C,** The recipient site is prepared. **D,** The grafts are placed in the recipient sites using specially designed instruments. **E,** Minigrafts are used in successive rows behind the hairline towards the crown of the head. *(Courtesy Brian W. Davies, MD.)*

lose hair according to the familiar male pattern baldness. Females loose their hair all over in a generalized manner. There are usually no isolated areas of baldness or thinned hair. Thin hair compared with baldness is not surgically treated. The hair is thin all over, including the usual donor sites. Hair grafts can be placed, but the result may not show measurable difference. Rogaine is usually the treatment of choice. Some women prefer to try wigs or hair extensions.

Women with a male pattern type of hair loss are better transplant candidates because they are more likely to show a positive result. Women undergo the same procedure as men, but they are able to cover up the grafted sites with longer and more hair.

Women who have had browlifts or facelifts can have complications that involve diminished scalp or hairline. Browlifts and facelifts both employ incisions within the hairline. Hair

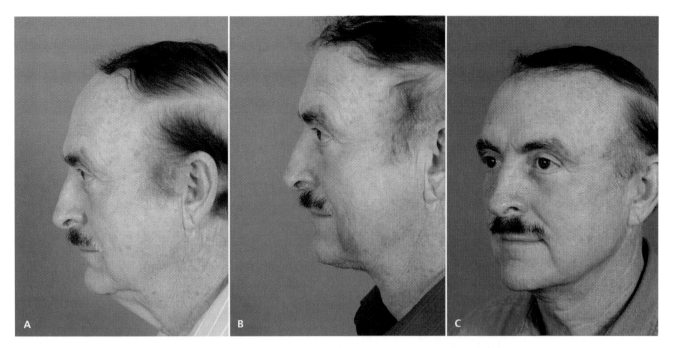

Fig. 9-44 Direct neck skin excision, upper eyelid blepharoplasty, and initial stages of hair transplantation removes years. **A,** Preoperative. **B,** One month postoperative. **C,** Six months postoperative. *(Courtesy Brian W. Davies, MD.)*

transplantation may be beneficial in correction of hair loss caused by closing the wound under tension. Thinning hair or hair loss can occur if the follicles are transected. These procedures can cause elevation of the hairline, which may be improved with hair grafting.

Bibliography

Brothers DB et al: Comparison of the furlow double opposing Z-plasty with the Wardill-Kilner procedure for isolated clefts of the soft palate, *Plast Reconstr Surg* 95(6):969, 1995.

Guter EP et al: The forehead lift, *Plast Surg Nurs* 13(4):188, 1993.

Jelks GW, Jelks EB: Preoperative evaluation of the blepharoplasty patient, *Clin Plast Surg* 20(2):213, 1993.

Maksud DP, Anderson RC: Psychological dimensions of aesthetic surgery, *Plast Surg Nurs* 15(3):137, 1995.

Mooney KM: External ear reconstruction with autogenous rib cartilage, *Plast Surg Nurs* 15(2):92, 1995.

Oostrom CA et al: Median cleft of the lip and mandible: case reports, a new embryologic hypothesis and subdivision, *Plast Reconstr Surg* 97(2):313, 1996.

Psillokis JM: *Subperiosteal approach for surgical rejuvenation of the upper face,* New York, 1994, Thieme Medical Publishers.

Ramirez OM: Endoscopic subperiosteal browlift and facelift, *Clin Plast Surg* 22(4):639, 1995.

Strohecker B: Cutis laxa: etiology, pathophysiology, characteristics, and management, *Plast Surg Nurs* 15(4):201, 1995.

Tebbetts JB: Blepharoplasty: a refined technique emphasizing accuracy and control, *Clin Plast Surg* 20(2):329, 1992.

Thompson HG, Reinders FX: A long-term appraisal of the unilateral complete cleft lip repair: one surgeon's experience, *Plast Reconstr Surg* 96(3):549, 1995.

Turpin IM: The modern rhytidectomy, *Clin Plast Surg* 19(2):383, 1992.

Wirt SW et al: Cleft lips and palates: a multidisciplinary approach, *Plast Surg Nurs* 12(4): 140, 1992.

Zorem HA, Resnick JI: Operative technique for transconjunctival lower blepharoplasty, *Clin Plast Surg* 20(2):351, 1992.

10   Breast Surgical Procedures

Breast surgery is performed for aesthetic, functional, and comfort reasons. Aesthetically, the breasts are viewed as a feminine beauty symbol. When present in equal weight bilaterally, they contribute to a sense of physical balance from a functional standpoint. If they are exceedingly large, they can be uncomfortable. If one or both breasts are underdeveloped, deformed, or missing, a woman may feel a diminished sense of self-esteem. In the presence of illness, such as cancer, breast surgery can be a life saver. Male patients can also have breast disease or disproportionate breast size.

ANATOMY AND PHYSIOLOGY OF THE BREAST

The breasts, or mammary glands, are cone-shaped secretory tissue structures located bilaterally on the anterior chest wall, encased by adipose tissue. Anatomically, each mammary gland is contained within the superficial fascia extending from the sternum to the mid-axillary line directly overlying the pectoral fascia. The upper outer quadrant, known as the *tail of Spence,* is the thickest portion extending into the axillary region. The glandular portions of the breast are arranged in lobular formations consisting of 12 to 20 pyramidal lobules (acini) divided by fibrous connective tissue septa known as *Cooper's suspensory ligaments* forming a ductal system. The lobules branch into alveoli that are lined with milk-secreting cells known as *lactiferous ducts.* These open into centrally directed mammary papilla, draining into temporary milk reservoirs known as *ampullae.* The openings merge to the surface of the breast forming the nipple, which is encircled by the pigmented contractile smooth muscle of the areola. The nipple consists of erectile tissue and muscle fibers covered with epithelium that have sphincterlike properties that control milk flow (Fig. 10-1).

Cooper's ligamental septa extend from the pectoral fascia to the skin supporting the glandular tissue lobes, blood and lymphatic vessels, and adipose tissue. These ligaments also define the shape of the breast and the position of the mammary tissue on the anterior chest wall.

The arterial blood supply arises laterally from the thoracic branches of the axillary, intercostal, and internal mammary arteries. The venous drainage forms an anastomotic circle around the base of the nipple with branches draining the circumference of the gland terminating in the axillary and internal mammary veins. The largest vessels are the internal thoracic and innominate veins.

The lymphatic drainage of the breast follows the venous drainage of the breast. The lateral and inferior portions of the breast drain along the thoracoacromial and lateral thoracic vessels toward the axilla, which handles 75% of the lymphatic flow. The medial portions drain along the anterior intercostal vessels toward the internal thoracic nodes, which lie along the internal thoracic artery parallel to the sternum. The small superior portion of the breast drains toward the supraclavicular nodes. Innervation is from the anterior and lateral cutaneous nerves of the thorax.

The most significant function of the mammary gland is milk production. Beginning at puberty, the mammary glands develop under the influence of estrogen and progesterone secretion. Estrogen stimulates the growth of the ductal system within the breast and increases the fat distribution, whereas progesterone stimulates the alveoli of the secretory cells to develop. The mammary glands reach their maximum development during pregnancy because estrogen and progesterone blood levels are elevated for a period of months. Hormonal influences cause the ductal system to proliferate and the secretory cells of the alveoli to enlarge.

NURSING CARE CONSIDERATIONS OF THE PATIENT IN BREAST SURGERY

Patients planning breast surgery should be educated about the procedure, risks, potential complications, and expected realistic outcomes. Sensation and nipple erection response can be altered, and breast feeding may not be a future option. Ideal candidates are of normal weight and are not immediately premenstrual or currently menstruating. Cyclic hormonal changes associated with menses affect the glandular tissue of the breast, increasing the risk of bleeding.

BREAST EXAMINATION AND THE PERIOPERATIVE PATIENT

Breast self examination (BSE) is extremely important in early detection of abnormalities of the breast. The best time to perform the BSE is every month immediately after menstruation. The perioperative nurse should include the BSE in the patient's postoperative teaching because the routine is still important regardless of the type of surgical procedure performed. Functional breast cysts are more common during peak hormonal activity associated with ovulation and may be mistaken for abnormal masses. Menopausal women also should examine their breasts monthly at the same time each month. Performing the examination at the same time each month is easier to remember if menstrual cycles are absent. Women on estrogen

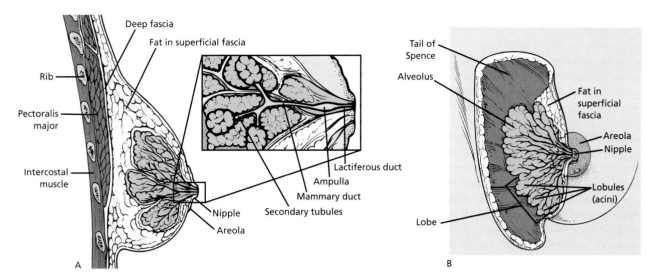

Fig. 10-1 The right breast. **A,** Saggital view of mammary gland. **B,** Frontal view of mammary gland.

replacement therapy may note some breast tissue enlargement after a period of use. Males have less breast tissue, but should examine their breasts for irregularities on a routine basis.

Breast examination includes direct visualization and palpation. Visually, the breasts should appear symmetrical without dimples or surface indentations. The patient should be observed in direct and indirect lighting in both sitting and supine positions. While sitting, the patient should be instructed to sit up straight with hands on hips, followed by slightly bent forward, and finally with both hands raised in the air over the head. Some men and women seek breast alteration procedures based on visual asymmetry, size, and degree of tissue ptosis.

To palpate the left breast, the left arm is raised and the left hand is placed behind the head. Using the fleshy portion of the middle three fingers of the right hand, press gently against the breast in a circular fashion against the ribs starting at the nipple working outward until the entire breast and adjacent axilla have been palpated. Keep the fingers together. If a lump or mass is felt, compare it with the same area on the opposite breast. If both regions feel similar, then this is probably normal breast tissue. The same procedure is repeated on the opposite breast with the opposite hand. After palpating the breast tissue, gently squeeze the nipples between the fingers to observe for any discharge. Bilateral clear or milky discharge is frequently hormonal and not usually a surgical problem, but unilateral bloody discharge indicates the need for further investigation. Benign tumors are usually firm and well circumscribed. Carcinomas are less well defined and may feel more attached to adjacent tissue. Any questionable areas should be reported to the physician (Fig. 10-2).

Breast examination by a clinician or the patient should be performed in both sitting and supine positions. Some masses are more distinct in the supine position, whereas others are felt better in the upright position. In patients whose breasts are exceptionally large, complete the examination in right and left lateral positions to examine the outer half of each breast.

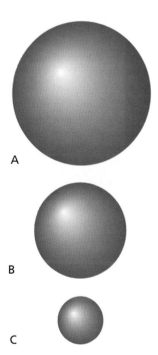

Fig. 10-2 Average size lumps found by self breast examination. **A,** Woman not practicing BSE. **B,** Woman practicing occasional BSE. **C,** Woman practicing monthly BSE.

Patient education is important. The patient who is having breast augmentation, reduction, or reconstruction may still develop tumors, cysts, or cancerous lesions. The patient should be taught how to do a BSE after any surgical procedure that alters the shape of the breast. Postoperative breast examination procedure does not vary significantly from preoperative examination. Scars or capsular contractures may alter the landscape of the breast. The patient should become accustomed to the changes in breast contour and texture and should be able to identify any changes that develop subsequent to the surgical procedure. Lumps are often more firm, glandular tissue, but they should be monitored by the patient and physician on a regular basis. It may be useful to instruct the patient to draw a simple diagram indicating any area on the breast that feels firmer or different. A brief descriptive note describing how the tissue feels facilitates comparison with previous examinations.

Mammography

Mammography has been useful in the identification of malignancies of the breast. Baseline mammograms should be performed between 35 and 40 years of age and every 2 years thereafter or as recommended by a healthcare provider. Women 50 years of age or older should have a yearly mammogram. Patients with breast implants should continue to have routine mammography as advised by their physicians. The mammography technician should be informed of any history of breast surgery, particularly augmentation with implants. Pulling the breast tissue over in front of the implant and displacing the implant posteriorly (Eklund view) may enhance the amount of glandular tissue imaged (Fig. 10-3). Submuscular placement may be easier to image than subglandular. Craniocaudal and mediolateral oblique views should be performed. Four views may be taken of each augmented breast making the procedure somewhat more costly than routine mammography. Implant rupture during mammography is uncommon but can happen. The procedure may be uncomfortable, but the patient should be educated about the postoperative changes in tissue appearance and the potential for the implant to obscure a breast lesion.

Ultrasound, fine needle aspiration, magnetic resonance imaging (MRI), and computer axial tomography (CAT) are performed if more conclusive testing of suspicious tissue is needed. Ultrasound may be helpful in detecting implant leaks missed by x-ray examination. Some leaks are only detected on direct visualization. Stereotactic biopsy is available in many facilities for precise tissue sampling.

Breast Cancer

One of eight women will develop breast cancer in her lifetime. It is most common over 30 years of age, usually between 40 and 50 years of age. Treatment usually involves surgical breast tissue removal (mastectomy) and sometimes chemotherapy and radiation. The fear of having cancer is an emotional stressor, but mastectomy causes emotional and physical deformity. A woman may experience devastating effects on her sexual function, self-esteem, and body image. The emotional distress may vary between individuals. Physical beauty is important to both younger and older women. Functionally, a woman of childbearing age is deprived of breast feeding. For many patients, mastectomy and reconstruction can be performed in one procedure conserving self-esteem and body image. It is important for the patient's oncologist to develop a plan of care in conjunction with the general surgeon and the plastic surgeon to provide the best outcome. Table 10-1 illustrates the types of mastectomy procedures and the extent of tissue loss.

Immediate reconstruction does not usually interfere with postoperative oncologic treatments. Reconstruction may be delayed to avoid poor healing and wound complications if radiation therapy and chemotherapy will be used. Some plastic surgeons wait up to 1 year after these therapies before they will

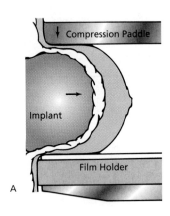

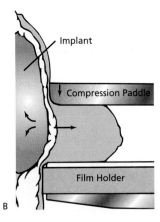

Fig. 10-3 A, Diagram showing the effect of standard mammographic compression being applied to the entire breast and prosthesis. The implant bulges forward, compressing the breast tissue between the implant and the skin. **B,** Modified view obtained by pushing the implant posteriorly and applying compression only to the breast tissue anterior to the implant.

Table 10-1 **Surgical Procedures for Breast Cancer**

PROCEDURE	TISSUE LOSS
Lumpectomy	Tumor and surrounding tissue are excised.
Segmental mastectomy	A wedge of the breast including the tumor and lobe of tissue is removed.
Simple mastectomy	All breast tissue is removed but nothing else.
Modified radical mastectomy	All breast tissue, axillary lymph nodes, and sometimes the pectoralis minor muscle are removed.
Radical mastectomy	All breast tissue, axillary lymph nodes, and muscles of the chest wall (including the pectoralis major) are removed.

begin reconstructive surgery if wound healing is in question. Autologous tissue breast construction enables the patient to have a reconstructed breast without implants and can supply a dermal and epidermal source for missing tissue.

Breast Cancer and the Augmented Breast

Breast cancer in a woman who has had previous augmentation with implants usually presents in a palpable form with lymph node involvement. This advanced stage could be due to the masking effect of the implant during screening mammography. When cancer is detected in an augmented breast, it is preferable to perform a total mastectomy rather than a breast-preserving procedure.

Of two million women in the United states who have had breast augmentation mammoplasties with silicone implants, approximately 200,000 have developed breast cancer. The silicone implants are not the cause of the cancer.

BREAST PTOSIS

Breast ptosis is the drooping of the female breast, which may appear in early adulthood, usually after childbirth and breast feeding, but it is more common in middle age. The elasticity of the dermis is lost as a result of aging or repeated engorgement during breast feeding. Loss of breast tissue is caused by age, atrophy, or rapid weight loss. Categories of breast ptosis include the following:

- *First degree:* The nipple lies at the level of the submammary fold and above the lower contour of the gland.
- *Second degree:* The nipple lies below the level of the submammary fold but above the lower contour of the breast.
- *Third degree:* The nipple lies below the submammary fold at the level of the lower contour of the breast.

Ptosis correction involves the removal of excessive skin, repositioning of the nipple, and plication of the breast tissue to produce a more anterior projection of the breast. Correction is performed in a very similar fashion to reduction mammoplasty. However, breast bulk is not removed; only redundant skin is excised and the breast mound is tightened and elevated. Ptosis correction may be performed in combination with breast reduction, augmentation, or reconstruction in order to achieve bilateral breast symmetry (Fig. 10-4).

BREAST REDUCTION MAMMOPLASTY

Breast reduction was described as early as 1922 when American surgeon Max Thorek discussed the possibility of amputating breast tissue, sculpting the residual, and performing a free nipple transfer. During the same decade, Lexer, Biesenberger, and Joseph described varying methods of breast reduction and nipple transpositioning.

In 1960, Strombeck devised a procedure using a Wise pattern for skin marking and nipple vascular preservation on a horizontal dermal breast pedicle. This was then modified by McKissock, Penn, and other plastic surgeons.

Hypertrophic breast tissue, macromastia, or giantomastia can cause back, neck, and shoulder pain. Women with pendulous breasts complain of ill-fitting clothing, grooves in their

shoulders from bra straps, and constant rashes of the inframammary folds. Mobility, balance, and posture are adversely affected. Psychologically, self-consciousness and sensitivity to thoughtless comments about having large breasts alters perception of self-image. Hormonal imbalance and familial tendencies contribute to the condition.

Objectives of reduction mammoplasty include relief of symptoms caused by heavy breast tissue, improved self-image, preserved nipple sensation, and aesthetic appearance of the breasts. Other indications for reduction include unilateral balancing after a contralateral mastectomy or removal of supernumerary breasts and nipples. Teenagers younger than 16 years of age who undergo a reduction mammoplasty are at risk for recurrent symptoms secondary to maturational breast development after the procedure.

Procedural considerations of reduction mammoplasty include the following:

- Absence of postoperative complications
- Viable transposition of the nipple-areolar complex
- Sufficient reduction of breast tissue volume
- Alteration of lactation potential in childbearing-age females
- Equalization of breast sizes
- Aesthetically acceptable results for the patient
- Minimal scarring
- Prevention of tissue loss caused by circulatory changes
- Prevention of blood loss

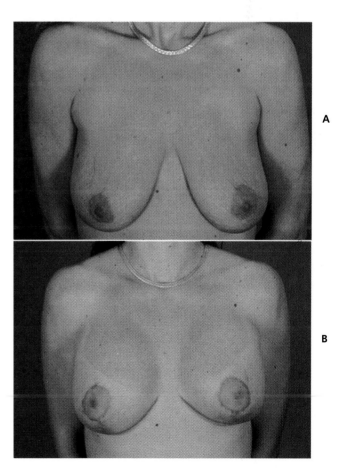

A

B

Fig. 10-4 Mastopexy. **A,** Preoperative. **B,** Postoperative. *(Courtesy Brian W. Davies, MD.)*

Marking Technique for Reduction Mammoplasty

Before induction of general anesthesia, the patient is placed in the upright standing position with arms at her side. If marked while seated, she may be inadvertently leaning to one side and cause the marking to be inaccurate. The marking procedure should be performed in a warm, private environment. First, a central vertical line is drawn starting at the sternal notch, through the xiphoid, and ending at the umbilicus. Bilaterally, additional vertical lines are drawn from the middle of the clavicle down the mid-axis of each breast to the top of the existing nipple. A diagonal line from the sternal notch to the future nipple site is marked and measures approximately 19 to 21 centimeters. The new nipple placement should fall between the middle and lower third of the humerus at the level of the inframammary fold (Fig. 10-5).

A keyhole-shaped template with flexible-extendible arms is used to determine placement of the nipple-areolar complex. It is positioned, and the inner angles are traced with surgical marking pens to create incisional outlines. The keyhole template is placed so that the top of the new areola will be directly opposite the center of the inframammary fold in the middle axis of the breast. The keyhole arms are angled apart and held at varying angles depending on the desired cup size (Fig. 10-6):

- B-cup: 120-degree angle
- C-cup: 90-degree angle
- D-cup: 60-degree angle

The length of the keyhole arm for the vertical incision is also varied according to the desired cup size:

- B-cup: 4 cm
- C-cup: 5 cm
- D-cup: 6 cm

The vertical incisions are usually 6 centimeters or less. Longer incisions cause an excessively high nipple placement on the upper aspect of the breast. The inframammary fold is marked with a small equilateral triangle extending superiorly in the center of the incision. The inframammary incision is kept short both medially and laterally. Markings for these are joined with a curvilinear line from the end of the arm of the keyhole to the medial and lateral extent of the inframammary incision. The incision is kept as short as possible to prevent dog-ear closure.

Surgical Procedure for Breast Reduction

After induction of general anesthesia, the keyhole markings are scored with a sharp implement such as the reverse edge of the scalpel or a sterile 14-gauge needle. Scoring the incision lines preserves the accuracy of the measurements and prevents guessing if the prep solution washes away the ink markings. The patient is positioned either in a 30 to 40 degree semi-Fowler's position or supine.

The potential for blood loss may be decreased by injecting a mixture of 100 cc of 1% lidocaine with 1:100,000 units of epinephrine in 1000 cc of normal saline. This concentration is injected subcutaneously along the incision lines, down to the pectoralis fascia. The maximum volume of this solution should not exceed 10 cc/kg of body weight per breast.

A circular marking template referred to as a *cookie cutter* or *nipple washer* is used to mark the existing areola to fit the newly fashioned keyhole pattern. Some surgeons dip the rim of the marker into a colored surgical dye, such as methylene blue, and carefully apply the inked imprint to the nipple-areola complex.

Deepithelialization of the superficial skin layers of the breast is performed as illustrated in Fig. 10-7, *A*. Strict attention is paid to the integrity of the position of the dermal bridge superior and inferior to the areola (Fig. 10-7, *B*). Electrocautery is used to dissect the vertical bipedicle. The incision is carefully carried vertically down to the chest wall starting from the inframammary line and directed superiorly. Small bleeders are cauterized.

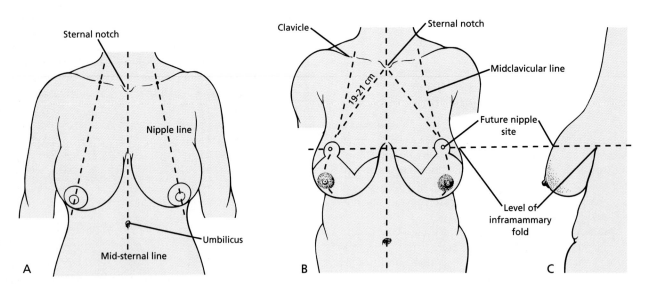

Fig. 10-5 Measuring the breasts for bilateral symmetry of nipple placement. **A,** Landmarks for breast reduction. **B,** Patient marking for breast reduction. **C,** Side view of inframammary fold level.

Superiorly, breast tissue is removed to accommodate a folded pedicle. The lateral skin pedicle containing subcutaneous fat and breast tissue is developed according to the anticipated breast size. The residual lateral breast tissue not attached to the skin is then dissected from the pectoral fascia and is removed as a unit. This is the largest amount of breast tissue to be removed (Fig. 10-7 *C*). Each portion is carefully weighed and recorded according to removal site. The tissue is separated into left and right containers. After the pedicle flap is formed, the residual breast tissue is removed from beneath

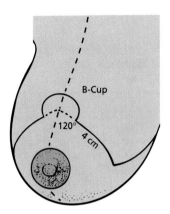

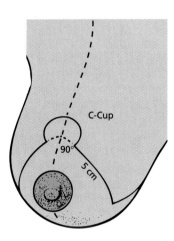

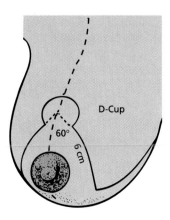

Fig. 10-6 Marking for the appropriate cup size for breast reduction.

the skin flaps. The superior portion of the central pedicle is trimmed to aid in placement of the pedicle during closure. The wound is then irrigated with warm normal saline, and hemostasis is achieved by cautery. A wound drain is positioned along the chest wall under each breast.

Before final closure, the breasts are compared for symmetry, and any adjustments are made. Closure begins by approximating the three points of the keyhole creating an inverted "T" closure (Fig. 10-7, *D*). The skin approximation should not be tight at closure. Tension on the suture line can create vascular embarrassment and poor wound healing. Suturing begins medially from the sternum to 1 inch from the vertical limb and then laterally to the same point. The skin is closed using a subcuticular suture technique with absorbable suture material. The vertical incisions are closed in the same two-layer fashion.

The nipple is closed last using several everting sutures at the dermis level and subcuticular sutures either by the interrupted or continuous running method (Fig. 10-7, *E*).

Breast dressings

Wound closure strips are placed along the suture lines followed by a fluff gauze absorbent pressure dressing. Some surgeons use xeroform gauze over the suture lines. A front closure elasticized surgical bra is applied for support. Underwires are avoided because they may interfere with healing of the inframammary incision. The patient is encouraged to wear a supportive bra 24 hours per day for 6 to 8 weeks.

The tissue specimens are weighed and labeled separately according to breast side. These should be sent to pathology for gross and microscopic inspection. Incidental malignancies have been found in reduction mammoplasty specimens (Figs. 10-8 and 10-9).

Postoperative antibiotics and analgesia are prescribed. The drains are removed approximately 24 to 36 hours after the procedure depending on the amount of drainage.

Strenuous exercise is avoided for 4 to 6 weeks. Walking is encouraged as soon as possible. A mammogram may be taken 1 month after the procedure to observe for any adverse tissue changes with a follow-up mammogram 12 to 18 months later. This set of mammograms can set a postsurgical baseline to delineate altered tissue response caused by surgery and neoplastic changes.

In giantomastia, the breast is severely distorted. Mammoplasty using the inferiorly based pedicle with the nipple-areolar complex is difficult and yields poor results, such as nipple necrosis and loss. Amputation of the breast with a free nipple transplantation and an inferiorly based pyramidal parenchyma flap adds fullness and less risk of nipple loss.

GYNECOMASTIA

Gynecomastia is a common condition of bilateral or unilateral breast enlargement found in males. The condition may be idiopathic or related to normal puberty (between the ages of 14 and 17) (Fig. 10-10). Resolution usually takes place within 2 years. In athletes over 40 years of age, it may be a side effect of anabolic steroid abuse. It is also caused by primary hypogonadism,

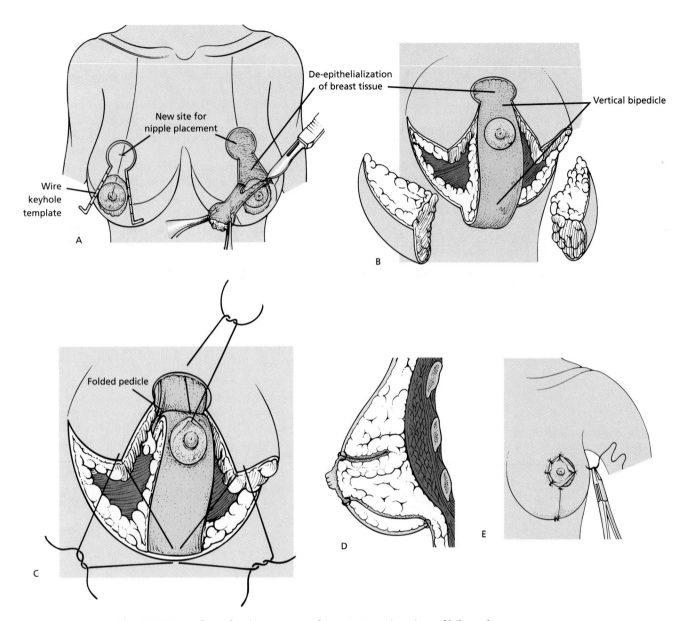

Fig. **10-7** Steps for reduction mammoplasty. **A,** Anterior view of bilateral mammary glands. Wire keyhole template in place on patient's right breast. (Note marking of new location for nipple replacement.) Deepithelialization of left breast is performed by sharp dissection. **B,** Deepithelialization is complete, and segments of mammary gland are removed. Vertical bipedicle is formed. **C,** The superior portion of the bipedicle is folded on itself and sutured in place. Closure points are aligned with sutures for reconstruction of reduced breast. **D,** Lateral view of completed and closed reconstruction of reduced breast. **E,** Frontal view of breast with closure completed. Nipple attachment in process. (Wound drain not shown)

hyperestrogenism, growth hormone, androgen deficiency, or an underlying neoplasm that produces sex hormones or corticosteroids. Underlying systemic disorders such as liver disease, thyrotoxicosis, and renal failure are other known causes. Drugs such as estrogen or marijuana can cause male breast enlargement. Studies have shown that men with gynecomastia have denser and more extensive body hair than normal and have experienced early maturation and childhood obesity.

Gynecomastia in younger males is usually more glandular, and in older males it is more adipose.

Gynecomastia may consist of a glandular button under the areola, diffuse tissue hypertrophy, or diffuse hypertrophy with extreme amounts of redundant skin. Surgical treatment is based on the location and type of tissue in the male breast. Avoid the use of the term male menopause in patient teaching. Males do not menstruate and therefore are not subject to menopause.

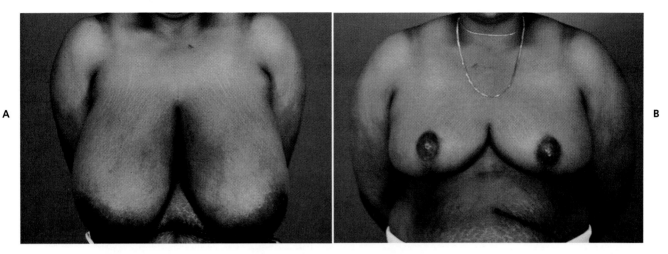

Fig. 10-8 Reduction mammoplasty. Note grooves in shoulders from bra straps. **A,** Preoperative. **B,** Postoperative. *(Courtesy Brian W. Davies, MD.)*

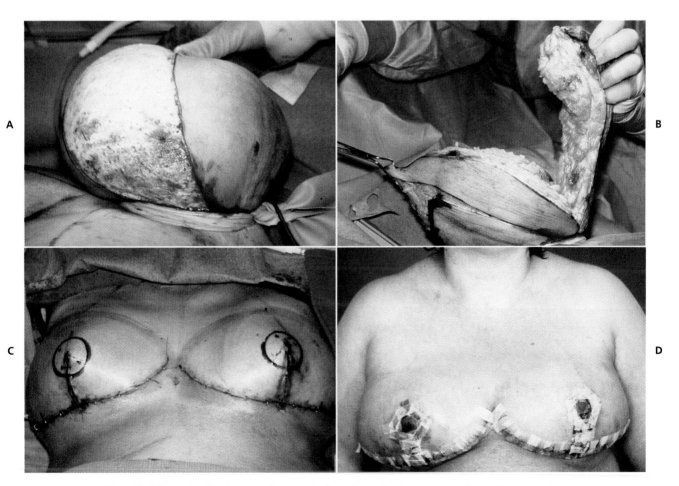

Fig. 10-9 Dr. Brian Davies tourniquet technique for reduction mammoplasty. *(Courtesy Brian W. Davies, MD.)*

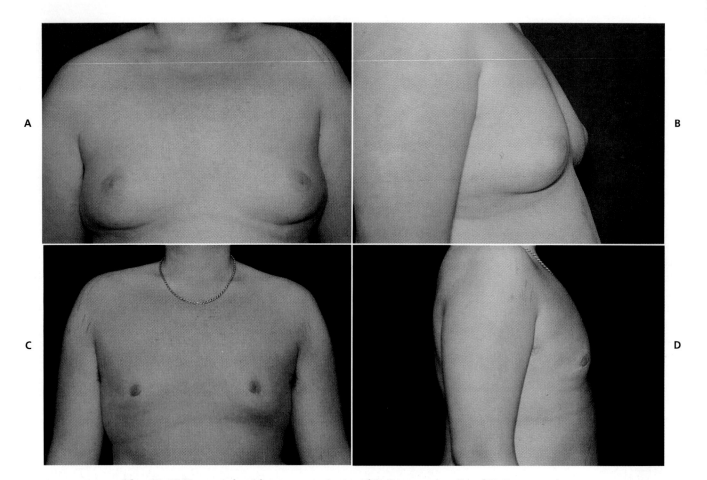

Fig. 10-10 Young male with gynecomastia. **A and B,** Preoperative. **C and D,** Postoperative. *(Courtesy Brian W. Davies, MD.)*

The first choice of therapy for gynecomastia is to treat the underlying cause and thereby reverse the gynecomastic state. Should this fail, careful removal of excess adipose or glandular tissue either through the conventional method of breast reduction or by breast liposuction has been successful. Relief of the symptoms will also alleviate the psychologic aspects of having abnormally large breasts, especially in puberty.

Liposuction for Gynecomastia

For adipose gynecomastia, a suction cannula is introduced through a small incision made at the anterior axillary pilar area and on the right side of the inframammary fold or through a periareolar incision (Fig. 10-11). The tissue is suctioned through the liposuction cannula from where the contour is full until a well-defined contour is created. Some fat is left under the skin. This method does not work as well for the highly glandular tissue of young males. Excision of parenchymal tissue from under the nipple areola complex is also performed.

Occasionally, a drain may be inserted through a lateral stab wound or through the incision. The wound is closed using a subcutaneous closure and is dressed with an absorbent dressing. A breast binder is applied after the procedure and may be worn for 6 weeks.

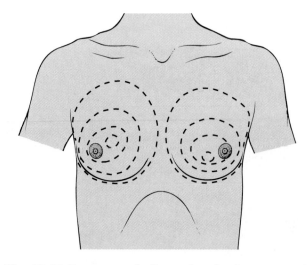

Fig. 10-11 Contour map for liposuction of male gynecomastia.

Liposuction procedures yield a lower incidence of postoperative complications and a higher degree of patient satisfaction. The advantages of the axillary approach are that breast tissue can be removed without large scars, and the postoperative recovery period is shorter and less painful.

Surgical excision is usually performed in larger types of gynecomastia. The results are not as satisfactory because of residual breast hypertrophy, redundant skin, scarring, and complications with nipple-areolar placement. A periareolar approach may be preferred, or for some patients a mastectomy with nipple reconstruction may produce more pleasing results.

BREAST AUGMENTATION, CONSTRUCTION, AND RECONSTRUCTION

Historically, breast augmentation, construction, and reconstruction involved the injection or insertion of various foreign substances (including paraffin, oils, dimethylpolysiloxane [silicone], and rubber) or implantation of prosthetic silicone, saline pouches, or living tissue flaps. Many forms of breast enlargement have become controversial because of potential risks associated with materials used for the procedure. Plastic surgical breast procedures have been refined in recent years to include increased aesthetics and safety for the patient.

Some augmentation procedures can be performed under monitored local anesthesia (MAC) or intravenous conscious sedation (IVCS). More complex reconstructive procedures require the use of general endotracheal anesthesia.

Indications for Breast Augmentation, Construction, or Reconstruction

The rationale for altering the size or contour of breast tissue is aesthetically and psychologically premised. Society has placed great value on the female breast as a symbol of femininity and beauty. Surgical enlargement, construction, or reconstruction is useful for patients who have experienced the following:

- *Mastectomy or partial mastectomy:* For cancer or fibrocystic disease, either bilateral or unilateral
- *Electively:* For the patient who has feelings of low self-esteem and self-confidence to attain a better proportioned figure (Fig. 10-12)
- *Breast hypoplasia:* Also known as Poland's syndrome, including absence or hypoplasia of the ipsilateral pectoral musculature
- *Breast asymmetry:* One breast larger than the other (Fig. 10-13)
- *Postpartum breast involution:* With tissue atrophy
- *Gender dysphoria:* Patient seeking transsexual surgery
- *Amastia:* Unilateral or bilateral developmental absence of the mammary glands including the nipple; unilateral amastia is also associated with the lack of the corresponding pectoral muscles

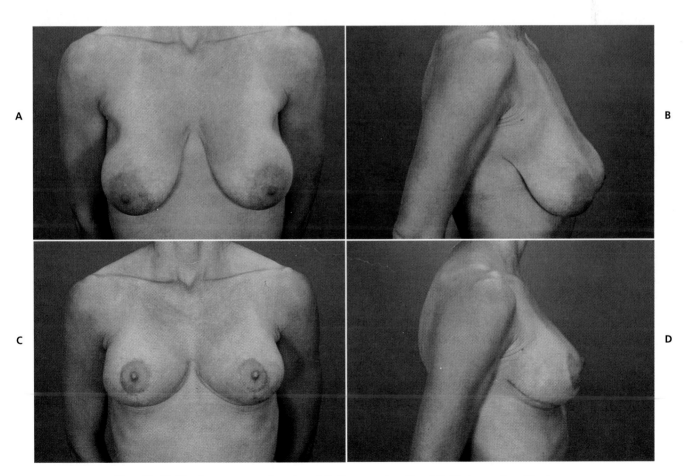

Fig. 10-12 Elective augmentation. **A and B,** Preoperative. **C and D,** Postoperative. *(Courtesy Brian W. Davies, MD.)*

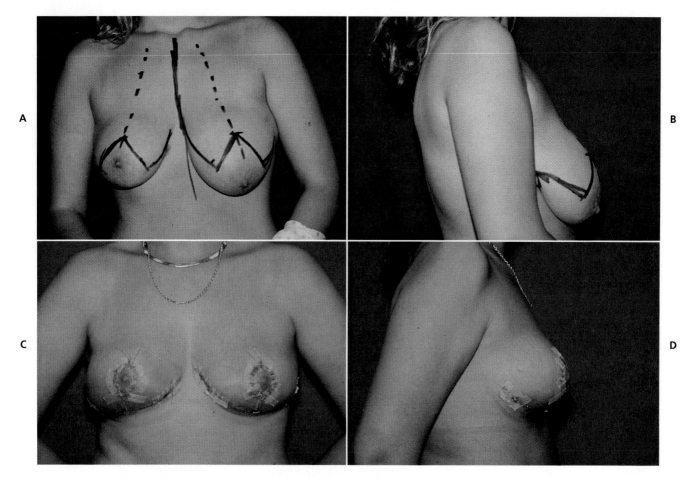

Fig. 10-13 Correction of breast asymmetry and equalization mastopexy. **A and B,** Preoperative. **C and D,** Postoperative. *(Courtesy Brian W. Davies, MD.)*

- *Athelia:* Bilateral or unilateral absence of nipples
- *Supernumerary breasts:* Extend from the axilla in tail of Spence to the groin

Preparing for breast implants

Tissue expansion

Tissue expansion for breast augmentation involves stretching existing chest wall tissue, causing redundancy of the epidermis and dermis sufficient in size to accommodate an underlying prosthetic device or to resurface an area equal in size of a defect (Fig. 10-14). A pocket is created under the pectoralis muscle and maintained to contain a future permanent breast implant. A temporary balloon-type device is positioned in the subpectoral pocket (Fig. 10-15). Progressive inflation with sterile saline causes the overlying tissue to expand over a period of weeks to months. When expansion is complete, the device is deflated and removed. The stretched pocket over the chest wall is ready to receive a permanent mammary implant. The expander stimulates the growth of a fibrous capsule. Implants placed subpectorally have a lower incidence of contracture formation.

A permanent, expandable implant device can be placed during an augmentation procedure. It is progressively expanded with sterile saline. Once the expansion is complete, the expanded device is left in place to serve as a mammary prosthesis. This type of implant is most often used for breast reconstruction after mastectomy.

Inflation procedure. A localized or remote self-sealing port is used to inflate the expander. Some ports have a metallic rim that is easily located with a small magnetic "finder" (see Fig. 8-31). When wound healing is satisfactory, unadulterated sterile saline is injected 10 to 14 days after implantation through the port with a small gauge needle until the skin overlying the prosthesis feels taut (Fig. 10-16). The patient is instructed to return to the facility on an outpatient basis once or twice per week for additional saline instillation until the desired volume has been reached. At this point the expander will be intentionally overinflated by as much as several hundred milliliters and maintained at this level for up to 4 months. The result is a breast that looks more natural.

During the ongoing process of saline inflation of the tissue expander, the skin color and integrity is monitored. Tissue discoloration may indicate interruption of blood supply and potential injury to the expanded area. Expanders and implants are contraindicated in the presence of active infection. Metallic magnetic rims can interfere with MRI tests and

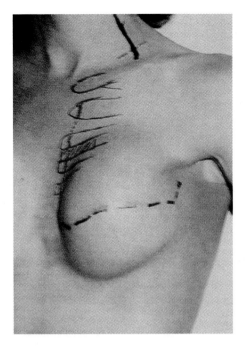

Fig. 10-14 Tissue expander in place after mastectomy. *(Courtesy Brian W. Davies, MD.)*

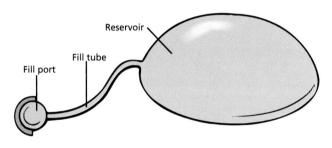

Fig. 10-15 Tissue expander.

should not be used in patients with pacemakers, drug infusion devices, implantable defibrillators, or other automatic sensing devices. The magnetic fields can adversely affect interfunctioning.

Advantages of tissue expansion for breast surgery
- The device can be placed at the time of mastectomy.
- Tissue transplantation is not performed.
- Expanded tissue is the same color and texture and nonhair bearing.
- Minimal anesthesia is needed.
- Hospitalization is not necessary.
- The patient may return to work within 3 to 5 days.
- Complications are minimal.
- Tissue expansion can be used in combination with muscle flap reconstruction.

Contraindications for tissue expansion
- Radiated tissue will not expand and may break down.
- Patients who have undergone a classical radical mastectomy may not have sufficient tissue for expansion.
- Excessive scar tissue may inhibit expansion.

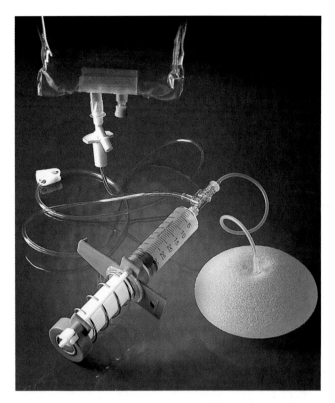

Fig. 10-16 Mammary fill kit. *(Courtesy McGhan Medical Corporation, Santa Barbara, California.)*

- Vascular or lymphatic drainage is insufficient.
- Patient has unrealistic expectations.

Augmentation Mammoplasty

Several surgical approaches are available for augmentation mammoplasty with implants. These involve varying degrees of surgical manipulation and different types of instrumentation. Augmentation with implantation is often performed as an ambulatory procedure under local or general anesthesia. IVCS is commonly used, and an intercostal block may be performed to supplement pain management.

Breast augmentation implants may be positioned subglandularly (under the breast tissue) or subpectorally (under the chest muscle). The patient and her physician determine which method is used based on the aesthetic appearance of the breast before the procedure, the expectations of the patient, and the desired bra cup size (Fig. 10-17).

Breast Implants

Breast implants in use for elective augmentation are filled with saline. The food and drug administration (FDA) closely regulates the use of a silicone-filled prosthesis to a clinical-trial status only. Breast implants are contoured into tear drop shape or round with a smooth or textured surface (Figs. 10-18 and 10-19). The fill valve location on saline implants varies according to style and manufacturer.

The FDA requires logging of all implants. Refer to Chapter 8 for information about recording implants.

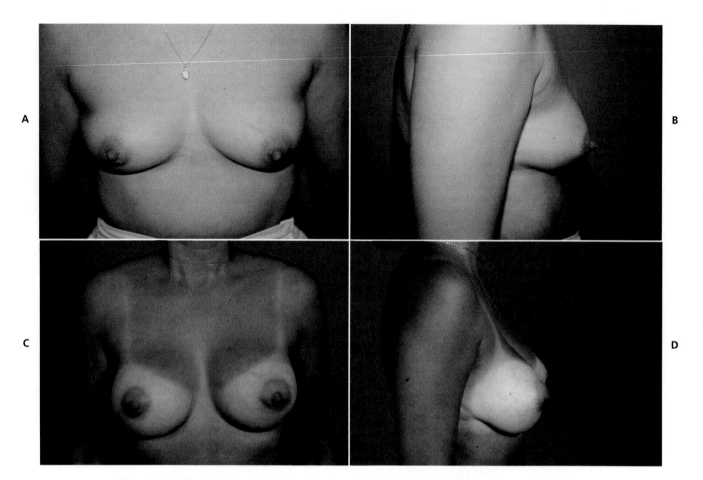

Fig. 10-17 Elective breast augmentation. **A and B,** Preoperative. **C and D,** Postoperative. *(Courtesy Brian W. Davies, MD.)*

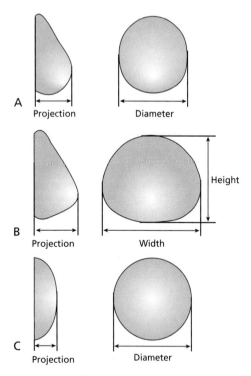

Fig. 10-18 Shapes of breast implants. **A,** Smooth oval. **B,** Contour profile. **C,** Round.

Incisional Approaches for Breast Implant Placement (Fig. 10-20)

Periareolar

The incision is within the pigmented areolar ring. In women with dark complexions, the incision should be made just outside the nipple-areola complex, especially if they have extremely dark areolae. The resultant scar tissue may be a lighter color than the areola. In lighter complexions, the scar is usually more aesthetic and less noticeable than with other methods.

Inframammary

The incision is made just above the inframammary fold. It offers good visualization of the surgical field and varies in length from 3 to 5 cm depending on the size of the implants. The scar is more noticeable than with other methods.

Transaxillary

The incision is made in the axilla in either the submammary or subpectoral plane. Visualization is poor. Implants are placed retropectoral. An endoscope can be used for placement.

Periumbilical

The incision is made supraumbilical. Implants are placed using an endoscope and tunneling instrument. Patients experience less discomfort, shorter recovery, and less scarring with this method. Sensation is not altered.

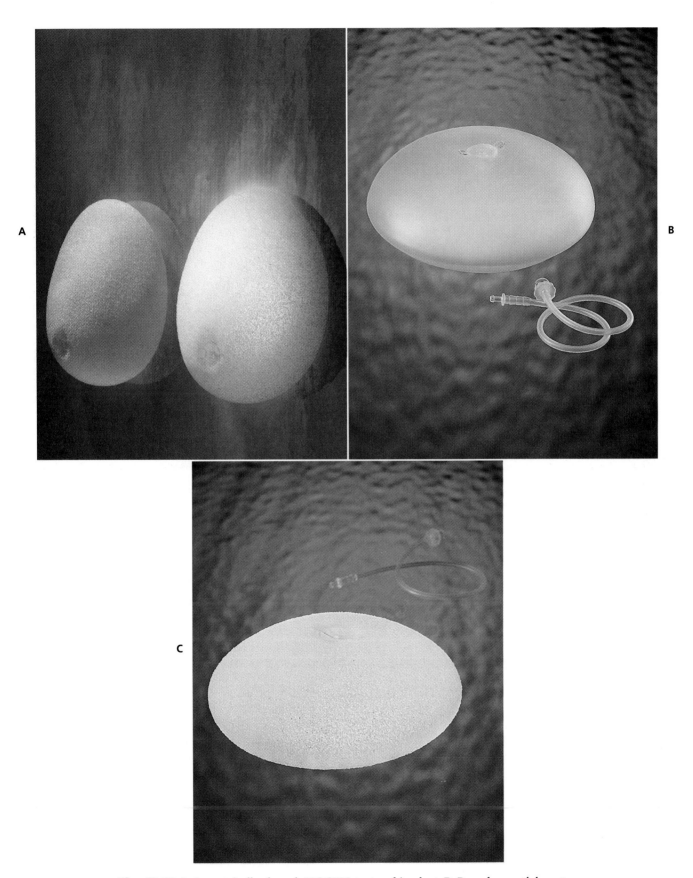

Fig. 10-19 **A,** Anatomically-shaped, BIOCELL textured implant. **B,** Round, smooth breast implant. **C,** Round BIOCELL textured implant. *(Courtesy McGhan Medical Corporation, Santa Barbara, California.)*

Breast Implant Placement Options

Subglandular (submammary)

A 5 to 6 cm inframammary incision is made, and a pocket is created using blunt, sharp, electrosurgical dissection between the mammary gland and the pectoral muscles. The dimensions of the pocket are usually made slightly larger than the implant to allow for placement of the implant without buckling, wrinkling, or rupture. The implant is inserted by gentle digital pressure until it lies flat in the pocket. The inframammary incision is closed with a subcutaneous closure. This is the oldest method of prosthetic placement and is still popular. Risk of lateral displacement is decreased with this method. The incidence of capsular contracture is greater with this method than with subpectoral or submuscular placement.

Subpectoral

The implant is placed behind the pectoralis major superiorly and in either a subglandular, subfascial, or subcutaneous plane at the inferior border. The aesthetic result is a natural appearance.

Submuscular

The implant is placed beneath the pectoralis major, pectoralis minor, serratus anterior, rectus abdominis, and the external oblique muscles. Smooth-walled implants with complete muscle coverage have fewer capsular contractures. The aesthetic result is a less natural appearance, but the borders of the implant are look smoother. The risk of hematoma is

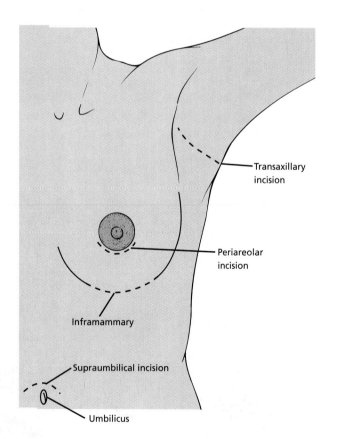

Fig. 10-20 Incisions for placement of augmentation prosthesis.

decreased in this less vascular placement. Routine mammography is less complex when this method is used.

Endoscopic Placement of Breast Implants

Advantages of endoscopic placement of breast implants include smaller hidden scars, decreased recovery time, minimal pain, and decreased surgical and anesthetic time. The main disadvantages of endoscopic implant placement are financially based. The instrumentation is very expensive, and the implantation procedure should be performed in a hospital operating room (OR) or an ambulatory center. Endoscopic placement is contraindicated in breast ptosis because a mastopexy may be necessary. Multiple abdominal surgeries may have caused excessive scar tissue and could cause complications with endoscopic placement. Implants are placed subglandularly with this method because submuscular dissection is complex with this instrumentation.

After marking the planes of the chest and anterior body surface, an incision is made to the fascial layer with a #15 blade, and a tunneling endotube is inserted. The umbilicus and the axilla are the most common incisional sites. The endotube is progressed to the breast between the subcutaneous and fascial layers. Placement is checked with video-assisted endoscopy. A sizer is rolled and inserted through the lumen to the desired subglandular space. The sizer is positioned, and the endotube is withdrawn. Expansion of the sizer creates the pocket. The sizer is expanded 150% of the desired final pocket dimensions and left in place while the same procedure is performed on the opposite side. After the tissue is stretched, sizers are deflated and withdrawn. The actual implants are then placed and filled with saline. The fill tubes are removed, and the tunnels are milked for excess blood and air to eliminate dead space. The deep tissues are closed with interrupted stitches, and the skin is closed with a subcuticular closure. Compression wrap dressings are placed over the tunneled tissue, and the breasts are dressed superiorly causing the breast tissue to be depressed downward. The patient returns to the office for follow-up the next day. A surgi-bra is placed at that time and is to be worn 24 hours a day for the next 4 weeks (Fig. 10-21).

Complications of breast augmentation with implants

Regardless of prosthetic placement site, the potential for capsular contracture within 6 months of implantation caused by foreign-body reaction is possible. Any type or style of breast prosthesis can result in contracture. When smooth-walled prosthetics are used, breast massage may be performed after the procedure as recommended by the surgeon as a preventative measure. Treatment consists of releasing the contracture with capsulotomy or capsulectomy under general anesthesia. Closed capsulotomy may result in rupture of the implant. Some physicians will convert a submammary implant to a submuscular position during an open capsulectomy for better results. Capsular contractures are classified according to the degree of postoperative deformity. The Baker grade scale includes the following:

- *Class I:* The augmented breast is as soft as an unaffected, nonaugmented breast.
- *Class II:* The augmented breast is less soft, and the implant is palpable but not visible.

- *Class III:* The augmented breast is firm, the implant is palpable, and distortion is visible.
- *Class IV:* The augmented breast is hard and painful, and the distortion is pronounced.

Sensory changes are commonly seen and usually abate in 6 to 12 months. Extremes of sensation may include pain or numbness. This may be permanent or temporary. Nipple sensation can be affected if the nerve has been divided during lateral dissection.

Malpositioning or asymmetry is possible. Implants may "ride high" when initially placed but settle into a more natural position over several months. In some patients, a second repositioning procedure may be necessary.

Other complications include hematoma and hypertrophic scars. Hematomas should be drained to prevent the potential for infection. Hypertrophic scar tissue can be revised after the procedure and is commonly seen in inframammary incisions. Device failure includes leaking or rupture of the implant. Rupture, leak, or extrusion of silicone is not always detectable by x-ray examination, ultrasound, or MRI. Endoscopy has been used successfully to detect leaks. Infection is always a risk with any invasive surgical procedure.

Explantation of breast implants

Explantation of implants is performed either through an open procedure or endoscopically. In some cases, silicone implants are removed during capsulectomy encased within the capsular scar to prevent spillage. Many are replaced with a saline-filled implant.

Some reconstruction procedures are performed using the patient's own muscle tissue in the form of a vascular pedicle flap taken from the abdomen, the back, or other adjacent site.

Some patients who have experienced complications prefer to return to their preimplant breast size and refuse any further augmentation procedures. Psychologic improvement is noted in these patients after explantation. Patients who undergo further reconstruction after explantation with a muscle flap or saline implants have also shown improvement in their physical and emotional state of health.

BREAST RECONSTRUCTION

Some patients prefer breast reconstruction with autologous tissue. This type of reconstruction is often done immediately after mastectomy unless radiation therapy is indicated. The patient must be willing to accept the scars that result from autogenous tissue flaps. Several flap site options are available to the patient:

- Free muscle flap reconstruction using the axillary vessels as the blood supply
- Transverse rectus abdominis myocutaneous (TRAM) flap with a blood supply from the anastomosed mammary vessels and the thoracic vessels; this pedicle-flap is buried allowing for better perfusion of the transpositioned tissue
- External oblique myocutaneous flap used to cover large chest wall defects after mastectomy for advanced breast tumors; many of these patients have received external beam radiation and/or chemotherapy
- Pectoralis major flaps
- Latissimus dorsi flaps utilized as a pedicled, deepithelialized dermis and fat flap; sufficient to support the thoracodorsal vessels, leaving the major part of the muscle functionally intact

TRAM Flap

The TRAM flap is used for breast reconstruction in patients who have adequate amounts of lower abdominal fat relative to their body size (Fig. 10-22). A section of anterior rectus sheath is dissected free with an intact neurovascular supply attached by a stalk to an island of abdominal fat covered with abdominal skin (Fig. 10-23). The incision extends transversely from the iliac crest on one side to the iliac crest on the opposite side. Dissection of the rectus abdominis flap is performed carefully to protect neurovascular integrity of the tissue. Circulation at the flap can be checked during the procedure by sterile Doppler auscultation.

A presternal tunnel is made, and the flap is carefully rotated and passed through to its new position (Fig. 10-24). The neurovascular stalk is protected from vascular occlusion and stretching. The deep epigastric artery and the thoracodorsal

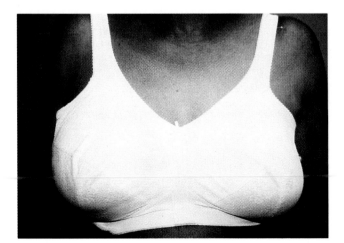

Fig. 10-21 Breast dressing support. Used after reconstruction, augmentation, and reduction. *(Courtesy Brian W. Davies, MD.)*

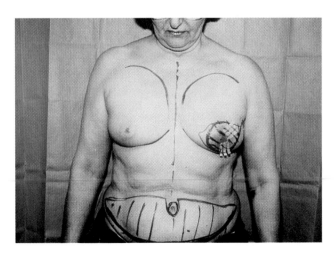

Fig. 10-22 Marking technique for TRAM flap breast reconstruction. *(Courtesy Brian W. Davies, MD.)*

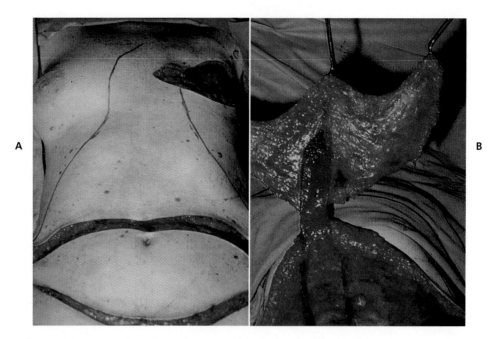

Fig. 10-23 A, A section of anterior rectus sheath dissected free. **B,** Intact neurovascular supply. *(Courtesy Brian W. Davies, MD.)*

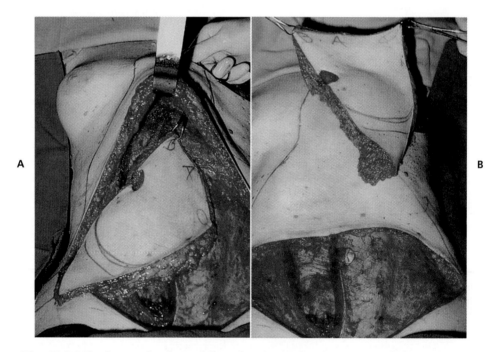

Fig. 10-24 Flap is rotated and passed through to its new location. *(Courtesy Brian W. Davies, MD.)*

artery are anastomosed under the microscope to augment the blood supply. The skin island is seated into the mastectomy defect. The tissue is deepithelialized and trimmed to fit (Fig. 10-25).

The use of autologous tissue allows the surgeon to sculpt the shape of the neobreast. A sterile scale may be used to determine the weight of the tissue in proportion to the flap size needed. The surgeon may use liposuction or sharp dis-

section to refine the contour of the breast to obtain a specific aesthetic result. Double reconstruction is performed in the same manner as the single pedicle dissection with the exception that the flap is divided in the midline and each flap is refashioned individually (Fig. 10-26, *A*). Surgery and anesthesia times are increased because of the time needed to dissect and divide the muscle flap, anastomose the vascular supply, and close the abdominal and breast site wounds (Fig. 10-26, *B*).

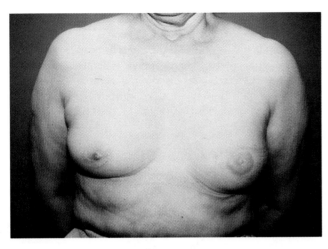

Fig. 10-25 Completed TRAM flap reconstruction. *(Courtesy Brian W. Davies, MD.)*

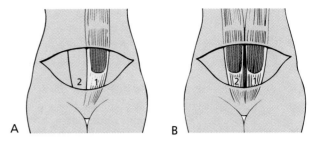

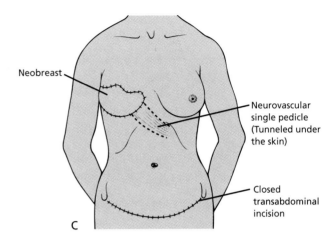

Fig. 10-26 TRAM flap. **A,** Sites of TRAM flaps. **B,** Single TRAM flap in position.

The patient will experience a decrease in abdominal strength caused by the removal of the rectus abdominis muscle; however, other abdominal muscles compensate for the loss. The possibility of a herniation developing at the site of muscle removal on the abdomen is minimized by the use of implantable mesh over the fascia. The mesh support adds to aesthetic aspects of the abdominoplasty, which is performed as a result of the use of a TRAM flap.

The skin of the neobreast may be a slightly different shade than the tissue of the chest wall in that area. Unwanted hair growth is also a possibility because the skin island was proximal to the pubis. Breast sensation and response to stimulation does not return. Patients seem to adapt readily to the "new breast" because it has a natural appearance and feel.

This procedure is recommended for patients who have received radiation therapy before and/or after mastectomy. The added benefit of a skin island helps to create wound cover at the mastectomy site. Nipple-areolar complex reconstruction is performed at a later date (commonly 6 weeks) to give the new tissue a chance to settle.

Contraindications to a TRAM flap include previous TRAM flap procedure, abdominoplasty, multiple abdominal procedures, ventriculoperitoneal shunt, herniorrhaphy with inplantable mesh, or liposuction.

Preoperative patient preparation

The patient is advised to stop smoking for at least 3 months before the surgical procedure. Studies have shown that smoking adversely affects circulation and oxygen supply to the flap. Aspirin and anticoagulant therapy is discontinued at least 2 weeks in advance. Before the procedure, methylprednisolone sodium may be given IV and continued through the first day after the procedure to minimize edema and prevent thromboembolism. Antibiotics may be started before the procedure and continued for several days after. In patients who are allergic to penicillin, erythromycin may be administered.

The patient is involved in the formulation of a postoperative plan of care because compliance is critical to the outcome of

the procedure. Analgesia is delivered through a patient-controlled analgesic (PCA) pump.

Intraoperative patient care considerations

Patients undergoing a TRAM will be placed in a modified semi-Fowler's position to relieve the stress from the abdominal musculature. The feet and legs are slightly elevated to prevent the patient from sliding down on the table. A gel pad should be placed under each pressure point. Antiembolism stockings or alternating compression hose should be applied to the patient's lower legs. An indwelling Foley catheter should be used because of the prolonged length of the procedure. Care is taken to prevent hypothermia. Irrigation and IV fluids should be warmed before use. The skin prep is performed with an approved antiseptic solution.

Tissue and sponges should be weighed. The wound will be irrigated with heparinized solution to prevent microembolization. Blood salvage equipment can minimize the need for blood-loss replacement. Closed-wound suction drains will be placed in the abdominal wound and at the neobreast. Nipple-areola reconstruction is performed at a later date.

Postoperative patient care considerations

The patient is maintained in the modified semi-Fowler's position from the OR table to a division bed. This position is maintained for 24 hours after the procedure. The flap site is checked frequently with a Doppler monitor. Changes in flap color, swelling, or bleeding is reported to the surgeon immediately.

On the first day after the procedure, the patient is assisted out of bed and encouraged to ambulate. Mobility may be difficult because the abdominal musculature has been altered. Coughing is avoided because it may interrupt the integrity of the mesh. Deep breathing and yawning can help prevent pulmonary complications.

The Foley catheter is removed, and the diet is advanced as tolerated. The patient uses a PCA pump until the IV is removed, usually 24 to 36 hours after the procedure. The drains are removed when the drainage is less than 25 ml per day. A long-line bra without underwires may be worn to support the breast mound and the abdominal tunnel site. The patient is discharged on the fifth or sixth day after the procedure.

NIPPLE RECONSTRUCTION

Nipple absence or deformity is corrected by creating a tissue advancement to simulate a nipplelike structure, areolar tattooing with iron oxide and titanium dioxide pigments, resculpting, or free nipple grafts (Figs. 10-27 and 10-28).

Nipple Surgical Procedures

The position of a nipple on the breast is determined by matching the position of the nipple on the opposite breast or by measuring a 19 to 21 cm diagonal distance from the sternal notch to the midclavicular line. Figure 10-5, A-C illustrates the measurement of nipple placement. Nipple dimensions are derived from the size of the original or remaining nipple. If nipple-areolar complexes are to be resized, a measuring "cookie cutter" or "washer" is used as a template. Many sizes are available. The surgeon also determines the nipple tip diameter and projection (Fig. 10-29).

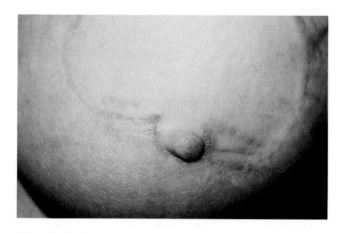

Fig. 10-27 Nipple projection reconstruction. *(Courtesy Brian W. Davies, MD.)*

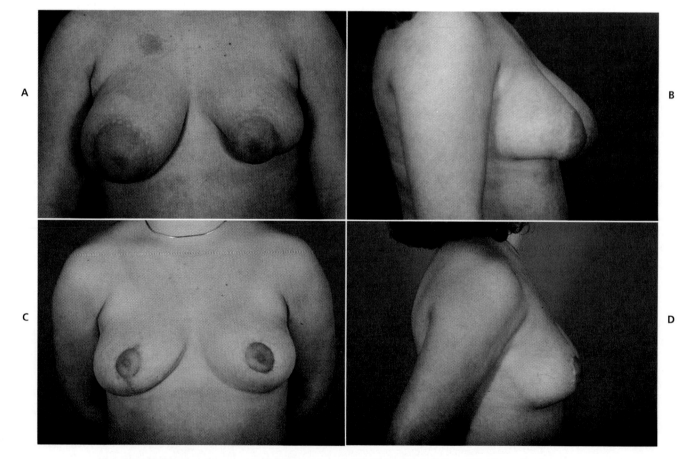

Fig. 10-28 Tuberous breast nipple deformity. **A and B,** Preoperative. **C and D,** Postoperative. *(Courtesy Brian W. Davies, MD.)*

Nipple-areolar complex reduction

A sizing template is inked and placed over the center of each areola to mark the new dimensions. Additional incision lines are marked along the rim of the existing areola and extended laterally and medially to form an ellipse. The incision is made on each areola along the newly created margin circumferentially. Deepithelialization is performed from the new margin to the distal edge of the areola. The old areolar tissue is circumscribed and excised. The wound edges are approximated and closed with interrupted sutures (Fig. 10-30).

Correction of nipple inversion deformity

In technique I, a traction suture is placed through the inverted nipple tip to cause eversion. The areola around the base of the nipple projection is circumferentially incised and undermined. Small wedges of deepithelialized areolar tissue are excised at three or four points along the radius of the complex. The radial incisions are closed from the periphery to the base of the nipple with interrupted sutures. A purse string is placed around the base of the projection. The traction suture is released (Fig. 10-31). Other techniques require incision of muscular and fibrous layers between the ducts. Care is taken to not occlude the ducts if the patient wants to breast feed at a later date.

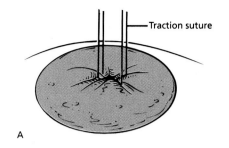

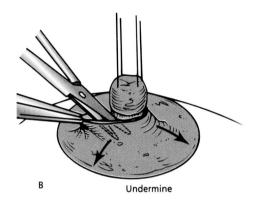

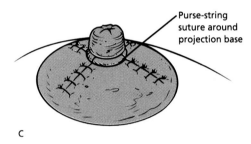

Fig. 10-31 Correction of nipple inversion deformity. **A,** Traction sutures are applied to inverted nipple tip. **B,** Base of nipple to periphery of areola is undermined, and wedges of deepithelialized areola are excised. **C,** Wedges are closed and a purse string is placed around the base of elevated nipple tip to maintain raised position.

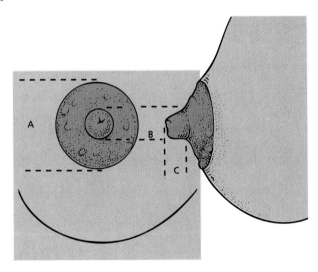

Fig. 10-29 Measurement parameters for nipple repair or creation. **A,** Areolar diameter. **B,** Nipple tip diameter. **C,** Nipple tip projection (height).

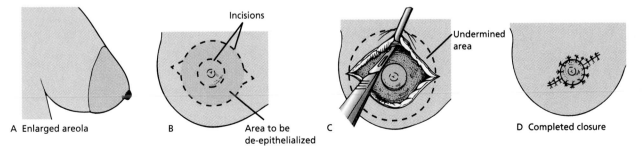

Fig. 10-30 Steps in nipple reduction procedure. **A,** Large areola of tuberous breast. **B,** Outlines for excisional deepithelialization of excess areolar tissue. **C,** Periphery is undermined after excision of excess areola. **D,** Finished closure of reduced nipple.

Neoconstruction of nipple-areolar complex

Placement of the nipple-areolar complex is measured according to the midclavicular and midsternal axis. Local tissue advancement is performed for propeller flap, tube flap, or skate flap nipple creation. The diameter is marked with a circular template. The circumference of the areolar margin is incised. Three small, triangular dermal wedges are excised and deepithelialized. The central portion remains attached to the adipose base, and a traction suture is applied centrally to elevate the nipple tip projection (Fig. 10-32, *A-C*). The vertical edges are approximated to maintain the projected surface. A purse string is placed around the base of the projection, and excess dermal tissue is excised (Fig. 10-32, *D*). A full-thickness graft is taken from a site that closely matches the tissue of the original areola. Some surgeons graft portions of the contralateral nipple. The graft is sutured into position with interrupted stitches (Fig. 10-32, *E and F*).

Micropigmentation

Nipple graft sites may vary, but some tissue may require pigmented tattooing. The plastic surgeon or a certified nurse tattoo artist performs this procedure 1 month after the procedure. The nipple projection is tinted a deeper shade than the areola to minimize the fading process. This gives the nipple tip a better contrast if the projection recedes. Subsequent touch-ups may be needed if the color fades (Fig 10-33).

Free nipple grafts

Patients who require resection of 1500 to 2000 g of breast tissue may not be candidates for pedicled nipple repositioning. Pedicles in excess of 30 cm may result in nipple loss caused by folding or torsion of the circulation. Free nipple grafting may be indicated.

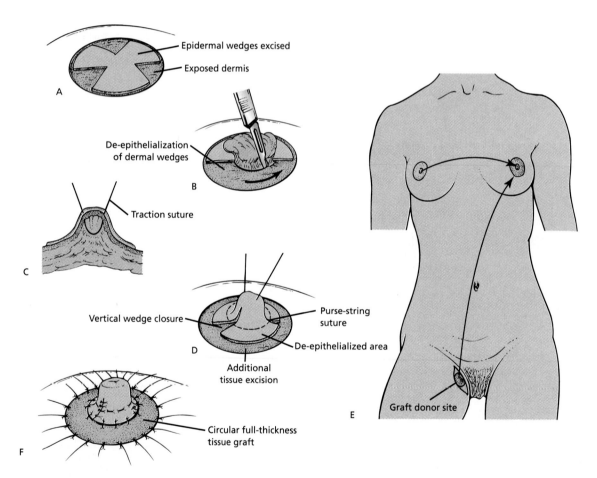

Fig. 10-32 Creation of nipple. **A,** Circumferential incisional demarcation of nipple periphery with removal of dermal wedges. **B,** Secondary dermal wedges are deepithelialized from the peripheral rim toward the intact center. **C,** A traction suture is used to elevate the central future nipple tip. **D,** Traction is applied to the future nipple tip as the wedges are approximated to create a permanent projected surface. A purse string is applied around the base to secure the elevation. Excess deepithelialized tissue is excised. A peripheral dermal ring remains. **E,** Possible full-thickness donor site areolar color match may be found in the labial folds. **F,** Donor graft is measured, cut, and secured to dermal ring of neonipple-areolar complex.

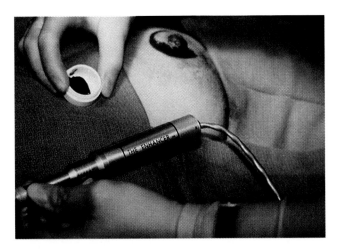

Fig. 10-33 Dermapigmentation. *(Courtesy Brian W. Davies, MD.)*

Nipple Dressings

Even, firm contact of the newly reconstructed or grafted nipple to the recipient bed is essential for blood supply and survival. Immobilization is necessary for the graft to take to the underlying tissue. The nipple is secured with a tie-over bolster dressing technique to prevent seroma.

Bibliography

Ahn CY, Shaw WW: Regional silicone-gel migration in patients with ruptured implants, *Ann Plast Surg* 33(2):201, 1994.

Abramo AC: Axillary approach for gynecomastia liposuction, *Aesthetic Plast Surg* 18(3):265, 1994.

Beer GM, Kompatscher P: Endoscopic plastic surgery: the endoscopic evaluation of implants after breast augmentation, *Aesthetic Plast Surg* 19(4):353, 1995.

Bensimon RH, Bergmeyer JM: Improved aesthetics in breast reconstruction: modified mastectomy incision and immediate autologous tissue reconstruction, *Ann Plast Surg* 34(3):229, 1995.

Beraka GJ: Autologous secondary breast augmentation with pedicled transverse rectus abdominis musculocutaneous flaps, *Ann Plast Surg* 34(3):242, 1995.

Brenner P et al: Male reduction mammoplasty in serious gynecomastias, *Aesthetic Plast Surg* 16(4):325, 1992.

Brown H et al: Variables affecting symmetry of nipple-areola complex. *Plast Reconstr Surg* 96(4):846, 1995.

Cahan AC et al: Breast cancer after breast augmentation with silicone, *Ann Surg Oncol* 2(2):121, 1995.

Camirand A, Doucet J: Subpectoral breast augmentation under local anesthesia, *Can J Plast Surg* 3(2):79, 1995.

Chajchir A et al: Endoscopic augmentation mammoplasty, *Aesthetic Plast Surg* 18(4):377, 1994.

Davies BW et al: Reduction mammaplasty: a comparison of outpatient and inpatient procedures, *Aesthetic Plast Surg* 20(1):77, 1996.

Eklund GW: Mammographic compression: science or art? *Radiology* 181(2):339, 1991.

Eklund GW et al: Improved imaging of the augmented breast, *Am J Roentgen* 151(3):496, 1988.

Glass AR: Gynecomastia, *Endocrinol Metab Clin North Am* 23(4):825, 1994.

Gold AH: Elliptical breast reconstruction: an improved and simplified technique, *Ann Plast Surg* 28(6):516, 1992.

Hall FM et al: Mammography of the augmented breast, *Am J Roentgen* 153(5):1098, 1989.

Harouche EF: The double dermal keyhole pattern for breast reconstruction, *Plast Reconstr Surg* 96(6):1452, 1995.

Hart D: Women and saline breast implant surgery, *Plast Surg Nurs* (15)3:161, 1995.

Heddens CJ: Postoperative survey of reduction mammoplasty patients, *Plast Surg Nurs* 13(3):148, 1993.

Hollos P: Breast augmentation with autologous tissue: an alternative to implants, *Plast Reconstr Surg* 96(2):381, 1995.

Katez P: Reduction mammoplasty, *Plast Surg Nurs* 12(2):51, 1992.

Koger KE et al: Reduction mammoplasty for gigantomastia using inferiorly based pedicle and free nipple transplantation, *Ann Plast Surg* 33(5):561, 1994.

Kossovsky N, Friedman CJ: Silicone breast implant pathology: clinical data and immunologic consequences, *Arch Pathol Lab Med* 118(7):686, 1994.

Kruse BD et al: Breast imaging and the augmented breast, *Plast Surg Nurs* 12(3):109, 1992.

Logothetis ML: Women's reports of breast implant problems and silicone-related illness, *J Obstet Gynecol Neonatal Nurs* 24(7):609, 1995.

McCain L: Counseling the woman with silicone breast implants, *Plast Surg Nurs* 12(2):61, 1992.

McMahan JD et al: Lasting success in teenage reduction mammoplasty, *Ann Plast Surg* 33(3):227, 1995.

Monteiro DT: Secure dressing after nipple-areolar reconstruction, *Ann Plast Surg* 35(2):220, 1995.

O'Hanlon DM et al: Unilateral breast masses in men over 40: a diagnostic dilemma, *Am J Surg* 170(1):24, 1995.

Patrizi I et al: Immediate reconstruction after radical mastectomy for breast carcinoma with Becker-type expander prosthesis, *Minerva Chir* 48(9):453, 1993.

Romano JJ et al: Free nipple graft reduction mammoplasty, *Ann Plast Surg* 28(3):271, 1992.

Samdal F et al: Surgical treatment of gynecomastia: five years experience with liposuction, *Scand J Plast Reconstr Surg Hand Surg* 28(2):123, 1994.

Serletti JM et al: Efficacy of prophylactic antibiotics in reduction mammoplasty, *Ann Plast Surg* 33(5):476, 1994.

Simler AG: Endoscopic augmentation mammoplasty: the umbilical approach, *Plast Surg Nurs* 14(3):149, 1994.

Spear SL, Arias J: Long-term experience with nipple-areola tattooing, *Ann Plast Surg* 35(3):232, 1995.

Strombler RE: Breast implants and the FDA: past present, and future, *Plast Surg Nurs* (13)4:185, 1993.

Stone J, Dowden RV: Breast implant endoscopy, *AORN J* 59(5):1007, 1994.

Troilius C: Total muscle coverage of breast implant is possible through transaxillary approach, *Plast Reconstr Surg* 95(3):509, 1995.

Vasconez HC, Holley DT: Use of TRAM and latissimus dorsi flaps in autogenous breast reconstruction, *Clin Plast Surg* 22(1):153, 1995.

Waltman N: Treatment options for the patient with breast cancer, *Plast Surg Nurs* 14(1):15, 1994.

Wickman M: Rapid versus slow tissue expansion for breast reconstruction: a three-year follow-up, *Plast Reconstr Surg* 95(4):712, 1995.

Williams JK et al: TRAM flap breast reconstruction after radiation treatment, *Ann Surg* 221(6):756, 1995.

Clinical Standards of Plastic Surgical Nursing

STANDARDS OF CARE

Standard 1. Assessment and collection of data

The plastic surgical nurse initiates assessment of the patient seeking plastic surgery to determine pertinent data about health history and current health status, which is documented, retrievable, and communicated.

Statement

Health data are collected systematically and continuously, using appropriate assessment techniques such as interview, observation, physical assessment, and review of prior records. Presented problems are ranked by priority as indicated by the patient's present condition and needs. Utilizing the scientific method, reviews of the patient's current health status are systematically documented and recorded in a retrievable form. The data collection process includes significant others and appropriate health care providers. Scientific data are reported to other health care professionals as appropriate and recorded in the patient's permanent record.

Outcome

The client is assessed on initial interview and regularly thereafter, based on symptomology and risks for complications. Perception of health status and immediate suitable goals are identified. Patient information and its sources are guarded as confidential.

Standard 2. Nursing diagnosis and analysis of assessment data

The plastic surgical nurse analyzes assessed data and formulates nursing diagnoses and individual plan of care.

Statement

Nursing diagnoses are derived, ordered by priority, validated with the patient's significant others and appropriate health care providers, and comprehensively documented and communicated as needed to facilitate the plan of care and expected outcomes.

Outcome

Nursing priorities are clearly established. Documented diagnoses are amenable to nursing intervention. Diagnostic statements reflect current nursing practice that facilitates ongoing patient care by all nursing professionals concerned with the plan of care.

Standard 3. Expected outcome identification specific to the patient

The plastic surgical nurse documents a plan of care describing nursing intervention and attainable outcomes.

Statement

Outcomes are derived from the diagnosis and documented as measurable goals with projected time estimates. Realistically related to the patient's present and potential capabilities as well as available resources, patient outcomes are formulated with the appropriate health care providers and significant others and include suggestions for continuity of care. The patient is an informed participant whenever possible.

Outcome

The patient and significant others acquire knowledge of known physiologic and psychological responses to the contemplated surgical intervention. The individual's present and potential physical capabilities and behavior patterns are established as congruent with anticipated outcomes. Plans for continuance of care are documented and reflect a logical sequence of nursing activities to attain outcomes. The plan of care respects the patient's rights and desires and makes adequate provision to protect patient confidentiality.

Standard 4. Planning that prescribes intervention to attain expected outcome

The plastic surgical nurse designs and implements a plan of care based upon nursing diagnosis and realistic, measurable outcomes.

Statement

Nursing interventions and outcomes are documented throughout the permanent record to assess care specific to the patient's individual needs. The plan of care uses nursing process and is collaborated with other health care providers; nursing and patient actions are analyzed as ongoing assessment and communicated to the health care team. Confidentiality is maintained.

Outcome

A documented plan of care reflects the nursing process that prescribes nursing intervention to attain outcomes specific to the needs and desires of the individual patient.

Standard 5. Evaluation toward the attainment of outcome

The plastic surgical nurse reviews and evaluates nursing intervention, and reassesses the plan of care to attain desired outcomes of individual patient goals.

Statement

Well-formulated, realistic outcomes focus nursing care. Patient responses to interventions are evaluated with regard to outcome. Systematic and ongoing assessment of data are used to revise diagnosis, outcome, and plan of care as needed. Revisions to the plan of care are determined by written record, observation, patient response, and perception, and are communicated to appropriate care providers. Outcome attainment is regularly assessed and reconsidered with the nursing diagnosis and patient goals. Such ongoing reassessment allows modification of the plan as the patient progresses toward wellness.

Outcome

The patient is a full participant on the health care team, and significant others are included in the nursing process as appropriate. Nursing action effectiveness is reevaluated and new goals devised and implemented as necessary. Improved concepts of self care, patient participation, patient education, and health promotion are treated as basic parts of the outcome. Effectiveness is demonstrated by the patient's recognition of progress and satisfaction of attainable goals and outcomes.

STANDARDS OF PROFESSIONAL PERFORMANCE
Standard 1. Quality of care

The plastic surgical nurse provides quality care based on professional nursing practice and encompassing accepted components of analysis, interpretation, and implementation, consistent with Patient's Bill of Rights and State Nursing Practice Act(s).

Statement

Quality nursing care is provided to the plastic surgical patient within an environment conducive to its effective administration. The needs of the patient are met in a manner compliant with local, state, and federal statutes and quality assurance guidelines. Desired outcomes or probability of undesired outcome are communicated to the patient as part of the plan of care.

Outcome

The quality of care reflects the values and priorities of plastic surgical nursing as outlined in these *Standards of Clinical Practice*. The patient remains the unalterable focus of the patient care-centered nursing process, which activates appropriate changes in the plan of care and overall health care system.

Standard 2. Performance appraisal

The plastic surgical nurse accepts responsibility for professional autonomy and performance by peer review, continued education, and skill development.

Statement

As part of a continuous process, self-evaluation of each individual nurse's practice relates to applicable professional standards and statutes. The plastic surgical nurse functions within the limits of educational preparation and experience as related to specific responsibilities. The plastic surgical nurse seeks knowledge and skills appropriate to the practice setting through ongoing educational activities. Professional sharing of knowledge and skills with other members of the health care team provides constructive feedback.

Outcome

Plastic surgical nurses accept accountability for their practice and participate within peer review to achieve goals identified by performance appraisal. Constructive feedback is encouraged regarding professional and practice development.

Standard 3. Education

The Plastic Surgical Nurse acquires and maintains current knowledge in nursing to improve clinical skills and offer optimum quality care to the plastic surgical patient.

Statement

The plastic surgical nurse pursues knowledge and skills appropriate to the practice setting through ongoing education and maintains competency in the skills required for professional licensing and/or certification; and actively seeks practical experience to maintain and refine clinical skills.

Outcome

Continued education in pursuit of self-improvement and high proficiency in current practices in plastic surgical nursing ensures the plastic surgical nurse's effective contribution to all aspects of health care delivery, particularly an uneventful surgical experience for the plastic surgical patient.

Standard 4. Collegiality

The plastic surgical nurse demonstrates collegiality by communication and mutual professional acceptance.

Statement

The plastic surgical nurse communicates with health team members and is a resource to other providers, follows the policies and procedures of the practice setting as appropriate, and actively engages in activities that share clinical expertise and encourages a multidiscipline approach to care of the plastic surgical patient.

Outcome

The plastic surgical nurse contributes to an environment that supports the delivery of quality nursing care and communication among all nursing specialties.

Standard 5. Ethics

The plastic surgical nurse acts as an advocate for the patient, guided by Nursing Codes and Standards, and ensures that all patient-related decisions and actions are taken in an ethical manner.

Statement

While delivering patient care in a nonjudgmental or discriminating manner, the plastic surgical nurse acknowledges the patient's right to be engaged as the focus and as a team player in the plan of care. Required data from any source concerning the patient are safeguarded as confidential. With constant sensitivity to patient diversity and individuality, the nurse serves as patient advocate and confidant.

Outcome

Ethical Standards of Plastic Surgical Nursing Performance are compatible with ANA Medical/Surgical Practice Standards. They also comply with Standards of Nursing Practice of the Association of Operating Room Nurses. These are standards consistent with standards of practice recognizing patients' rights to be the focus and active participants in their plan of care. Ethical decisions are formulated with the available resources as appropriate to the plastic surgical patient and the plan of care.

Standard 6. Collaboration

The plastic surgical nurse functions as a member of a multidiscipline team promoting health and wellness.

Statement

The plastic surgical nurse consults with peers regarding patient care and the role of nursing care providers, and seeks referral networks suitable to the continuation of care for the patient as appropriate. The nurse communicates with the patient regarding the nurse's role in the plan of care.

Outcome

Nursing performance is reflected by the plastic surgical nurse's cooperation with community resources and referrals appropriate to the needs of the patient. Plastic surgical nurses assist the patient and significant others in securing services available to health-related needs.

Standard 7. Research

The plastic surgical nurse values and utilizes research in nursing practice.

Statement

The plastic surgical nurse participates in ongoing research to identify concerns and facilitate problem-solving activities appropriate for development and performance specific to nursing, implementation, and outcomes. In varied practice settings, the nurse offers input to the development of policies and procedures and organizes fostering inquiry for the improvement of patient care.

Outcome

Nursing care is enhanced by the increased knowledge and skills of the provider. Patient education and community awareness regarding plastic surgical nursing is heightened.

Standard 8. Resource utilization

The plastic surgical nurse identifies appropriate resources considering safety, effectiveness, and cost in planning the delivery of patient care.

Statement

The plastic surgical nurse identifies necessary and appropriate resources and selects, supervises, and coordinates provision of necessary and appropriate health care services.

Outcome

Patient and significant others are guided and assisted in the identification and acquisition of necessary and appropriate services available for health and wellness-related needs. Established goals are identified to provide a data base and rationale for change in resource allocation.

References/Readings

American Nurses Association. (1991). *American Nurses Association standards of clinical nursing practice.* Washington, DC: Author.

American Nurses Association, Committee on Nursing Practices and Guidelines. (1995). *Manual to Develop Guidelines.* Washington, DC: Author.

American Society of Plastic and Reconstructive Surgical Nurses. (1987). *Standards of plastic surgical nurses.* Pitman, NJ: Author.

Association of Operating Room Nurses, Inc. (1995). *Standards & recommended practices.* Denver, CO: Author.

Association of Operating Room Nurses. (1981). *Standards of perioperative practice.* Kansas City, MO: Author.

Brunner, L., & Suddarth, D. (1984). *Medical surgical nursing.* Philadelphia: J.B. Lippincott Company.

Carpenito, L. (1983). Nursing diagnosis: *Application to clinical practice.* Philadelphia: J.B. Lippincott Company.

Dermatology Nurses Association. (1993). *Dermatology scope of practice* and *dermatology nursing standards of clinical nursing practice.* Pitman, NJ: Author.

Goodman, T. (Ed.). (1988). *Core curriculum for plastic and reconstructive surgical nursing.* Pitman, NJ: American Society of Plastic and Reconstructive Surgical Nurses, Inc.

Goodman, T. (Ed.). (1996). *Core curriculum for plastic and reconstructive surgical nursing* (second edition). Pitman, NJ: American Society of Plastic and Reconstructive Surgical Nurses, Inc.

Oxford English Dictionary. (1971). New York: Oxford University Press.

Soukhanov, A.H. (Ed.). (1992). *The American heritage dictionary.* New York: Houghton Mifflin Company.

Sullivan, J.M., & Mann, R.J. (1994, December). Clinical practice guidelines: Implications for use. *Dermatology Nursing,* pp. 413-418.

Young, W. (1987). *Introduction to nursing concepts.* Scarborough, Ontario: Prentice Hall Canada.

Key Terms

As does most professional and technical communication, these Standards rely upon words of art and specialized language to convey information with precision and clarity. To facilitate understanding and compliance, readers will find explicated here the terms central to the intent of this document.

ASSESSMENT:
A systematic, dynamic process by which the nurse, through interaction with the patient, significant others, and health care providers, collects and analyzes data about the patient. Data may include these dimensions: physical, psychologic, sociologic, spiritual, cognitive, functional ability, developmental, economic, and lifestyle.

CRITERIA:
Relevant, measurable indicators of the standards of clinical nursing practice.

DIAGNOSIS:
A clinical judgment about the patient's response to actual or potential health conditions or needs. Diagnoses provide the basis for determining a plan of care to achieve expected outcomes.

EVALUATION:
The process of determining the patient's progress toward the attainment of expected outcomes and the effectiveness of nursing care.

GUIDELINES:
Systematically developed statements based on available scientific evidence and expert opinion.
A process of patient care management that has the potential of improving the quality of clinical and consumer decision making.

HEALTH CARE PROVIDERS:
Individuals with special expertise who provide health care services or assistance to patients. They may include nurses, physicians, psychologists, social workers, nutritionists/dieticians, and various therapists. Providers may also include service organizations and vendors.

IMPLEMENTATION:
Activities such as intervening, delegating, coordinating. Patient, significant others, or health care providers may be designated to perform interventions within the plan of care.

NURSING:
The diagnosis and treatment of human responses to actual or potential health problems. (ANA, Nursing: A Social Policy Statement)

OUTCOMES:
Measurable expected patient-focused goals.

PATIENT:
Recipient of nursing action.

PLAN OF CARE:
Comprehensive outline of care to be delivered to attain expected outcomes.

SIGNIFICANT OTHERS:
Family members and/or those persons important to the patient.

STANDARD:
Authoritative statement enunciated and promulgated by the profession and by which the quality of practice, service, or education can be judged.

STANDARDS OF CARE:
Authoritative statements that describe a competent level of clinical nursing practice demonstrated through assessment, diagnosis, outcome identification, planning, implementation, and evaluation.

STANDARDS OF NURSING PRACTICE:
An authoritative statement that describes a level of care or performance common to the profession of nursing by which the quality of nursing practice can be judged. Standards of clinical nursing practice include both standards of care and standards of professional performance.

STANDARDS OF PROFESSIONAL PERFORMANCE:
Authoritative statements that describe a competent level of behavior in the professional role, including activities related to quality of care, performance appraisal, education, collegiality, ethics, collaboration, research, and resource utilization.

Adapted from ANA standards of clinical nursing practice, Washington, DC, American Nurses Association, 1991.

Index

A

Abdomen
  anatomy and physiology of, 110
  rotational flap from, *84*
Abdominal flap in abdominoplasty, 111-112, *112*
Abdominal suction-assisted lipectomy, 105, *106*
Abdominoplasty, 108-113, *110*
  anatomy and physiology in, 110
  complications of, 113
  indications and contraindications for, 110-111
  intraoperative care for, 111, *111*
  postoperative care for, 112-113
  preoperative care for, 111
  procedure of, *111*, 111-112, *112*
  reverse, 111
Abducens nerve, 144
ABPS; *see* American Board of Plastic Surgery
Absorbable sterile suture, 59
Accreditation Association for Ambulatory Health Care, 23
Accreditation of free-standing center, 23-24
Acrylic implant(s), 125
Acyclovir for herpetic lesions, 62
Adhesion in wound healing, 57
Adhesive strip(s), 60
Adipocyte(s), 98
Adipose gynecomastia, *170*, 170-171
Adipose tissue, 46t, 47, 98, *99*
Administrative issues, 23
Advancement flap, *83*, 84
  in cleft palate repair, *154*, 154
Aeromonas hydrophilia of leech, 87, 88
Aesthetic surgery
  otoplasty in, 149-152, *151*, *152*
  reconstructive versus, *2*, 2-3
  rhinoplasty in, 146-149, *147*, *148*, *149*, *150*
Afferent nerve, 46t, 49
Age
  suction-assisted lipectomy and, 99, *100*
  wound healing and, 51
Agglutination in inflammatory response, 51
AHA; *see* Alpha hydroxy acid
Alar base reduction, 149, *150*
Alcohol, ethyl, for skin preparation, 43t
Alexandrite laser, 66t
Alginate dressing, 60t
Allergic reaction to local anesthesia, 26, 27t
Allograft(s), 79
  bone, 118-123, *122*
  in burn treatment, 92
  cartilage, 124
Alloplastic implant(s), 124-126
Alpha hydroxy acid, 63, 71, *71*
Alveolus, 153, *153*
Amastia, breast augmentation in, 171
American Association for Accreditation of Ambulatory Surgery facilities, 23
American Board of Plastic Surgery, 19
American Society of Plastic and Reconstructive Surgeons, 13
  on certification, 19
  on clinical photography, 7

American Society of Plastic and Reconstructive Surgical Nurses, 13, 14, *16*
Amino amide anesthetics, 26, 26t
Amino ester anesthetics, 26, 26t
Amniotic membrane in burn treatment, 92
Ampullae, 162
Amputation, traumatic, 130-131, *131*, *132*
Analysis of assessment, 185
Anastomosis(es)
  of amputated digits, 130, *131*
  in toe-to-hand transfer, 131, *132*
Androgenic alopecia, 159
Anesthesia, 25-30, 37-38
  for blepharoplasty, 144
  for carpal tunnel release, 128-129
  for chemical peel, 62
  for cleft lip and palate repair, 153
  for collagen injection, 114
  complications of, 30
  for dermabrasion, 65
  epidural, 28
  for graft procurement, 79
  for hand surgery, 130
  monitoring of, 27-28, *28*
  for otoplasty, 151
  for pediatric patient, 29-30
  for photothermolysis, 66
  regional, 28-29
  for rhinoplasty, 148
  for rhytidectomy, 137
  for suction-assisted lipectomy, 102-104, *104*
  for tissue expansion, 116
Ankle, liposuction of, 105
Antihelical deformity, 152
Antimicrobials
  in burn treatment, 92
  in skin grafting, 82
  in skin preparation, 43t
AORN; *see* Association of Operating Room Nurses
Apocrine glands, 48-49
Aponeurosis, 110
Appraisal, performance, 186
Areola, 46t, 162
Argon laser, 66, 66t
Arm
  compression garment for, *109*
  innervation of, 126, *128*
  postburn reconstruction of, 95
Arrector pilli, 48
Artery(ies)
  of breast, 162
  of ear, 150
  of epidermis and dermis, 49
  of face, 134, *136*
  of hand, 126, *127*
ASPRS; *see* American Society of Plastic and Reconstructive Surgeons
ASPRSN; *see* American Society of Plastic and Reconstructive Surgical Nurses
Assessment
  definition of, 188
  standards of, 185
Association of Operating Room Nurses, 14
Athelia, 172
Ativan; *see* Lorazepam

Augmentation
  breast, *33*, 171-177
  breast cancer and, 165
  implants in, 173-177, *174*, *175*, *176*, *177*
  indications for, *171*, 171-172, *172*
  mammoplasty in, 173, *174*
  preparation for, 172-173, *173*
  marking for, *41*
Auricle, 150-151
Autograft(s), 79, 113
  bone, 118-123, *122*
  in burn treatment, 92
Autologous fat injection, 113, 115
Autologous implant, 113, 118, 123, 124
Axillary nerve block, 29
Azelaic acid in skin lightening, 69

B

Back compression garment, *109*
Backhaus towel forceps, *8*
Baker-Gordon solution in chemical peel, 63
Baldness, 156; *see also* Hair replacement
Bames, 136
Bard Parker knife handle, *8*
Basal cell carcinoma, 72t, 72-73, *73*, *74*
Basosquamous cell carcinoma, 73
BCC; *see* Basal cell carcinoma
Benign skin lesion(s), 72t
Bettman, 136
Bicarbonate
  in liposuction, 104
  in local anesthesia, 26, 26t
Bier block, 29
BIOCELL textured implant, *175*
Bioceramic implant, 125
Bioglass implant, 125
Biologic dressing, 92
Biopsy of skin lesion, 76, *76*
Bipedicle flap, 84
  in reduction mammoplasty, 167, *168*
Blair-Rollet retractor, *8*, *9*
Bleach, skin, 69
Bleeding
  in rhytidectomy, 140
  in wound healing, 57, *58*
Blepharoplasty, *32*, *34*, *35*, 137, *139*, 141-146, *143*
  anatomy and physiology in, 143-144, *144*
  anesthesia for, 144
  browlift and, 141, *142*
  complications of, 145-146
  in geriatric patient, *38*
  hair transplantation and, *161*
  indications for, 143
  intraoperative care for, 144
  postoperative care for, 145, *146*
  preoperative care for, 144, *144*
  procedure of, 144-145, *145*, *146*
Blister, burn, 91
Blood flow
  in abdominal wall, 110
  in breast, 162
  in ear, 150
  in graft, 79
  in hand, 126, *127*
  in tissue flap, 82

Blunt cannula, 106, *107*
Body image, 36, 117
Body surface area, 91, *91*, 92
Body temperature, 37
Bolster dressing, 82, *83*
Bone(s), 49-51
  anatomy of, 118, *121*
  grafts of, 118-123, *121*, *122-123*
  of hand, 126, *127*
  healing of, 118
Bovine collagen injection, *114*, 114-115
Bra compression garment, *109*
Breast(s)
  anatomy and physiology of, 162, *163*
  asymmetry of
    augmentation in, 171, *172*
    implants in, *121*
  cancer of, 164t, 164-165
Breast implant(s), 118, *121*, 173, *174*, *175*
  breast cancer and, 165
  complications of, 176-177
  incisional approaches for, 174, *176*
  mammography and, 164, *164*, 164, *164*
  placement of, 176, *177*
    markings for, *41*
  preparing for, 172-173, *173*
  silicone in, 124-125
Breast self examination, 162-163, *163*
Breast surgery, 162-183
  anatomy and physiology in, 162, *163*
  augmentation in, *33*
    breast cancer and, 165
  examination in, 162-165, *163*, *164*, 164t
  mastopexy in
    equalization, *172*
    in ptosis, 165, *165*
    transabdominal myocutaneous flap in, *42*
  nursing care for, 162
  ptosis in, 165, *165*
  reconstruction in, *177*, 177-180, *178*, *179*
    nipple tattoo and, *70*
    transabdominal myocutaneous flap for, *42*
  reduction mammoplasty in, 165-171
Breslow's classification of melanoma, 76
Browlift, *35*, 137, *138*, *139*, *140*, 140-141, *141*, *142*
Brown dermatome, 81, *82*
BSA; *see* Body surface area
BSE; *see* Breast self examination
Bullet cannula, 106, *107*
Bupivacaine hydrochloride, 26, 26t
Burn(s), 89-96
  assessment of, 89-90
  classification of, *90*, 90-91, *91*, *93*
  complications of, 95-96, *96*
  nursing considerations for, 93
  in pediatric patient, 89
  physiologic approach to, 93-95, *94*
  psychologic considerations in, 89
  split-thickness skin graft in, 79
  treatment of, 91-92
  wound of, 57
Burrow's triangle, *83*, 84
Buttocks, liposuction of, *102*, 105